Safe and Effective Exercise for Overweight Youth

Melinda S. Sothern

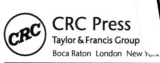

CRC Press
Taylor & Francis Group
Boca Raton London New York

CRC Press is an imprint of the
Taylor & Francis Group, an **informa** business

CRC Press
Taylor & Francis Group
6000 Broken Sound Parkway NW, Suite 300
Boca Raton, FL 33487-2742

First issued in paperback 2019

ISBN-13: 978-1-4398-7288-8 (hbk)
ISBN-13: 978-0-367-37865-3 (pbk)

Library of Congress Cataloging-in-Publication Data

Sothern, Melinda.
   Safe and effective exercise for overweight youth / Melinda S. Sothern.
      pages cm
      Summary: "Drawing on the recommendations of leading health and fitness organizations, this timely book develops a 20-week exercise program to assist children in achieving a healthy weight. Providing specific recommendations for intensity, duration, frequency, and modality of exercise for patients with significant obesity and chronic health issues such as hypertension, asthma, and diabetes, it covers aerobic exercise, strength training, flexibility training, motivation techniques, tracking techniques, measurements for health and fitness outcomes, and future trends in exercise research for overweight youth"-- Provided by publisher.
   Includes bibliographical references and index.
   ISBN 978-1-4398-7288-8 (hardback)
   1. Obesity in adolescence. 2. Obesity in children. 3. Reducing exercises. 4. Reducing diets. I. Title.

RJ399.C6S68 2014
616.3'9800835--dc23
                                       2013047330

Visit the Taylor & Francis Web site at
http://www.taylorandfrancis.com

and the CRC Press Web site at
http://www.crcpress.com

Safe and Effective Exercise for Overweight Youth

DEDICATION

This book is dedicated to Dr. Charles Brown my "partner in crime," or so he calls me. Charlie, as he likes to be called, was instrumental in the integration of nutrition and exercise science into medical school education. His efforts were vital to raising the awareness of physicians nationwide to the importance of healthy nutrition and regular exercise to the prevention and management of chronic diseases, such as obesity and related comorbidities, especially in youth.

Charlie first began integrating his concepts for nutrition and exercise into professional sports as the New Orleans Saints team physician internist, where he served from 1967 to 2000. In 1988, he helped write the newly formed "Drugs of Abuse and Alcohol Policy" for the National Football League. Charlie then served as a member of this committee until his resignation in 2009. He was also a hero in the fight against smoking in public places. Charlie served as the chairman of the Steering Committee of the Louisiana Cancer Research Center Tobacco Free Living Initiative. Under his guidance, the state of Louisiana passed the Clean Indoor Air Act, which prohibits smoking in public buildings and restaurants.

Charlie joined the Louisiana State University Health Sciences Center (LSUHSC) as a faculty member in 1998 while I was conducting research in the Department of Pediatrics. I already knew Charlie because he was the oncologist for one of my family members who survived melanoma under his care. It was during this time that he and I discussed our similar philosophies and passion for nutrition and exercise science, and collaborated on my very first research abstract.

After Charlie joined the LSUHSC faculty, he and I worked together for more than a decade to bring the dream of a research and educational wellness center to the university. I am pleased to share that we now have a premier exercise and wellness facility at the LSUHSC, which serves the medical students, faculty, staff, and their families. More important, the center serves as a health promotion education resource to all while also providing state-of-the-art exercise instruction to members and research study participants. Trained and experienced staff members are available to help with the implementation of research studies examining the benefits of nutrition and exercise to the prevention of obesity and related comorbidities. Charlie also led the efforts to establish the Jim Finks Endowed Chair in Health Promotion, which provides research funding for students and graduate assistants, and helps to support the development of new projects for junior faculty. The availability of these resources has made it possible for us to conduct innovative translational research in the social, behavioral, environmental, biological, and molecular factors related to metabolic and inflammatory disease and to study the impact of exercise and nutrition on this process in children and adolescents.

The expansive reach of Charlie's efforts over the years cannot be measured. His dedication and passion for disease prevention through health promotion nationally and, especially in the state of Louisiana, resulted in major initiatives to improve public health through policy, research, and education. I am so grateful to be his colleague and partner, but more important to call Charlie my friend.

CONTENTS

Chapter 5 MOTIVATING OVERWEIGHT CHILDREN TO INCREASE PHYSICAL ACTIVITY

Chapter 6 PUTTING IT ALL TOGETHER

Chapter 7   MONITORING PROGRESS

Chapter 8 MEASURING HEALTH AND FITNESS OUTCOMES

PREFACE

This textbook, *Safe and Effective Exercise for Overweight Youth,* encompasses decades of scientific research and clinical experience. The recommendations contained within are based on current scientific evidence and my personal clinical experience working with thousands of overweight and obese children and adolescents for 24 years. The contents provide accurate, scientifically sound, and practical guidance that clinical health care providers, educators, public health, and fitness professionals may utilize to promote physical activity in overweight and obese children of all ages, including those with significant obesity and chronic health conditions, such as hypertension, asthma, and type 2 diabetes. The text also provides a current best practices model for implementing clinical- and recreational-based physical activity interventions for preventing and managing pediatric obesity based on decades of research experience by leaders in the field. In addition, this text complements the *Handbook of Pediatric Obesity: Clinical Management*, which I coedited along with psychologist T. Kristian von Almen, PhD, and pediatrician Stewart Gordon, MD, and was published in 2006.

In preparation for writing this book, I spent 2 years gathering information in an effort to update the tailored exercise prescriptions contained within, which were designed specifically to age, level of obesity, and medical condition. I discovered in this process that the original exercise guidelines that I developed in collaboration with Dr. Mark Loftin, and which were based on physiologic and metabolic testing in his laboratory at the University of New Orleans, are still applicable today. In this regard, the scientific evidence actually followed our initial exercise testing findings and resulting intervention design, as our early observational studies were repeated and conducted in more rigorous scientific designs by other researchers. The results of these subsequent studies continually supported our initial hypothesis: *Children with increasing levels of obesity are physiologically and metabolically impaired during exercise, especially weight-bearing modalities.* This is especially relevant in younger children with comorbidities such as asthma, insulin resistance, and type 2 diabetes, and even more pertinent in those with musculoskeletal problems or disorders. As such, the results of our exploratory research became the conduit for future more rigorous scientific studies that now support current U.S. guidelines for physical activity in overweight and obese youth.

In the initial exercise curriculum, which was designed based on the results of our research, we established two major goals for managing overweight conditions in children: (1) increasing overall energy expenditure by raising daily activity levels and improving body movement awareness through fitness counseling, including motivational techniques based on social cognitive theory (Bandura, 1986); and (2) improving cardiopulmonary endurance, muscular strength, and flexibility by engaging in a structured and tailored moderate-intensity, progressive exercise program. The first goal was accomplished by motivating the child to replace sedentary behavior with short bursts of light to moderate activities, such as twisting while watching television, dancing to a favorite song, shooting hoops outside, riding a bike to a friend's house, or stretching on the floor throughout the day while educating him or her on how the body responds to movement. Children thus gained the physiologic and kinesthetic awareness necessary to adopt physical activity patterns that promote long-term health. This goal was intended to be promoted in parallel with the second goal. The second goal was accomplished by establishing weekly short-term goals for intensity, duration, and frequency based on information from our laboratory findings, which provided upper level limits of ability for each obesity category, that is, level 1 (red) severely obese (more than 20 percent of the 95th percentile BMI or an absolute BMI greater than 35 kg/m^2 [Kelly et al., 2013; U.S. Centers for Disease Control and Prevention, 2012]), level 2 (yellow) obese (more than

95th–99th percentile BMI), level 3 (green) overweight (more than 85th–95th percentile BMI), and level 4 (blue) healthy weight or maintenance (less than 85th percentile BMI). Children were encouraged to select activities that they enjoyed from a list of options with an intensity and modality (weight-bearing or non-weight-bearing activities) appropriate for their individual overweight level. Goals for how long and often they should exercise became more challenging as they progressed through the program. These recommendations eventually were utilized to develop an individualized exercise program, which was translated for home use in the book, *Trim Kids: The Proven 12-Week Plan That Has Helped Thousands of Children Achieve a Healthier Weight* (2001) with coauthors T. Kristian von Almen, PhD, and Heidi Schumacher, RD.

Our original recommendations remain appropriate for healthy weight, overweight, obese, and severely obese youth with and without comorbidities. Current research, however, indicates that light activity, in particular, including activities that require the body weight to be supported (weight-bearing activities) are advantageous for improving metabolic health in overweight and obese children. In a recent review of decades of research (see Chapter 10), it was concluded that exercise prescriptions in overweight and obese youth should consider a multistep strategy. In this case, sedentary activities initially are replaced with light activities that are enjoyable and unstructured, such as table tennis, billiards, darts, archery, fishing, or playing in a pool. Then intensity gradually is increased over time by selecting moderate and then vigorous activities in such a way that U.S. guideline goals to include 60 minutes of moderate- to vigorous-intensity activity eventually are met. Thus, the original goal of increasing overall energy expenditure by raising daily activity levels is now more specific as the recommendations in this text also include options for light-intensity activities, which are specific to age, obesity level, and medical condition, during the first few weeks of the program. Light to moderate exercise is supported by a multitude of researchers as overweight and obese children can exercise at this intensity for long periods without fatigue, thus enabling youth to burn calories and fat (see Chapters 1 and 10). This, in turn, improves metabolic health, promotes the attainment of a healthy body weight, and reduces the risk of developing obesity comorbidities.

HOW TO USE THIS BOOK

Chapters 1–5 provide an overview of the existing scientific literature in support of individualized, tailored exercise prescriptions for overweight and obese children with and without comorbidities. This information provides the basis of support for the specific recommendations contained in Chapters 6–9. Chapters 2–5 also contain exercise instructions, illustrations, and sample lesson plans to improve cardiopulmonary endurance, muscular strength, power and endurance, and muscular flexibility.

Chapter 6 applies the existing scientific literature to specific guidelines for prescribing exercise to overweight children along with verbal cues or "talking points," clinical reminders, and handouts to assist health care providers with discussing the most appropriate exercise modality, intensity, frequency, and duration for each child's individual needs. At the end of the chapter, a 40-week exercise curriculum, including lesson plans, is provided, which can be implemented in clinical, recreational, or home-based settings. This curriculum contains the complete exercise intervention from the comprehensive, multidisciplinary approach that my colleagues and I utilized successfully for more than two decades to assist children in achieving a healthier weight. Our hands-on, clinical setting provided the optimal laboratory in which to discover what is unique about obese children and to identify specific approaches and activities for promoting improved health through increased physical activity and structured exercise.

Chapter 7 discusses the importance of regular medical and self-monitoring and also provides easy tools and techniques that health care providers can use to track the child's progress, including forms, handouts, talking points, and reminders. Chapters 8 and 9 provide detailed clinical and field protocols to assist with the measurement of health and fitness outcomes. Chapter 9 also describes realistic expectations and presents the current U.S. recommendations for promoting physical activity and fitness in youth. Chapter 10 provides a summary of current studies to support future research in the area of physical activity to prevent and manage pediatric obesity.

Each chapter contains printable forms that can be used in clinical practice or community and field settings. These forms also may be downloaded from our website at http://publichealth.lsuhsc.edu. In addition, this website provides links to exercise instructional videos that are based on the color-coded four-level approach, and a link to an educational series from Louisiana Public Broadcasting Company as well as updates from our current studies, Trim Teens and Trim Tots.

SUMMARY

Many professionals lack the time to keep up to date on such a rapidly changing field of pediatric exercise science as it relates to the prevention and treatment of obesity and chronic disease. Medical, public health, recreational, and exercise professionals need a solid, readily available resource to consult when developing exercise plans for overweight and obese children. More important, colleges, universities, and medical schools need an authoritative manual on the subject of childhood obesity to better prepare health care and educational professionals on the appropriate care and counseling of physical activity and exercise for obese youth. *Safe and Effective Exercise for Overweight Youth* provides a state-of-the-art, scientifically supported, and clinically relevant source of information to research, medical, educational, public health, and recreational professionals, which is essential to the design of appropriate exercise interventions for obese youth. The text condenses all of the available scientific literature and recommendations into a prescriptive, comprehensive guide and hopefully will serve as a valued resource to universities, hospitals, recreational and educational facilities, clinics, and physician offices.

The success or failure of children to achieve a healthy weight is a responsibility that is shared by both the family and the health care professional. This textbook will provide the necessary information and tools for you to become proficient in matching or tailoring physical activity recommendations to the medical, physical, and emotional needs of developing children. When paired with your dedication, positive approach, time, and energy, the most appropriate care can be provided to overweight and obese children and adolescents.

REFERENCES

Bandura, A. (1986). *Social Foundations of Thoughts and Actions: A Social Cognitive Theory.* Englewood Cliffs, NJ: Prentice-Hall.

Kelly, A. S., Barlow, S. E., Rao, G., Inge, T. H., Hayman, L. L., Steinberger, J., et al. (2013). Severe obesity in children and adolescents: Identification, associated health risks, and treatment approaches—A scientific statement from the American Heart Association. *Circulation*, 128(15), 1689–1712.

Sothern, M., Gordon, S., von Almen, T. K. (Eds.). (2006). *Handbook of Pediatric Obesity: Clinical Management.* Boca Raton, FL: Taylor & Francis.

Sothern, M., von Almen, T. K., Schumacher, H. (2001). *Trim Kids: The Proven Plan That Has Helped Thousands of Children Achieve a Healthier Weight.* New York, NY: HarperCollins.

U.S. Centers for Disease Control and Prevention. (2012). Overweight and obesity: Consequences. Retrieved June 9, 2012, from http://www.cdc.gov/obesity/childhood/basics.html.

ACKNOWLEDGMENTS

Because this textbook summarizes a large part of my life's work, I would first like to acknowledge and thank the most influential person in my life, my father, James M. Sothern, professor, geologist, musician, visual artist, author, folklorist, organic farmer, and cultural, wetlands, and coastal preservationist (aka, the *Cajun Naturalist*), who at a very young age made me believe I was the best of everything—the smartest, brightest, fastest, and funniest. He also led me to believe that I could do absolutely anything I set my mind to, no matter how challenging, as long as I worked hard and knew deep inside that I could do it. My father taught me to love and cherish all things in nature, especially small things—animals, plants, children. More important, he instilled in me the belief that I was responsible for taking care of and protecting those most vulnerable, especially children. This is what led me to an initial career in youth aquatic sports and eventually in pediatric medicine—the ideal that those who are young and small are to be protected and allowed to be children and to experience all that childhood offers (e.g., play, exploration, running until out of breath). I also would like to thank my father for allowing me to explore the world with his blessing, wise words of caution, and assurance that I could always come home. And, notably, he did not promote typical female career goals, but rather he encouraged me to seek advanced education and opportunities typically held by men. He did this from the time I was born, and it is why I became a "tomboy" and eventually pursued a career in sports medicine, public health education and research, and pediatric exercise physiology.

Second, I would like to thank my mentor, Dr. Mark Loftin, who was the most instrumental person in my academic development. He took my passion for helping children seriously and was especially helpful and encouraging as I transitioned from teaching and coaching to pediatric exercise physiology research. I remember my first research paper during my graduate studies at the University of New Orleans (UNO), which was full of references to popular-press family, health, and fitness magazines. Dr. Loftin allowed me to present to the class without criticism, but, later, he pulled me aside in his always-laughing voice and steered me in the right direction (e.g., research journals housed in the library). Once I learned where to find the scientific literature, all I wanted to do was explore the research contained in those journals. And, to this day, I still thoroughly enjoy poring through the research, now conveniently online.

I especially would like to acknowledge *Trim Kids* developers and coauthors, Heidi Schumacher, RD, and T. Kristian von Almen, PhD, for their support, collaboration, and friendship for more than 20 years. Without their dedication and commitment to overweight and obese children, my research and this textbook would not have been possible.

I would like to express my gratitude to my current mentors, Dr. Eric Ravussin, who inspired and challenged me to transition from clinical intervention work to mechanistic explorations and who became a dear friend, as well as Dr. Sarah Moody Thomas, who is probably unaware of how much her mentorship helped to shape my current career. She taught me temperance and patience as well as how to be poised and professional even when faced with difficult challenges. I am grateful to the Dean of the Louisiana State University Health Sciences Center (LSUHSC), School of Public Health (SPH), Dr. Terri Fontham, and the Clinical Director of the Pennington Biomedical Research Center (PBRC), Dr. Donna Ryan, who remain the ultimate role models for young female clinicians and scientists. I wish to thank and acknowledge the LSUHSC Director of Communications, Leslie Capo, whose expertise, unyielding determination, and hard work at the LSUHSC continue to provide me with opportunities to translate important pediatric obesity, exercise, and physical activity scientific findings to the public.

I also appreciate the guidance, support, and continued opportunities for collaboration provided by Drs. John Udall, Oded Bar-Or (deceased), Michael Goran, Dianne Ward, William Dietz, Frank Greenway, Robert Newton, Stephanie Broyles, Peter Katzmarzyk, Donald Williamson, Claude Bouchard, George Bray, Stewart Gordon, Lauren Keely Carlisle, Sandra Hunter (deceased), Larry Webber, Steve Nelson, Edward Trapido, Stewart Chalew, Arlette Soros, Alphonso Vargas, Ricardo Sorensen, Robert Suskind, Julia Volaufova, Jovanny Zabaleta, Cruz Velasco, Richard Scribner, Tung Sung Tseng, Marc Bonis, Henry Nuss, Hamid Boulares, Donna Williams, Stephen Phillippi, Joan Wightkin, Leslie Lewis, Augusto Ochoa, and John Estrada.

I would like to especially thank the editorial team at Taylor & Francis/CRC Press, Randy Brehm and Kari Budyk, for understanding the importance of this publication and for their patience and support during the development of the manuscript.

I gratefully acknowledge the research, editorial, computer, and clerical support of my student workers, Amanda Arguello, Alexandria Augustus, and Lauren Griffiths, and graduate assistant, Maura Mohler. And I would like to express my gratitude to my former research associate, Brian Bennett, for his dedication and commitment during the SILLY and MET studies; my current research associate, Nicole Pelligrino, for her expert coordination of the behavioral counseling and exercise interventions in my ongoing research studies; Ann Clesi, for her coordination of our preschool obesity prevention studies and research office needs; and Betty Gonzales, for continued business office support. I sincerely appreciate the continued support and guidance of the LSUHSC SPH administration, faculty, and staff, and the Department of Pediatrics, the PBRC, the UNO, and The Obesity Society. I am grateful to the American Academy of Pediatrics, the American College of Sports Medicine, the U.S. Centers for Disease Control and Prevention, the U.S. Surgeon General, and the National YMCA for their continued commitment to supporting physical activity as a vital and important part of pediatric obesity prevention and management.

On a personal note, I am very grateful to my husband, Dave, who helped me to raise my children even while I traveled extensively as part of my obligation as a research scientist, educator, and clinician, and who provided encouragement every step of the way. To my mother, Jerry (deceased), and sister Becky (deceased), whom I still miss so much, and my sisters Rachael, Wilma, and Julie, my brother Jim, and childhood friend Dena, who have been my best friends throughout my life and offered support when I most needed it.

Most important, I would like to acknowledge my children, Samantha and Allyson, who sacrificed so much during their childhood so that their mother could achieve graduate degrees—thus affording me the opportunity to realize my career goals—and who, to this day, provide me with so much love and encouragement, are just a joy, and are the most valuable gifts in my life.

ABOUT THE AUTHOR

Melinda S. Sothern, PhD, CEP, is a licensed clinical exercise physiologist and currently serves as academic program director and professor with tenure at the Louisiana State University (LSU) Health Sciences Center (HSC), School of Public Health in New Orleans, Louisiana, and the Prevention of Childhood Obesity Laboratory at the LSU Pennington Biomedical Research Center in Baton Rouge. She is a recipient of the Jim Finks Endowed Chair in Health Promotion in Behavioral and Community Health Sciences and maintains an adjunct appointment in the Department of Pediatrics, School of Medicine, LSUHSC. Dr. Sothern's research is widely published in a multitude of peer-reviewed scientific journals and in two scientific textbooks, *The Handbook of Pediatric Obesity: Clinical Management* (Taylor & Francis, 2006) and *The Handbook of Pediatric Obesity: Etiology, Pathophysiology and Prevention* (Taylor & Francis, 2005). She also senior-authored a popular press book for parents of overweight children to use in conjunction with their pediatrician or family physician entitled *Trim Kids* (HarperCollins, 2001). The *Trim Kids* program is recognized by the National Cancer Institute as a Research-Tested Intervention Program and is acknowledged by the U.S. Surgeon General for its community dissemination in The YMCA centers in Louisiana. Dr. Sothern was the 2009 recipient of The Obesity Society's Oded Bar-Or Award for Excellence in Pediatric Obesity Research. In 2008, she received the Cecil J. Picard Award for Excellence in Education to Prevent Childhood Obesity in Louisiana, and was selected as one of the Top Ten Female Achievers in New Orleans by *New Orleans* magazine. She recently cofounded and chaired the Louisiana Childhood Obesity Research Consortium (LA CORC).

Dr. Sothern is currently serving as principal investigator on two National Institutes of Health (NIH)–sponsored studies entitled *Molecular and Social Determinants of Obesity in Developing Youth* (NIMHD) and *Obesity and Asthma: Determinants of Inflammation and Effects of Intervention* (NIMHD). She also serves as principal investigator of a Louisiana Office of Public Health Maternal and Child Health–sponsored study, *An Intervention to Promote Environmental Changes in Pre-School Centers to Prevent Childhood Obesity* (NAP SACC), and co-investigator/scientist on another NIH-sponsored grant, *Community-Academic Partnership to Address Health Disparities in New Orleans* (NIMHD). Dr. Sothern previously served as a principal investigator on two other NIH-sponsored studies entitled *Exploring Mechanisms of the Metabolic Syndrome in African American and Caucasian Youth* (NICHD) and *Insulin Sensitivity in Children with Low Birth Weight* (NICHD) and as co-investigator on the NIH-sponsored study, *Anthropometric Assessment of Abdominal Obesity and Health Risk in Children and Adolescents* (RC1), and another NIH-sponsored, 6-year study entitled *Increasing Physical Activity Patterns in Adolescent Girls: The TAAG Study,* with seven other sites nationwide. She previously directed the physical activity intervention of the NIH-sponsored study, *Environmental Approaches for the Prevention of Weight Gain: The Wise Mind Study,* and served as co-principal investigator or mentor of three additional NIH-funded studies: (1) *Environmental Determinants of Physical Activity in Parks* (K01), (2) *Training Translational Researchers in Louisiana* (COBRA), and (3) *Measurement of Sedentary Behavior in African American Adults* (K01). Dr. Sothern also served as consultant to several NIH-funded projects, including a school-based study entitled *LA Health* at the LSU PBRC.

Dr. Sothern coauthored a position paper and serves as faculty for the Academy of Nutrition and Dietetics pediatric weight management certificate program. She is considered a national spokesperson for overweight youth and has been featured extensively in national and international television, radio, and print media, including *Good Morning America, The Today*

Show, CNN International, NPR Radio, Fox News TV, *48 Hours,* Nickelodeon TV, *The Oprah Show,* Discovery Channel, Yorkshire TV British Broadcasting Co., *USA Today, Associated Press—World News, Washington Post, Wall Street Journal, National Geographic, LA Times, Parents Magazine, Parenting, Better Homes and Garden, Prevention Magazine, Psychology Today,* WebMD, and many others.

Dr. Sothern led her field in establishing standardized guidelines for prescribing exercise for children with increasing levels of obesity and is best known for her work in promoting active play as a means of preventing and treating childhood obesity. In acknowledgment of her achievements, she received the University of New Orleans Dr. Vane Wilson Award in recognition of excellent work and service in the field of human performance and health promotion in May 2000. She has been a member of the American College of Sports Medicine (ACSM) and The Obesity Society for more than 20 years, is a fellow and former council member of The Obesity Society, and previously served as a member of the Annual Scientific Program Planning and Education committees. In 2007, Dr. Sothern served as chairman of the Publications Committee and supervised the transition of the scientific journal entitled *Obesity* to publication in the Nature Publishing Group. She is currently an associate editor for the journal, *Obesity,* and serves on the editorial board of the journal, *Childhood Obesity.* She previously served as associate editor for the journals *Pediatric Obesity* and *Childhood Obesity* for 4 years. She cofounded the Pediatric Obesity Interest Group, which is now formally integrated into The Obesity Society as the Pediatric Obesity Section.

Dr. Sothern was a scientific presenter for The Obesity Society Distinguished Lecture Series in 2004, the Southeast ACSM Distinguished Lecturer in the fall of 2007, and was chosen as the Delta Omega Honorary Society in Public Health Faculty inductee for outstanding public health performance in scholarship, teaching, research, and publications in October 2007. In June 2011, she provided the keynote lecture for the 2011 U.S. Public Health Service Commissioned Officer Scientific and Training Symposium and delivered an invited lecture for the 2012 American Academy of Pediatrics Annual Scientific Meeting. Dr. Sothern also served as a member of the American Heart Association/Clinton Foundation Advisory Board and is currently a scientific advisory board member for the Windward Islands Research and Education Foundation, St. George's University, School of Medicine, Grenada. She is a member of the scientific advisory committee for the Louisiana Report Card on Physical Activity and Health for Children and Youth and for the United States Report Card on Physical Activity for Children and Youth.

During the past 24 years, Dr. Sothern has presented more than 250 invited scientific lectures or presentations to universities, medical centers, and scientific meetings. She is a reviewer for the NIH and for numerous pediatric, obesity, behavioral science, and exercise scientific journals and she provides scientific advice to several major national and international corporations, including Gerber Foods, Kraft Foods, Nestle International, Knoll Pharmaceuticals, Health Nutrition Technology, Susan Dell Foundation, the Disney Corporation, and others.

Chapter 1

PROFILE OF THE OVERWEIGHT CHILD: IMPLICATIONS FOR EXERCISE PRESCRIPTION

Over the past three decades the number of obese children ages 6 to 11 years has tripled and the prevalence of obese preschool-age children has doubled (Singh, Siahpush, & Kogan, 2011). Furthermore, approximately 17% or 12.5 million of U.S. children and adolescents ages 2 to 19 years old are obese. Physical inactivity has been recognized as a major contributing factor to the obesity epidemic, yet a large portion of the U.S. child and adolescent population do not engage in the recommended moderate and vigorous physical activity (MVPA) (Hills, King, & Armstrong, 2007; Tomporowski, Lambourne, & Okumura, 2011). This observation is due to several factors, including a lack of opportunity to participate in physical activity (Curtis, Hinckson, & Water, 2012); an overemphasis on academics, which promotes extended periods of sedentary time during the school day (Kalish & Sabbagh, 2007; McCurdy et al., 2010; Milteer et al., 2012); and diminished safe outdoor environments because of increased crime, overdevelopment, and blighted properties (Molnar et al., 2004; Singh et al., 2011). These challenges lead to an obesity-promoting environment, which negatively affects multiple sectors of society that struggle to identify solutions (Huang, Grimm, & Hammond, 2011; Sothern et al., 1999a). Thus, promoting the addition of daily physical activity into the lives of obese children continues to be a frustrating experience for most families and pediatric health care professionals (Kiess et al., 2001; Sothern et al., 2010). Further adding to this negative state of affairs is a lack of consistent professional guidelines for exercise therapy. Recently, general physical activity guidelines were established for sedentary youth, which in many cases includes overweight and obese children and adolescents (Strong et al., 2005; U.S. DHHS, 2008) and the American Heart Association included broad-based suggestions for tailoring exercise to obese populations in a recent publication (Daniels et al., 2009). In addition, Brambilla, Pozzobon, and Pietrobelli (2011) recently published an extensive review paper concerning the favorable impact of exercise to metabolic disease prevention in youth, which included suggestions for exercise intensity and modality. To date, however, no one professional medical or scientific organization has provided specific recommendations for intensity, duration, frequency, or modality of exercise for the management of pediatric obesity (American Academy of Pediatrics [AAP], Committee on Sports Medicine, 1990; American College of Sports Medicine [ACSM], 2010; Daniels et al., 2009; Eisenmann, 2011; Faigenbaum et al., 2009; Ganley et al., 2011; Kitzmann et al., 2010; Sothern, 2001; Sothern et al., 2006; U.S. Preventive Services Task Force, 2010; Washington, Bernhardt, Gomez, Johnson, et al., 2001). Pediatric health care professionals, thus, must rely on the available scientific literature when determining initial exercise recommendations for overweight and obese children and adolescents with varied family and medical histories.

FACTORS THAT LIMIT PHYSICAL ACTIVITY IN CHILDREN

AGE AND STAGE OF DEVELOPMENT: DO CHILDREN RESPOND DIFFERENTLY THAN ADULTS?

Research indicates that young children have an intrinsic need to be physically active (Bailey et al., 1995; DiNubile, 1993; Stucky-Ropp & DiLorenzo, 1993). More important, physical activity is essential for healthy growth and development in youth (Milteer et al., 2012). Large motor skills (e.g., running, skipping, hopping, the "butterfly") are associated with better cognitive and executive functioning (and reading ability) later in life (Davis, Tomporowski, et al., 2011; Hillman et al., 2006; Hills et al., 2007; Kalish & Sabbagh, 2007). Unfortunately, there are several barriers and environmental risk factors that limit adequate opportunities for infants, toddlers, and preschool-age children to be physically active, including the following: (1) more than 2 hours of screen time per day, (2) restricted play spaces, (3) disproportionate use of strollers, infant seats, etc., (4) safety concerns,

(5) poorly designed neighborhoods that limit opportunities for walking, (6) parental work demands, and others (Gunner et al., 2005; Milteer et al., 2012). Thus, parents must develop ways to encourage playtime from infancy through the childhood years. Figure 1.1 details developmentally appropriate structured, unstructured, and sedentary activity guidelines for infants, toddlers, and preschool-age children.

Figure 1.2 provides suggestions for increasing physical activity for parents of infants, toddlers and preschool-aged children. Additional suggestions and activities for younger children may be found in Chapter 6 of this textbook.

Developmentally appropriate physical activity during childhood is associated with better academic achievement, lower absenteeism, and decreased behavior problems (Castelli et al., 2007; Davis et al., 2007; Davis, Tomporowski, et al., 2011). Interestingly, obesity during childhood is not shown to share the same relationship (Leblanc et al., 2012). Despite this essential need for movement, even young children are more likely to chose sedentary pursuits if the selected activity or exercise is too challenging (Sothern, 2002, 2004; Sothern & Gordon, 2005; Sothern, Hunter, et al., 1999; Sothern et al., 2006; VanVrancken-Tomkins & Sothern, 2006). Thus, exercise techniques must be appropriate to both the physical and emotional development level of the child (Davis, Tomporowski, et al., 2011; Hillman et al., 2006; Hills et al., 2007; Kalish & Sabbagh, 2007).

In general, running activities of long durations cannot be sustained by younger children because of their immature metabolic systems (Bar-Or & Rowland, 2004). Obesity during early childhood exacerbates this phenomenon (Sothern, 2001, 2002; VanVrancken-Tomkins & Sothern, 2006). But, if provided the opportunity, young children, even those overweight, will perform relatively large volumes of intermittent physical activity (Bailey et al., 1995; DiNubile, 1993; Stucky-Ropp & DiLorenzo, 1993). One reason for this is that young children are distracted easily and are incapable of focused activity for long periods of time, which contributes to the sporadic nature of their physical activity (Bailey et al., 1995; Milteer et al., 2012). Adults can engage in long-duration exercise easily because of their enhanced ability to concentrate. Although most individuals engage in activity because they enjoy the effort, children need activity to be fun in order for them to continue (Milteer et al., 2012; Sothern, 2001, 2002, 2004).

 Key Points: Developmentally Appropriate Physical Activity
Young children will engage in large volumes of intermittent, nonstructured physical activity if provided with an environment that promotes free play.

- Preschool years: General movement activities (e.g., jumping, throwing, running, climbing)
- Prepubertal (6–9 years old): More specialized and complex movements and anaerobic activities (e.g., tag, games, recreational sports)
- Puberty (10–14 years old): Organized sports and skill development
- Adolescence (15–18 years old): More structured health and fitness activities and refinement of skills

Sources: Adapted from Bailey et al., 1995; DiNubile, 1993; Stucky-Ropp & DiLorenzo, 1993.

The AAP recently published a position paper stating that "[p]lay is essential to the social, emotional, cognitive, and physical wellbeing of children beginning in early childhood." As such, supervised active play, especially outdoors is the most appropriate type of exercise for children during the preschool and elementary school years. Moreover, "it is essential that parents, educators, and pediatricians recognize the importance of lifelong benefits that children gain from play" (Milteer et al., 2012, p. e204).

	Structured physical activity	Unstructured physical activity	Sedentary and screen time
Infants (0–1 year)	◆ Encourage physical activity from birth, every day (moving arms, legs, reaching objects, etc.) ◆ Provide objects, toys, and games that encourage infants to move and do things for themselves	◆ Respect natural activity patterns (spontaneous and intermittent) ◆ Promote gross motor play (e.g., develop head control, sitting, crawling) and fun locomotor activities ◆ Provide a safe, nurturing and minimally structured play environment, inside and outside	◆ Avoid TV and electronic media ◆ Replace screen time with interactive activities that promote brain development: singing, talking, playing and reading together ◆ Avoid prolonged periods restrained in high chair, stroller, etc.
Toddlers (1–3 yrs)	◆ Provide 30 minutes of daily (cumulative) structured physical activity ◆ Activities should be fun and occur through physical activity, but also as part of games, transportation, and unplanned activities ◆ Encourage activity that helps child develop competence in movement skills (e.g., throwing, catching, or kicking a ball)	◆ Provide 60 minutes to several hours of daily unstructured physical activity, as part of play, games, transportation, and recreation ◆ Develop outdoor activity and unstructured exploration under adult supervision (e.g., walking in the park, free play)	◆ No more than 60 consecutive minutes of sedentary activity (except sleeping!) ◆ With children under 2, avoid spending time viewing TV or electronic media (DVDs, computer, electronic games) ◆ With children between 2 and 3, limit media time to no more than 1–2 hours per day of quality programming ◆ Do not put TV sets in bedrooms ◆ Encourage activities such as reading, athletics, hobbies, and creative play ◆ Encourage child to walk instead of using the stroller
Preschoolers (3–5yrs)	◆ Provide 60 minutes of daily (cumulative) structured physical activity ◆ Encourage activity that helps child develop competence in movement skills (e.g., throwing, catching, or kicking a ball) ◆ Focus on participation, not competition	◆ Provide 60 minutes to several hours of daily unstructured physical activity, as part of play, games, transportation, and recreation ◆ Ensure that free play is fun, safe, and allows for experimentation and exploration ◆ Include a few variables and instruction in unorganized play	◆ Limit media time to no more than 1–2 hours per day of quality programming ◆ Do not put TV sets in bedrooms ◆ Encourage activities such as reading, athletics, hobbies, and creative play ◆ Encourage child to walk instead of using stroller

Figure 1.1 Guidelines relating to physical activity and inactivity in infants, toddlers, and preschool-age children.*

*Selected and adapted from 2010 Active Healthy Kids Canada Report Card on Physical Activity for Children and Youth, page 7.

PLAYFUL INFANTS

Even the youngest babies like to play! Here are some fun ideas that you can do with your baby that will provide opportunities to let her explore the world. Babies need to stretch, roll, and have a safe area for activities to learn new skills as they grow.

- Place baby on a large blanket or rug on the floor over a generally large area to allow him to roll, creep, crawl, sit, and develop other large muscle activities.
- Place toys slightly out of reach to encourage the infant to work for them.
- Having "tummy time" is important for developing muscle strength for crawling and sitting, but don't leave your baby alone during tummy time.
- Play games such as "pat-a-cake" and "peek-a-boo" to support the growing infant's learning and motor skills.
- Give your baby the chance to see new places, to be held and rocked.
- Offer a variety of age-appropriate toys that will stimulate the senses, including toys that make sounds, have varied textures, and bright colors.
- Rattles, large blocks, bubbles, balls, pans, wooden spoons, small boxes, and soft stuffed animals are great toys.

BUSY TODDLER PLAY

Your growing toddler keeps you going! It seems like there is hardly a moment that he isn't climbing, running, hopping and jumping. That's good for him and gives you plenty of opportunity to make all of this activity fun! You can even share some simple household chores.

- Give your toddler lots of time for unstructured physical activity, including trips to a variety of places, such as playgrounds that provide children the opportunity to crawl around structures, climb, and balance on equipment.
- Play with soft inflatable balls, chasing bubbles, or digging in the soil with spoons are inexpensive and easy activities toddlers love.
- Play a variety of music for dance and movement to support development of a sense of rhythm and a creative sense of movement.
- Make musical instruments out of paper towels tubes to blow through.
- Have messy play with a garden hose or sprinkler.
- Make running with the child fun! For example, run like a monkey, walk like a spider, hop like a bunny, or stretch like a cat.
- Use scaled-down adult items like telephones, hammers, pots, pans, and brooms to foster imaginative play.
- Have a contest working in the yard or collect trash on a walk around the neighborhood.
- Purchase riding toys, scooters, push toys, large building blocks, cardboard boxes, trucks, doll strollers, or toy lawn mowers.

FANTASTIC PRESCHOOLER PLAY

Creative and fun! Preschoolers find excitement in everything! Tumbling, dancing to music, and playing with friends, your child is growing and finding so much to learn and do! Children learn by watching the most important people in their life—YOU! By showing your child how much fun being active is, you are a terrific example how to live a healthy and active life.

- Provide a variety of structured physical activity that may include supervised water play, group dance, ball play, scavenger hunts, group balance, and tumbling activities.
- Engage in rolling, skipping, and hopping games.
- Provide activities that allow for challenges in climbing, hanging, balancing, and sliding.
- Offer chalk for hopscotch, balls to roll on top of, large cars, trucks, and trains to create imaginary roads and towns.
- Teach your child games of tag, chase, "red rover," and hide-and-seek.
- Walk with your child to the library, park, or store.
- Take your child on an adventure hike, even if it is just around the block.
- Encourage activity and assign responsibilities around the house.
- Stimulate imagination and creativity with a sheet draped over the furniture to create a tent, fort, or playhouse.
- Purchase toys such as scooters, tricycles, and large balls.

With permission: *Journal of Pediatric Health Care*, 19(4).

Figure 1.2 Infants and young children at play.

Key Points: Children Are Not Little Adults

- Movement is required for cognitive development.
- Children enjoy unstructured physical activity (play).
- Play fosters healthy emotional development.
- Children cannot stay focused for long periods of time.
- Immature metabolic systems limit exercise duration.
- Children have lower oxygen uptake than adults.

Recent research identifies numerous benefits of exercise and the resulting increase in physical fitness in young children to academic achievement (Castelli et al., 2007; Davis et al., 2007; Davis, Tomporowski, et al., 2011; Donnelly & Lambourne, 2011; Grissom, 2005; London & Castrechini, 2011), thus supporting the integration of frequent opportunities for active play throughout the school day. Studies have demonstrated that, in particular, recess (regular unstructured physical activity during the school day) has cognitive, emotional, physical, and social benefits for young children (Murray, Ramstetter, & Council on School Health Executive Committee, 2013). In addition, there is actually no evidence that time spent in physical activity has a negative influence on student achievement; research indicates the contrary. Evidence reveals that appropriate levels of physical activity among children and youth, including sufficient time in MVPA, are related positively to increased on-task classroom behavior, cognitive development, and academic performance (Siedentop, 2009). Despite this finding, schools are reducing recess to accommodate additional time for academic subjects (Murray et al., 2013). The amount of time allotted for recess decreases with age and is less abundant among children of lower socioeconomic status and in the urban setting. Ironically, minimizing or eliminating recess may be counterproductive for academic improvement. Recess provides time away from rigorous cognitive tasks and, therefore, improves attention and productivity in the classroom. Furthermore, recess develops constructs and cognitive understanding through interaction and provides social and emotional peer interaction that develops communication and coping skills, such as negotiation, cooperation, sharing, problem solving, and self-control. Furthermore, recess provides time to practice movement and motor skills that contribute to the recommended 60 minutes of moderate to vigorous physical activity daily. Regardless of whether children play vigorously at recess, it provides the opportunity for children to use their imagination and be active in the mode of their choosing (Murray et al., 2013). Recess should occur at regular intervals and provide sufficient time for children to regain their focus before further instruction. Some advocate for structured recess, which is recess based on structured play, during which games and physical activities are taught and led by a trained adult. It is important to realize the social and emotional trade-off, which would limit the acquisition of developmental skills obtained during recess. There are ways to encourage physical activity without making structured, planned, adult-led games, such as providing safe, appealing equipment.

Key Points: Benefits of Exercise to Academic Achievement

- Exercise improves cognition and academic achievement (Woodcock-Johnson III) in overweight children.
- Objective measures of physical fitness are associated with higher academic achievement.
- Physically active classroom lessons improve standardized test scores.
- Overall physical fitness is a better predictor of academic achievement than obesity.

Sources: Adapted from Castelli et al., 2007; Davis et al., 2007; Davis et al., 2011; Donnelly & Lambourne, 2011; Grissom, 2005; London & Castrechini, 2011.

It is essential that children participate in exercise activities that promote the attainment of muscular strength and endurance (U.S. DHHS, U.S. Guidelines, 2008). The ability to participate in daily physical activities is limited in children with weak muscles. If properly administered, strength or resistance-training programs not only may be safe in youth but also may promote enhanced motor performance (Behringer et al., 2011) and help reduce the risk of injury during other physical activities (Faigenbaum & Myer, 2010). The developing musculoskeletal system of the preadolescent child must be considered when selecting activities to promote the development of muscular strength and endurance (Ganley et al., 2011; Sothern, 2001). The intensity and duration of an individual strength exercise bout (set) must be appropriate to the level of maturity of the growing bones and muscles (Faigenbaum et al., 2009; Ganley et al., 2011; Sothern 2002, 2004; Sothern, Loftin, Ewing, et al., 1999; VanVrancken-Tomkins & Sothern, 2006). The ACSM (2010, 2011), the National Strength and Conditioning Association (Faigenbaum et al., 2009), the AAP (1990; Washington, Bernhardt, Gomez, et al., 2001), and others (Behm et al., 2008) have all published statements in support of properly administered and supervised, developmentally appropriate muscular strength and endurance training in children and adolescents. It is suggested that a child be of a sufficient age to participate in sports activities before engaging in structured exercise to specifically improve muscular strength and endurance, which is typically 7–8 years of age (Faigenbaum et al., 2009). Trained professionals should consult these guidelines before designing a program specific to their patients' or students' needs. Table 1.1 provides a summary of recommendations to develop muscular strength and endurance in overweigh and obese children (Bar-Or & Rowland, 2004).

In addition, Chapter 3 provides specific information to aid in the development of muscular strength and endurance exercise programs for children of all ages and levels of obesity.

EXCESS ADIPOSITY: IS EXERCISE MORE DIFFICULT IN OVERWEIGHT CHILDREN?

Several factors distinguish the overweight and obese child from a healthy weight child. Compared with healthy weight children, obese children are reported to have greater physical activity restrictions, school problems, greater school absenteeism, depression, developmental delay, asthma, allergies, headaches, and ear infections as well as bone, joint, and muscle

Table 1.1 Guidelines for Resistance Training

Guidelines
1. Check for physical and medical contraindication.
2. Ensure experienced supervision, preferably by an adult, when using free weights or training machines.
3. Ascertain proper technique.
4. Warm up with calisthenics and stretches.
5. Begin a program with an exercise that uses body weight as resistance before progressing to free weights or weight-training machines.
6. Individualize training loads whether using free weights or machines.
7. Train all major muscle groups and both flexors and extensors.
8. Exercise the muscles through their entire range of motion.
9. Alternate days of training with rest days, limiting participation to no more than three times a week.
10. When using free weights or machines, progress gradually from light loads, high repetitions (more than 15), and few sets (two to three) to heavier loads, fewer repetitions (6–8), and three to four sets.
11. Cool down after training, using stretch exercises for major joints and muscle groups.
12. When selecting equipment, check for durability, stability, sturdiness, and safety.
13. Consider sharp or persistent pain as a warning, and seek medical advice.

Source: From Bar-Or, O., Rowland, T. W., *Pediatric Exercise Medicine: From Physiologic Principles to Health Care Application,* Human Kinetics, Champaign, IL, 2004. With permission.

problems (Halfon, Larson, & Slusser, 2013). Overweight and obese children also typically display advanced physical bone age and density (De Simone et al., 1995; Giuca et al., 2012; Johnson et al., 2012) and increased body mass and height (Frisch & Revelle, 1971; Johnson et al., 2012). Obesity also is associated with advanced sexual maturation in females (Austin et al., 1991; Biro et al., 2012; De Simone et al., 1995), with mixed results in males (Tinggaard et al., 2012). There are both advantages and disadvantages to the advanced age, maturation, and increased body size (Bar-Or & Rowland, 2004). Overweight and obese children have a technical advantage during physical activities and sports in which enhanced height and arm span provide an advantage, such as in football, volleyball, and basketball (Bar-Or & Rowland, 2004). In addition, because pediatric obesity is associated with advanced bone age and increased bone and muscle density (Austin et al., 1991), obese and overweight children and adolescents have an advantage over healthy weight children when participating in activities associated with muscular strength, such as weightlifting and shot put (VanVrancken-Tomkins, Sothern, & Bar-Or, 2006). Also, due to a higher ratio of fat to lean body mass, obese children are more buoyant than their healthy weight peers. This provides an advantage during water-based games, such as water polo, and other swimming activities, such as synchronized swimming or water ballet. Furthermore, obese children are more thermally insulated and, therefore, are able to perform for longer durations in cooler water. Despite these advantages, obesity in children is associated with low levels of physical fitness (Brambilla et al., 2011; Joshi, Bryan, & Howat, 2012; Nemet et al., 2003), reduced speed and agility (Cliff et al., 2012; D'Hondt et al., 2012; Schultz et al., 2009; Schultz et al., 2010; Schultz et al., 2011), and obese youth have a greater metabolic cost or energy expenditure than healthy weight children when engaging in similar activities (Bar-Or & Rowland, 2004; Brandou et al., 2005; Daniels et al., 2009; Drinkard et al., 2007; Goran et al., 2000; Loftin et al., 2005; Maffeis, 2008; Nassis et al., 2005; Norman et al., 2005; Sothern, 2001; Sothern et al., 1999b). Thus, obese children are often unable to perform certain physical activities as well as their normal-weight peers (Brambilla et al., 2011; Sothern, 2001; VanVrancken-Tomkins et al., 2006).

Key Points: Overweight Children Are Not Like Healthy Weight Children

- Physically compromised during weight-bearing aerobic exercise
- Metabolically compromised due to impaired fat oxidation and insulin sensitivity
- Biomechanically disadvantaged during walking and running
- Emotionally compromised due to teasing

Physical fitness, defined as an attribute that includes fitness components, such as cardiorespiratory endurance, muscle strength and endurance, flexibility, and body composition (Bovet, Auguste, & Burdette, 2007) is lower in obese versus healthy weight youth (Brambilla et al., 2011; Joshi et al., 2012). A recent study examined differences in physical fitness in children in the lowest versus the highest weight categories and compared the results to children with normal weight (Bovet et al., 2007). The authors reported a strong inverse relationship between excess body fat and physical fitness. The association was particularly present for physical fitness tests involving agility and ambulation in contrast to those requiring muscular strength and endurance (Bovet et al., 2007). Schultz and colleagues (2011) conducted a review of the available scientific literature and identified several physiological differences that may promote reduced physical activity in overweight and obese children. Musculoskeletal pain may occur in overweight children, especially in the lower extremities (Jacobson, 2006; Krebs et al., 2007). Moreover, the extra energy cost of moving a greater body mass results in breathlessness and fatigue during exercise sooner than in their normal-weight counterparts (Brandou et al., 2005; Daniels et al., 2009; Drinkard et al., 2007; Goran et al., 2000; Maffeis, 2008; Nassis et al., 2005; Norman et al., 2005; Schultz et al., 2009; Schultz et al., 2010; Schultz et al., 2011; Sothern, 2001; Sothern et al., 1999b).

Key Points: Excess Fat and Physical Activity in Youth

- Excess body fat in children does not necessarily reduce the ability to maximally consume oxygen:
  - Has a detrimental effect on submaximal aerobic capacity.
- Physical activity recommendations for obese youth should account for their limited exercise tolerance:
  - Should include realistic goals to encourage success.
- Physical training improves insulin sensitivity:
  - May counteract the decline in fat oxidation from calorie reduction.
- Recommend activities that keep demands below ventilatory threshold so that physical activity can be sustained.

Sources: Adapted from Brandou et al., 2005; Daniels et al., 2009; Drinkard et al., 2007; Goran et al., 2000; Nassis et al., 2005; Norman et al., 2005.

Similarly, Norman et al. (2005) determined that overweight and nonoverweight adolescents have similar absolute cardiorespiratory fitness but that the functional impairment observed in overweight adolescents is significantly associated with the increased energy demands needed to move their excess body weight (see Figure 1.3). For overweight adolescents, simply moving their lower limbs induced significantly greater absolute oxygen uptake and led to consumption of a significantly larger proportion of their cardiorespiratory reserve. In turn, this predicted poorer performance during sustained exercise (Norman et al., 2005). Salvadori et al. (1999) reported data in line with research suggesting that overweight and obese children have a relatively less efficient cardiac load, but the research also suggested that overweight and obese children's reduced work tolerance is linked with a reduced oxygen supply to the muscles. Maffeis et al. (1993) found that while walking at a speed of 5 km/hr, the obese child expended approximately 50% more energy then their normal weight control, and the additional cost was progressively higher with increased walking speed.

Gross motor competence and fundamental movement skills are negatively affected by excess body fat in children and adolescents (Cliff et al., 2012; Okely et al., 2004). Motor competence refers to the degree of skilled performance in a wide range of motor tasks as well as the movement coordination and control underlying a particular motor outcome (D'Hondt et al., 2012). Fundamental movement skills hold a similar meaning to motor competence; fundamental movement skills represent the foundational skills required to participate in many physical activities, and include locomotor skills (i.e., running, jumping, and hopping) and object-control or manipulation skills (i.e., running, jumping, and hopping) and object-control or manipulative skills (i.e., catching, throwing, and kicking). Cliff and colleagues (2012) compared the mastery of 12 fundamental movement skills and skill components between overweight and obese children and normal-weight children. For all 12 skills, the prevalence of mastery was lower among overweight and obese children compared with the normal-weight control, with the largest differences in running, sliding, hopping, dribbling, and kicking (Cliff et al., 2012). Another study reported that a group of 43 eight-year-olds with an average weight of 40 kg took twice as long as healthy weight children to get out of a lounge chair. In some of the children, assistance was required for them to stand up from the seated position (Riddiford-Harland, Steele, & Baur, 2006).

Obese Youth Have a Biomechanical Disadvantage

A group of 43 eight-year-olds with an average weight of 40 kg took twice as long as average-weight kids to get out of a lounge chair. Some even needed assistance.

"They have flatter feet, collapsed arches, . . . We think they are just more uncomfortable all the time." —Professor Steele

Source: From Riddiford-Harland et al., 2006.

Table 1.2 Overweight Youth Compared with Normal-Weight Youth (Mean Age: 12.4 years)

Parameter	N	Mean ± SD or range	Normal range
Percent fat	24	43.1 ± 27.1	<30
Cholesterol	50	170.8 ± 29.3	<170
LDL	31	123.5 ± 25.7	<110
VO$_2$ max	22	19.8 ± 4.4	45–53
Asthma	150	10.9–31.6%	10.5%
Liver fat	9	0.049 ± 0.04	0.022 ± 0.02
Low birth weight	177	3.4–29.6%	<10%
High birth weight	177	7.4–18.6%	<10%

Source: Adapted from Sothern, M. S., *Pediatric Clinics of North America*, 48(4), 995–1015, 2001.

In addition to physiologic, metabolic, and biomechanical differences (see Table 1.2), children who suffer from overweight and obesity face greater psychological challenges when engaging in physical activities with leaner children (Losekam et al., 2010; Salvy et al., 2012; Schwimmer, Burwinkle, & Varni, 2003). In one study examining quality-of-life factors, significantly obese children self-reported physical health, social, and school functioning scores, which were similar to terminally ill children with cancer (Schwimmer et al., 2003; see Table 1.3).

In addition, comorbidities associated with obesity place the child at greater risk during exercise (U.S. Centers for Disease Control and Prevention [CDC], 2012). Childhood obesity health effects include, but are not limited to, type 2 diabetes, coronary artery disease, asthma, and mental health conditions (Rahman, Cushing, & Jackson, 2011; Strong et al., 2005). Obese children and adolescents often demonstrate systemic hypertension at rest. Likewise, the level of resting blood pressure is related to the degree of adiposity. In addition, systolic blood pressure at maximal exercise typically correlates with resting values. Thus, greater levels of systolic pressure can be expected during exercise testing of obese youth (Pescatello et al., 2004). This makes it particularly challenging to those not trained in exercise science when selecting appropriate exercise modalities and intensities for obese children. Obesity also is shown to negatively affect asthma therapy in children with severe conditions (Carroll et al., 2006). In many cases, pediatric obesity increases the duration of therapy during severe asthma exacerbations. And, due to its inflammatory nature, childhood obesity is likely to negatively affect asthma control throughout the life of these individuals. Exercise, however, is shown to both protect against and provide therapeutic benefits to individuals with inflammatory diseases, such as asthma (Mathur & Pedersen, 2008; Pedersen & Saltin, 2006).

Metabolic disease is shown to follow obesity during childhood (Daniels et al., 2005). Obese children are at increased risk of developing type 2 diabetes at younger ages (American Diabetes Association, 2000; Riddell & Iscoe, 2006). There is a strong relationship between insulin sensitivity and level of physical activity (Brambilla et al., 2011). Recent investigations report significant improvements in metabolic health and increased insulin sensitivity in overweight and obese children and adolescents following both aerobic and resistance training (Davis, Gyllenhammer, et al., 2011; Davis et al., 2012; Fedewa et al., 2013; Shaibi, 2006; Zorba, Cengiz, & Karacabey, 2011). By improving both insulin sensitivity and glucose uptake

Table 1.3 Obese Children Are Emotionally Different from Healthy Weight Children and Similar to Children with Cancer

Self-report quality of life	Obese versus healthy odds ratio (95% confidence)	Obese versus cancer odds ratio (95% confidence)
Physical health score	5.0 (3.4–8.7)	1.0 (0.6–1.7)
Social functioning	5.3 (3.4–8.5)	1.8 (1.0–3.1)
School functioning	4.0 (2.4–6.5)	1.1 (0.6–2.0)

Source: Adapted from Schwimmer, J. B., Burwinkle, T. M., Varni, J. W., *JAMA*, 289(14), 1813–1819, 2003.

in skeletal muscle, physical activity may have the potential to reduce the incidence of type 2 diabetes in children and adolescents (Fedewa et al., 2013; McGavock, Sellers, & Dean, 2007; Ruzic, Sporis, & Matkovic, 2008).

RESPONSES OF THE OBESE CHILD TO EXERCISE

It is clear in the scientific literature that overweight children respond differently both physically and emotionally to exercise than children classified as normal weight (Brambilla

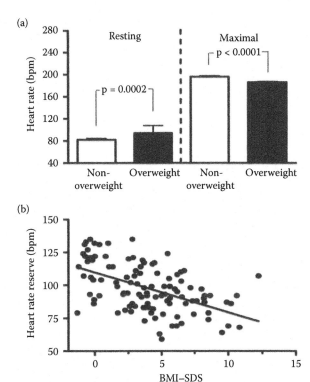

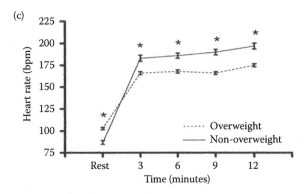

Figure 1.3 Resting and maximal heart rate (HR) during the cycle test. (From Norman, A. C., Drinkard, B., McDuffie, J. R., Ghorbani, S., Yanoff, L. B., Yanovski, J. A., *Pediatrics*, 115(6), e690–e696, 2005. With permission.)

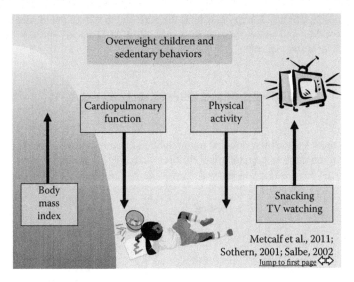

Figure 1.4 Sedentary behaviors follow the onset of obesity.

et al., 2011; French, Story, & Perry, 1995; Latner & Stunkard, 2003; Loftin et al., 2004; Loftin et al., 2005; Maffeis et al., 1993; Schultz et al., 2009; Schultz et al., 2010; Schultz et al., 2011; Schwimmer et al., 2003; Sothern et al., 1999b). During aerobic activities, these children exhibit higher cardiopulmonary values than healthy weight children (Loftin et al., 2003; Maffeis et al., 1993; Norman et al., 2005; Sothern, 2001; Sothern et al., 1999b) and lower over-all fitness levels (Joshi et al., 2012; Tomaszewski et al., 2011).

Overweight and obese children also have a greater metabolic cost or energy expenditure than healthy weight children when engaging in similar activities (Bar-Or & Rowland, 2004; Brandou et al., 2005; Goran et al., 2000; Maffeis, 2008; Sothern, 2001; Sothern et al., 1999b; VanVrancken-Tompkins et al., 2006). In addition, studies have shown that normal-weight children have a greater level of gross motor coordination over time than their obese or overweight counterparts (Cliff et al., 2012; D'Hondt et al., 2012; Morano et al., 2011). And, although exercise typically is associated with improved mental health, for example, reduced depression (Petty et al., 2009; Schwimmer, 2006) and enhanced self-worth (Ullrich-French, McDonough, & Smith, 2012), the weight criticism that overweight and obese children experience during physical activities offsets these benefits, and, in some instances, actually decreases sports enjoyment, perceived ability, and feelings of loneliness (Salvy et al., 2012).

A recent study examined the direction of the association between inactivity and obesity in children. The authors hypothesized that inactivity actually follows the development of obesity, rather than promoting an increase in body fat (Metcalf et al., 2011). The results indicated that percent of body fat was predictive of changes in physical activity over 3 years. The same

Table 1.4 Heart Rate during Walking in Children with Increasing Overweight Level (walking 3.5 mph)

	Body mass index	Maximum heart rate
Healthy weight	≤85th BMI	37.8% of max HR
Overweight	>85–≤95th BMI	47.8% of max HR
Obese	>95–≤99th BMI	65.4% of max HR
Severely obese	>20% of the 95th BMI or an absolute BMI >35kg/m²	85.3% of max HR

Source: Adapted from Sothern et al., 2001.

did not hold true, however, in the other direction as physical activity levels were not predictive of subsequent changes in body fat during the same period (Metcalf et al., 2011). This study confirms earlier research indicating that increases in weigh status deteriorate cardiopulmonary function, which results in reduced physical activity due to the increased physiological demand, metabolic demands, and biomechanical and psychological impairments (Maffeis, 2008; Norman et al., 2005; Salbe et al., 2002; Sothern, 2001; Sothern, Hunter, et al., 1999; Sothern et al., 1999b). This is followed by an increase in sedentary pursuits, such as television watching, which promotes snacking and further weight gain (Salbe et al., 2002; Sothern, 2001; see Figure 1.4).

Thus, efforts to reverse this inevitable trend toward increasing obesity should consider the limited exercise tolerance of sedentary, obese, or overweight children before selecting exercise modality, duration, frequency, and intensity (Brambilla, 2011, Brandou et al., 2005; Cliff et al., 2012; D'Hondt et al., 2012; Daniels et al., 2009; Drinkard et al., 2007; Norman et al., 2005; Sothern, 2001; Sothern et al., 2006).

AEROBIC PERFORMANCE

Excess body fat confounds the relationship between aerobic fitness, which is measured by maximal oxygen consumption (VO_2max) and age in both male and female children (Loftin et al., 2005; Sothern et al., 1999b). Thus, excess fat weight serves as a deterrent to exercise and body movement in general (Bray, 1994; Davis, Ettinger, & Neuhaus, 1990; Hills, 1994; McGoey et al., 1990; Sothern et al., 1999b). When overweight children are compared with normal-weight children during submaximal exercise, they exhibit higher cardiopulmonary values for a given work rate (Loftin et al., 2003; Loftin et al., 2005; Maffeis et al., 1993; Sothern, 2001; Sothern et al., 2006). It is not well understood whether this increase in cardiopulmonary stress per given work rate is due to reduced physical activity patterns in obese children, the metabolic consequences of the excess weight, or the impact of the additional weight on the modality of exercise.

Interestingly, Loftin and others have reported that increased body mass was associated with lower maximal heart rate in youth (Loftin et al., 2003). As a result, structured and vigorous, aerobic-type activity when prescribed to overweight children, regardless of the individual's age, stage of development, weight status, and medical condition may result in noncompliance or physical injury (Sothern, 2001; Sothern et al., 2006).

Studies using cycle (a non-weight-bearing exercise) as opposed to treadmill ergometry (a weight-bearing exercise) have yielded conflicting results (Loftin et al., 2004). Cooper et al. (1990) examined the oxygen uptake response in a sample of 18 overweight children ranging in age from 9 to 17 years during cycle ergometry. The authors reported normal O_2 kinetic responses when moving from rest to exercise. The overweight children, however, had significantly prolonged response kinetics when Ve and VCO_2 were observed. The authors concluded that overweight children might have normal fitness levels for their individual stages of development. Their findings should be interpreted cautiously, however, because responses may be different during cycle ergometry, as opposed to treadmill, when the excess body weight of the overweight subject is supported. This is evident when the results of Maffeis et al. (1994) are considered. They reported that VO_2max expressed in absolute values in overweight children was significantly greater than in nonoverweight children during treadmill testing, but it was not significantly different during cycle ergometry. When VO_2max was expressed relative to fat-free mass, however, no differences were observed between overweight and nonoverweight subjects during either walking or cycling protocols (Maffeis et al., 1993). The authors suggested that overweight children experienced no limitation in maximal aerobic power during weight-bearing or non-weight-bearing exercise. However, submaximal exercise results were not discussed (McGoey et al., 1990).

Zanconato et al. (1989) reported that VO_2max expressed in mL/kg/min was significantly greater in nonoverweight than in overweight children. In absolute terms, however, VO_2max

L/min was not significantly different between the two groups. In the same study, the performance run time and maximal work rate also were significantly lower in the overweight compared with the nonoverweight children. Recently, in a study examining metabolic health Ahn, McMurray, and Harrell (2013) reported a similar finding and recommended that aerobic fitness be expressed in units per kilogram of fat-free mass when examining associations between VO_2max and insulin resistance. Loftin et al. (2001) previously reported that when VO_2max values are adjusted for total body weight in children, a significant bias results. Thus, reporting VO_2max in absolute values or per kilogram of lean body weight reduces this bias. Using allometric scaling techniques also may be applied to reduce weight bias. Because of this bias and, because more research is needed in the obese child's response to aerobic exercise, pediatric health care professionals should exercise caution when interpreting exercise testing results.

ENERGY COST OF MOVEMENT

Because of excess weight, obese children may have a greater metabolic cost or energy expenditure for executing the same physical activity compared with normal-weight children (Bovet et al., 2007; Sothern, 1999). This greater cost of locomotion may explain why children may not perform as well as nonobese children during aerobic tasks (Bar-Or & Rowland, 2004). In a study by Volpe Ayub and Bar-Or (2003), the energy cost of walking was examined in obese and lean adolescent boys who were matched for total body mass. At the slow and moderate speeds, the obese and lean boys displayed similar energy cost. At the fastest speed, however, the obese adolescents displayed an energy cost that was 12% higher than the lean adolescents. Moreover, total body mass rather than adiposity explained a higher percentage of the variance in energy cost during all of the walking speeds.

Wasteful movements, particularly observed in the gait patterns of obese children, also increase the energy cost of locomotion (Bar-Or &Rowland, 2004; McGraw et al., 2000; Schultz et al., 2010). Hills and Parker (1992) observed the gait patterns of normal-weight and obese prepubertal children while walking at different velocities on a level surface. Even when the velocity was set at a comfortable pace, the obese children displayed a significantly lower cadence of steps per minute compared with the normal-weight children. During the faster, and especially slower speeds, obese children had even more difficulty walking. McGraw and colleagues (2000) examined differences in gait patterns and postural stability in obese and nonobese prepubertal boys. Similar to the study by Hills and Parker (1992), the obese boys displayed a significantly lower cadence, slower gait cycle, and reduced time in the swing phase, compared with the nonobese boys. With regard to postural stability, greater sway areas were observed especially in the medial and lateral direction in the obese boys. The authors concluded that this greater sway area was due to the excess weight rather than postural instability (McGraw et al., 2000).

MUSCULAR STRENGTH AND ENDURANCE

Numerous studies have examined the obese child's response to strength training. Sothern and colleagues (Sothern, Loftin, et al., 1999; Sothern et al., 2000) demonstrated that the inclusion of regular resistance training in a program to prevent and treat pediatric obesity in preadolescent children is not only feasible but also safe and may contribute to increased retention at 1 year. In another study, a meta-analysis examined 30 childhood obesity treatment studies that included an exercise intervention (LeMura & Maziekas, 2002). Significant improvements in body composition were associated with programs, including high-repetition strength training in conjunction with moderate intensity aerobic exercise. Thus, the combination of high-repetition resistance training, moderate aerobic exercise, and behavioral modification may be most efficacious for reducing body fat variables in overweight children. Because pediatric obesity is associated with advanced bone age and increased bone and muscle density (Austin et al., 1991), obese children achieve additional advantages when participating in strength training.

This is especially true given that research indicates that the enhancement of strength associated with resistance training is not accompanied by increased muscle size in pre-pubertal children (Blimkie, 1993).

Strength training may provide additional benefits and advantages to obese children. Most strength exercises are performed while the body weight is supported. In especially severely overweight youth, this may enhance performance. Although the excess fat weight is supported, the accompanying increased muscle and bone weight will enable more force to be generated (Sothern, 2001; VanVrancken-Tompkins et al., 2006). More research is needed, but it appears that strength and resistance training may be used safely to enhance the efforts to prevent and reverse childhood obesity in clinic-based interventions.

GROSS MOTOR COMPETENCE AND FUNDAMENTAL MOVEMENT SKILLS

Fundamental motor skills are critical to participation in most physical activities (Okely et al., 2004). Okely et al. (2004) examined the association between fundamental motor skills proficiency and body composition among children and adolescents. The following six skills were assessed: running, vertical jumping, catching, overhand throwing, forehand striking, and kicking. Body composition was assessed by waist circumference and BMI. An inverse linear association was observed among the overweight youth's ability to perform fundamental movement skills and degree of overweight. Moreover, the overweight youth were twice as likely as the nonoverweight youth to be in the lowest fundamental motor skills quintile (Okely et al., 2004). Similar results were observed when Graf and colleagues (2004) examined the correlation between BMI and gross motor development in first-grade children (mean age 6.70 years). In the overweight and obese children, BMI was correlated inversely with gross motor development and endurance performance. Thus, excess fat weight may negatively affect the fundamental motor skill performance of some children. These and other studies indicate that normal-weight children have superior gross motor coordination over time when compared with their obese and overweight counterparts (Cliff et al., 2012; D'Hondt et al., 2012). Adequate level of motor competence or fundamental movement skills is essential to the healthy development of children, but more important, these factors establish the foundation for an active lifestyle. Special attention is needed for overweight and obese children's motor skill improvement to eliminate the increasingly widening gap with their normal-weight counterparts and to ensure regular participation in physical activity (Cliff et al., 2012; D'Hondt et al., 2012). Pediatric health care professionals should provide opportunities for obese children to participate in activities that both consider and improve impaired fundamental motor skills.

PSYCHOLOGICAL CONSIDERATIONS

In addition to physiological differences, children who suffer from overweight or obesity face greater psychological challenges when engaging in physical activity. Regardless of their physical ability, overweight and obese children face social stressors, such as weight teasing and decreased self-efficacy, which result in greater levels of physical inactivity. Studies have consistently found that many youth, especially those who are overweight or obese, are less physically active, perceive physical activity more negatively, and find sedentary activity more reinforcing than physical activities when compared with normal weight youth (Salvy et al., 2012). Overweight or obese youth often are teased by their peers because of their physical appearances; they often are subjected to peer rejection, ostracism, and physical and verbal victimization; and these actions result in decreased physical activity in overweight, obese, and normal-weight youth (Losekam et al., 2010; Salvy et al., 2012). Research indicates that weight criticism during physical activity and other verbal, physical, and relational manifestations of victimization have been shown to be predictive of increased depressive symptoms, time spent alone, and feelings of loneliness as well as reduced sports enjoyment, children's perceived ability relative to their peers, and overall physical activity (Salvy et al., 2012).

Encouraging overweight and obese children to adhere to exercise programs is difficult because of the greater cardiopulmonary and biomechanical strain associated primarily with weight-bearing activity (Brambilla et al., 2011; Huttunen, Knip, & Paavilainen, 1986; Maffeis et al., 1993; Sothern, 2001; Sothern, Hunter, et al., 1999; Sothern et al., 1999b, 2006). The discomfort associated with transporting an overweight body may result in pain in the lower extremities, breathing difficulty, and premature fatigue, especially in severe conditions of obesity (Brambilla et al., 2011; Joshi et al., 2012; McGoey et al., 1990; Schultz et al., 2011; Sothern, 2001). In addition, recent data suggest that childhood obesity impairs fundamental motor skills (Cliff et al., 2012; D'Hondt et al., 2013). This, combined with a higher energy cost of locomotion, alters the obese child's perception of exercise difficulty (Sothern et al., 2006). Therefore, obese children may experience negative consequences to participation in activities considered appropriate for normal-weight children. Daily activities such as walking appear to be relatively easy, but an extremely complex biomechanical process occurs when the body weight is carried forward (Hills et al., 2002). Excess weight that must be carried during walking may adversely affect the gait pattern and posture of overweight and obese children (McGraw et al. 2000; Schultz et al., 2010; Schultz et al., 2011). Exercises to improve their gait pattern, posture, and balance should be considered when developing an exercise program for overweight, and especially severely obese, children (Hills & Parker, 1992). When designing exercise programs for obese children, the instructor should consider activities that are mastered easily. Such activities will ensure that students experience initial success when participating in physical activity if adherence to the program is desired (Sothern, 2001; Sothern, Hunter, et al., 1999; Sothern et al., 1999a, 2006).

APPROPRIATE EXERCISE FOR OVERWEIGHT AND OBESE CHILDREN

Most, but not all, physical activities if properly dosed and of appropriate intensity may be performed safely and successfully by obese children (Sothern, 2001; VanVrancken-Tompkins et al., 2006). Several factors inhibit obese children during physical activity, including awkwardness around normal-weight peers and limited speed and agility due to carrying excess fat weight. Therefore, it is important to consider the following factors when prescribing exercise to obese children. First, obese kids often are inhibited when expected to exercise together with normal-weight peers. In contrast, when their peers are all (or mostly) obese, they play and exercise with little or no inhibition. In settings in which exercise apparel is revealing, such as swimming activities, this is especially evident. Second, obese children are taller than their peers (especially during pre-, early-, and midpubertal years). And, although this gives them some advantage in sports where height and arm span are important (e.g., basketball, volleyball, shot put, discus, defensive or offensive line in football), their relative slowness and clumsiness limit their ability to excel in these competitive settings. In many case, however, they still can be useful to their team. Third, another type of activity in which the obese child can perform well is strength training. This may be due to advanced muscle development and bone age. Many strength exercises require the body to assume positions in which overall body weight is supported. In this case, obese children will perform equally if not superior to normal-weight peers. Finally, obese children have two advantages for water-based activities: They are more buoyant and are better thermally insulated. The buoyancy gives them a definite advantage to move or float in the water with less effort, which may boost their success in swimming and water games—a major contradistinction to land-based activities. Additionally, the better subcutaneous insulation is a definite advantage when the water is cool. In this environment, lean children will lose heat (and feel the cold) much faster than those with more fat (Sloan & Keatinge, 1973).

Several steps can be followed to motivate the obese child to be physically active. Chapter 5 discusses various motivational theories and models; however, specific physical factors can be addressed as well. Both parents and health professionals can help make physical activity enjoyable for the obese child. They can help identify local facilities for physical activity, including parks and swimming pools and community walking groups. Health professionals should teach the child how to listen to their body and exercise at their own pace (Hills & Byrne, 2004; Sothern et al., 2006). Pacing skills may not be inherent. Therefore, instruction should include methods to help children identify moderate versus vigorous activity and the resulting heat rate and breathing responses. Chapter 6 provides specific lesson plans to assist with this instruction as well as methods to help overweight and obese children develop pacing skills.

Weight-bearing activities should be limited at the start of a weight-loss program for obese children (Bar-Or & Rowland, 2004; Sothern, 2001; Sothern et al., 1999b, 2000, 2006; Vrancken-Tompkins et al., 2006). Deforche et al. (2003) reported that obese youth have poorer performances during weight-bearing tasks compared with the nonobese children. Swimming is an ideal, non-weight-bearing activity for obese children (Bar-Or & Rowland, 2004). Not only is swimming ideal for obese children because of their higher buoyancy and thermal comfort but also because their bodies are completely submerged, thus avoiding exposure to their nonobese peers.

INAPPROPRIATE EXERCISE FOR OVERWEIGHT AND OBESE CHILDREN

Exercise activities that require speed, quickness, and lifting one's body weight should not be part of the initial general prescription for overweight and obese children (Sothern, 2001; Sothern et al., 2006; Van Vranken-Tomkins et al., 2006). This is especially true of activities that require repeated attempts to lift the entire body. Therefore, overweight, and especially obese and severely obese, children will do poorly in sprinting and jumping, pull-ups, and ring dips on the parallel bars (Deforche et al., 2003). Activities such as stair climbing, jogging, and running should be given a low priority. The lower joints of obese children are compromised because of the excess fat weight during these activities. This can pose a threat to the child's joints, posture, and gait pattern (Brambilla et al., 2011; Hills et al., 2002; Jacobson, 2006; McGraw, 2000; Schultz et al., 2010, 2011). This is especially true in the obese, prepubertal child who has an increased risk of injury due to a reduction in joint flexibility caused by rapid growth in the long bones. Thus, non-weight-bearing activities, such as swimming, cycling, or resistance training, may provide the best option. In addition, the low levels of physical activity and reduced ability to participate in weight-bearing activities associated with musculoskeletal problems further place the overweight and obese child at risk for future osteoporosis and associated fractures later in life (Faigenbaum & Myer, 2010). Thus, it is important to consider alternative activities that do not require the weight to be supported during exercise but likewise to provide osteogenic stimulus during the pre- and postadolescent period of development. Resistance training provides the added benefit of producing mechanical strain, which may act concurrently with normal growth-related increases in bone development to maximize peak bone mass (Behm et al., 2008). As obese children will expend more energy performing physical activities of the same intensity as normal-weight children, they should not be prescribed running activities during which they must compete with normal-weight youth (Schultz et al., 2011).

SUMMARY

Exercise should be considered an essential adjunct to pediatric weight-management programs and efforts to prevent the onset of obesity in children (Sothern, 2004; Sothern et al., 1999a). Unfortunately, the positive effects of exercise training will be realized only if the obese child complies with the prescribed physical activities. It is imperative that careful consideration be given to selecting the most appropriate intensity, frequency, duration, and modality of

Table 1.5 Components of an Optimal Enhanced Activity Program for Juvenile Obesity

Use large muscle groups to achieve high-energy expenditure.
Move the whole body over distance (e.g., walking, skating, dancing, swimming).
Emphasize duration; deemphasize intensity.
Aim at energy equivalent of 10% to 15% total daily expenditure (e.g., 200–300 kcal) per session.
Include resistance training (particularly if program includes low-energy dieting).
Gradually increase frequency and volume (strive for daily activity, 30–45 min/day).
Consider the child's preference for activities.
Emphasize water-based sports and games.
Consider lifestyle changes, not merely regimented activities.
Let parents contract with the child to reduce sedentary activities (e.g., television).
Build in token remuneration.
Include other obese children in group activities (this reduces inhibition).
Remember, the key to compliance is fun, fun, fun!

Source: From Bar-Or, O., Rowland, T. W., *Pediatric Exercise Medicine: From Physiologic Principles to Health Care Application,* Human Kinetics, Champaign, IL, 2004. With permission.

exercise for each overweight or obese child (Daniels et al., 2009; Ganley et al., 2011; Sothern, 2011; Sothern et al., 2006). Exercise for overweight children should be appropriate to their specific physiologic and metabolic condition (Brambilla et al., 2011; Johnston & Steele, 2007; Maffeis, 2008; Norman et al., 2005; Sothern, 2001; Sothern et al., 2006). Activities should be based on well-established theories and principles to ensure successful motivation, a positive learning environment, and successful outcomes (Sothern, 2006). Activities must be appropriate to the child's emotional and physical development. Table 1.5 provides recommendations for an optimal enhanced activity program for obese children that may be safely and effectively used in the pediatric clinical setting. Detailed descriptions and illustrations of suitable exercises for overweight and obese children may be found in Chapters 2, 3, 4, and 6 of this textbook.

REFERENCES

Ahn, B., McMurray, R., Harrell, J. (2013) Scaling of VO$_2$max and its relationship with insulin resistance in children. *Pediatric Exercise Science,* 25(1), 43–51.

American Academy of Pediatrics, Committee on Sports Medicine. (1990). Strength training, weight and power lifting, and body building by children and adolescents. *Pediatrics,* 86(5), 801–803.

American Academy of Pediatrics, Committee on Nutrition. (2003). Prevention of pediatric overweight and obesity. *Pediatrics,* 112(2), 424–430.

American College of Sports Medicine. (2011). Position stand: Quantity and quality of exercise for developing and maintaining cardiorespiratory, musculoskeletal, and neuromotor fitness in apparently healthy adults: Guidance for prescribing exercise. *Medicine and Science in Sports and Exercise,* 43(7), 1334–1359.

American College of Sports Medicine. (2010). *ACSM's Guidelines for Exercise Testing and Prescription* (8th ed.) Philadelphia, PA: Lippincott Williams & Wilkins.

American Diabetes Association. (2000). Type 2 diabetes in children and adolescents. *Diabetes Care,* 23(3), 381–389.

Austin, H., Austin, J. M., Jr., Partridge, E. E., Hatch, K. D., Shingleton, H. M. (1991). Endometrial cancer, obesity, and body fat distribution. *Cancer Research*, 51(2), 568–572.

Bailey, R. C., Olson, J., Pepper, S. L., Porszasz, J., Barstow, T. J., Cooper, D. M. (1995). The level and tempo of children's physical activities: An observational study. *Medicine and Science in Sports and Exercise*, 27(7), 1033–1041.

Bar-Or, O. Rowland, T. W. (2004). *Pediatric Exercise Medicine: From Physiologic Principles to Health Care Application*. Champaign, IL: Human Kinetics.

Bar-Or, O. (unpublished data).

Behm, D., Faigenbaum, A., Falk, B., Klentrou, P. (2008). Canadian Society for Exercise Physiology position paper: resistance training in children in children and adolescents. *Applied Physiology, Nutrition, and Metabolism*, 33, 547–561.

Behringer, M., Vom Heede, A., Matthews, M., Mester, J. (2011). Effects of strength training on motor performance skills in children and adolescents: a meta-analysis. *Pediatric Exercise Science*, 23(2), 186–206.

Biro, F. M., Greenspan, L. C., Galvez, M. P. (2012). Puberty in girls of the 21st century. *Journal of Pediatric and Adolescent Gynecology*, 5(5), 289–294.

Blimkie, C. J. (1993). Resistance training during preadolescence: Issues and controversies. *Sports Medicine*, 15(6), 389–407.

Bovet, P., Auguste, R., Burdette, H. (2007). Strong inverse association between physical fitness and overweight in adolescents: a large school-based survey. *International Journal of Behavioral Nutrition and Physical Activity*, 4, 24.

Brambilla, P., Pozzobon, G., Pietrobelli, A. (2011). Physical activity as the main therapeutic tool for metabolic syndrome in childhood. *International Journal of Obesity*, 35(1), 16–28.

Brandou, F., Savy-Pacaux, A. M., Marie, J., Bauloz, M., Maret-Fleuret, I., Borrocoso, S., et al. (2005). Impact of high- and low-intensity targeted exercise training on the type of substrate utilization in obese boys submitted to a hypocaloric diet. *Diabetes Metabolism*, 31(4 Pt 1), 327–335.

Bray, G. (1994). The role of exercise in obesity: A personal view. In M. Wahlqvist (Ed.), *Exercise and Obesity* (pp. 7–9). London: Smith-Gordon.

Carroll, C. L., Bhandari, A., Zucker, A. R., Schramm, C. M. (2006). Childhood obesity increases duration of therapy during severe asthma exacerbations. *Pediatric Critical Care Medicine*, 7, 527–531.

Castelli, D. M., Hillman, C. H., Buck, S. M., Erwin, H. E. (2007). Physical fitness and academic achievement in third- and fifth-grade students. *Journal of Sport and Exercise Psychology*, 29(2), 239–252.

Cliff, D. P., Okely, A. D., Morgan, P. J., Jones, J. R., Steele, J. R., Baur, L. A. (2012). Proficiency deficiency: mastery of fundamental movement skills and skill components in overweight and obese children. *Obesity (Silver Spring, Md.)*, 20(5), 1024–1033.

Cooper, D. M., Poage, J., Barstow, T. J., Springer, C. (1990). Are obese children truly unfit? Minimizing the confounding effect of body size on the exercise response. *Journal of Pediatrics*, 116(2), 223–230.

Curtis, A. D., Hinckson, E. A., Water, T. C. (2012). Physical activity is not play: perceptions of children and parents from deprived areas. *New Zealand Medical Journal*, 125(1365), 38–47.

Daniels S., Arnett, D., Eckel, R., Gidding, S. S., Hayman, L. L., Kumanyika, S., et al. (2005). Overweight in children and adolescents: Pathophysiology, consequences, prevention, and treatment. *Circulation*, 11(15), 1999–2012.

Daniels, S. R., Jacobson, M. S., McCrindle, B. W., Eckel, R. H., Sanner, B. M. (2009). American Heart Association childhood obesity research summit: Executive summary. *Circulation*, 119(15), 2114–2123.

Davis, M. A., Ettinger, W. H., Neuhaus, J. M. (1990). Obesity and osteoarthritis of the knee: Evidence from the National Health and Nutrition Examination Survey (NHANES I). *Seminars in Arthritis and Rheumatism*, 20(3 Suppl 1), 34–41.

Davis, C. L., Tomporowski, P. D., Boyle, C. A., Waller, J. L., Miller, P. H., Naglieri, J. A., et al. (2007). Effects of aerobic exercise on overweight children's cognitive functioning: A randomized controlled trial. *Research Quarterly for Exercise and Sport*, 78(5), 510–519.

Davis, C. L., Tomporowski, P. D., McDowell, J. E., Austin, B. P., Miller, P. H., Yanasak, N. E., et al. (2011). Exercise improves executive function and achievement and alters brain activation in overweight children: A randomized, controlled trial. *Health Psychology*, 30(1), 91–98.

Davis, J. N., Gyllenhammer, L. E., Vanni, A. A., Meija, M., Tung, A., Schroeder, E. T., Spruijt-Metz, D., Goran, M. I. (2011). Startup circuit training program reduces metabolic risk in Latino adolescents. *Medicine and Science in Sports and Exercise*, 43(11), 2195–2203.

Davis, C., Pollock, N., Waller, J., Allison, J., Dennis, B., Bassali, R., Melendez, A., Boyle, C., Gower, B. (2012). Exercise dose and diabetes risk in overweight and obese children. *JAMA*, 308(11), 1103–1112.

De Simone, M., Farello, G., Palumbo, M., Gentile, T., Ciuffreda, M., Olioso, P., . . . De Matteis, F. (1995). Growth charts, growth velocity and bone development in childhood obesity. *International Journal of Obesity and Related Metabolic Disorders*, 19(12), 851–857.

Deforche, B., Lefevre, J., De Bourdeaudhuij, I., Hills, A. P., Duquet, W., Bouckaert, J. (2003). Physical fitness and physical activity in obese and nonobese Flemish youth. *Obesity Research*, 11(3), 434–41.

D'Hondt, E., Deforche, B., Gentier, I., De Bourdeaudhuij, I., Vaeyens, R., Philippaerts, R., Lenoir, M. (2013). A longitudinal analysis of gross motor coordination in overweight and obese children versus normal-weight peers. *International Journal of Obesity*, 237(1), 61–67. doi: 10.1038/ijo.2012.55. Epub 2012 Apr 17.

DiNubile, N. A. (1993). Youth fitness—problems and solutions. *Preventive Medicine*, 22(4), 589–594.

Donnelly, J. E., Lambourne, K. (2011). Classroom-based physical activity, cognition, and academic achievement. *Preventive Medicine*, 52(Suppl 1), S36–S42.

Drinkard, B., Roberts, M. D., Ranzenhofer, L. M., Han, J. C., Yanoff, L. B., Merke, D. P., et al. (2007). Oxygen-uptake efficiency slope as a determinant of fitness in overweight adolescents. *Medicine and Science in Sports and Exercise*, 39(10), 1811–1816.

Eisenmann, J.; for the Subcommittee on Assessment in Pediatric Obesity Management Programs, National Association of Children's Hospital and Related Institutions. (2011). Assessment of obese children and adolescents: A survey of pediatric obesity-management programs. *Pediatrics*, 128(Suppl 2), S51–S52.

Faigenbaum, A., Myer, G. (2010). Pediatric resistance training: Benefits, concerns, and program design considerations. *Current Sports Medicine Reports*, 9(3), 161–168.

Faigenbaum, A., Kraemer, W., Blimkie, C., Jeffreys, I., Micheli, L., Nitka, M., Rowland, T. (2009). Youth resistance training: Updated position statement paper from the National Strength and Conditioning Association. *Journal of Strength and Conditioning*, 23(Suppl 5), 60–79.

Fedewa, M., Gist, N., Evans, E., Dishman, R. (2013). Exercise and insulin resistance in youth: A meta-analysis. *Pediatrics*, 133(1), 1–12.

French, S. A., Story, M., Perry, C. L. (1995). Self-esteem and obesity in children and adolescents: A literature review. *Obesity Research*, 3(5), 479–490.

Frisch, R. E., Revelle, R. (1971). Height and weight at menarche and a hypothesis of menarche. *Archives of Disease in Childhood*, 46(249), 695–701.

Ganley, K., Paterno, M., Miles, C., Stout, J., Brawner, P., Girolami, G., Warran, M. (2011). Health-related fitness in children and adolescents. *Pediatric Physical Therapy*, 23(3), 208–220.

Giuca, M. R., Pasini, M., Tecco, S., Marchetti, E., Giannotti, L., Marzo, G. (2012). Skeletal maturation in obese patients. *American Journal of Orthodontics and Dentofacial Orthopedics*, 142(6), 774–779.

Goran, M., Fields, D. A., Hunter, G. R., Herd, S. L., Weinsier, R. L. (2000). Total body fat does not influence maximal aerobic capacity. *International Journal of Obesity and Related Metabolic Disorders: Journal of the International Association for the Study of Obesity*, 24(7), 841–848.

Graf, C., Koch, B., Kretschmann-Kandel, E., Falkowski, G., Christ, H., Coburger, S., Lehmacher, W., Bjarmason-Wehrens, B., Platen, P., Tokarski, W., Predel, H. H., Dordel, S. (2004). Correlation between BMI, leisure habits and motor abilities in childhood (CHILT-project). *International Journal of Obesity and Related Metabolic Disorders*, 28(1), 22–26.

Grissom, J. (2005). Physical fitness and academic achievement. *Journal of Exercise Physiology*, 8, 11–25.

Halfon, N., Larson, K., Slusser W. (2013) Associations between obesity and comorbid mental health, developmental, and physical health conditions in a nationally representative sample of US children aged 10 to 17. *Academic Pediatrics*, 13(1), 6–13.

Hillman, C. H., Motl, R. W., Pontifex, M. B., Posthuma, D., Stubbe, J. H., Boomsma, D. I., et al. (2006). Physical activity and cognitive function in a cross-section of younger and older community-dwelling individuals. *Health Psychology*, 25(6), 678–687.

Hills, A. (1994). Locomotor Characteristics of Obese Children. In M. Wahlqvist (Ed.), *Exercise and obesity* (pp. 141–150). London: Smith-Gordon.

Hills, A. P., Byrne, N. M. (2004). Physical activity in the management of obesity. *Clinics in Dermatology*, 22(4), 315–318.

Hills, A. P., Hennig, E. M., Byrne, N. M., Steele, J. R. (2002). The biomechanics of adiposity—structural and functional limitations of obesity and implications for movement. *Obesity Research*, 3(1), 35–43.

Hills, A. P., King, N. A., Armstrong, T. P. (2007). The contribution of physical activity and sedentary behaviours to the growth and development of children and adolescents: Implications for overweight and obesity. *Sports Medicine*, 37(6), 533–545.

Hills, A. P., Parker, A. W. (1992). Locomotor characteristics of obese children. *Child Care Health and Development*, 18(1), 29–34.

Huang, T., Grimm, B., Hammond, R. (2011). A systems-based typological framework for understanding the sustainability, scalability and reach of childhood obesity interventions. *Children's Health Care*, 40(3), 253–266.

Huttunen, N. P., Knip, M., Paavilainen, T. (1986). Physical activity and fitness in obese children. *International Journal of Obesity*, 10(6), 519–525.

Jacobson, M. (2006). Medical complications and comorbidities of pediatric obesity. In M. Sothern, T. K. von Almen, S. Gordon (Eds.), *Handbook of Pediatric Obesity: Clinical Management* (pp. 31–39). Boca Raton, FL: Taylor & Francis.

Johnson, W., Stovitz, S. D., Choh, A. C., Czerwinski, S. A., Towne, B., Demerath, E. W. (2012). Patterns of linear growth and skeletal maturation from birth to 18 years of age in overweight young adults. *International Journal of Obesity*, 36(4), 535–541.

Johnston, C., Steele, R. (2007). Treatment of pediatric overweight: an examination of feasibility and effectiveness in an applied clinical setting. *Journal of Pediatric Psychology*, 32, 106–110.

Joshi, P., Bryan, C., Howat, H. (2012). Relationship of body mass index and fitness levels among schoolchildren. *Journal of Strength and Conditioning Research*, 26(4), 1006–1014.

Kalish, C. W., Sabbagh, M. A. (2007). Conventionality and cognitive development: Learning to think the right way. *New Directions for Child and Adolescent Development*, Spring (115), 1–9.

Kitzmann, K. M., Dalton, W. T., III, Stanley, C. M., Beech, B. M., Reeves, T. P., Buscemi, J., et al. (2010). Lifestyle interventions for youth who are overweight: A meta-analytic review. *Health Psychology*, 29(1), 91–101.

Krebs, N., Himes, J., Jacobson, D., Nicklas, T., Guilday, P., Styne, D. (2007). Assessment of child and adolescent overweight and obesity. *Pediatrics*, 120(Suppl 4), S193–S228.

Kiess, W., Galler, A., Reich, A., Muller, G., Kapellen, T., Deutscher, J., Kratzsch, J. (2001). Clinical aspects of obesity in childhood and adolescence. *Obesity Research*, 2(1), 29–36.

Latner, J. D., Stunkard, A. J. (2003). Getting worse: The stigmatization of obese children. *Obesity Research*, 11(3), 452–456.

LeBlanc, M., Martin, C., Han, H., Newton, R., Jr., Sothern, M., Webber, L., et al. (2012). Adiposity and physical activity are not related to academic achievement in school-aged children. *Journal of Developmental and Behavioral Pediatrics*, 33(6), 486–494. doi: 10.1097/DBP.0b013e31825b849e

LeMura, L. M., Maziekas, M. T. (2002). Factors that alter body fat, body mass, and fat-free mass in pediatric obesity. *Medicine and Science in Sports and Exercise*, 34(3), 487–496.

Loftin, M., Sothern, M., Trosclair, L., O'Hanlon, A., Miller, J., Udall, J. (2001). Scaling VO(2) peak in obese and non-obese girls. *Obesity Research*, 9(5), 290–296.

Loftin, M., Sothern, M., VanVrancken, C., O'Hanlon, A., Udall, J. (2003). Effect of obesity status on heart rate peak in female youth. *Clinical Pediatrics*, 42(6), 505–510.

Loftin, M., Sothern, M., Warren, B., Udall, J. (2004). Comparison of VO_2 Peak during treadmill and bicycle ergometry in severely overweight youth. *Journal of Sports Science and Medicine*, 3, 254–260.

Loftin, M., Heusel, L., Bonis, M., Sothern, M. (2005). Oxygen uptake kinetics and oxygen deficit in obese and normal weight adolescent females. *Journal of Sports Science and Medicine*, 4, 430–436.

London, R. A., Castrechini, S. (2011). A longitudinal examination of the link between youth physical fitness and academic achievement. *Journal of School Health*, 81(7), 400–408.

Losekam, S., Goetzky, B., Kraeling, S., Rief, W., Hilbert, A. (2010). Physical activity in normal-weight and overweight youth: associations with weight teasing and self-efficacy. *Obesity Facts*, 3(4), 239–244.

Maffeis, C. (2008) Physical activity in the prevention and treatment of childhood obesity: Physio-pathologic evidence and promising experiences. *International Journal of Pediatric Obesity*, 3(Suppl 2), S29–S32.

Maffeis, C., Schena, F., Zaffanello, M., Zoccante, L., Schutz, Y., Pinelli, L. (1994). Maximal aerobic power during running and cycling in obese and non-obese children. *Acta Paediatrica*, 83(1), 113–116.

Maffeis, C., Schutz, Y., Schena, F., Zaffanello, M., Pinelli, L. (1993). Energy expenditure during walking and running in obese and nonobese prepubertal children. *Journal of Pediatrics*, 123(2), 193–199.

Mathur, N., Pedersen, K. (2008). Exercise as a mean to control low-grade systemic inflammation. In *Mediators of Inflammation*. Copenhagen, Denmark: Hindawi.

McCurdy, L., Winterbottom, K., Mehta, S., Roberts, J. (2010). Using nature and outdoor activity to improve children's health. *Current Problems in Pediatric and Adolescent Health Care*, 40(6), 102–117.

McGavock, J., Sellers, E., Dean, H. (2007). Physical activity for the prevention and management of youth-onset type 2 diabetes mellitus: Focus on cardiovascular complications. *Diabetes and Vascular Disease Research*, 4(4), 305–310.

McGoey, B. V., Deitel, M., Saplys, R. J., and Kliman, M. E. (1990). Effect of weight loss on musculoskeletal pain in the morbidly obese. *Journal of Bone and Joint Surgery* (British Volume), 72(2), 322–323.

McGraw, B., McClenaghan, B. A., Williams, H. G., Dickerson, J., Ward, D. S. (2000). Gait and postural stability in obese and nonobese prepubertal boys. *Archives of Physical Medicine and Rehabilitation*, 81(4), 484–489.

Metcalf, B. S., Hosking, J., Jeffery, A. N., Voss, L. D., Henley, W., Wilkin, T. J. (2011). Fatness leads to inactivity, but inactivity does not lead to fatness: A longitudinal study in children (EarlyBird 45). *Archives of Disease in Childhood*, 96(10), 942–947.

Milteer, R. M., Ginsburg, K. R., Council on Communications and Media, Committee on Psychosocial Aspects of Child and Family Health. (2012). The importance of play in promoting healthy child development and maintaining strong parent-child bond: Focus on children in poverty. *Pediatrics*, 129(1), e204–e213.

Molnar, B. E., Gortmaker, S. L., Bull, F. C., Buka, S. L. (2004). Unsafe to play? Neighborhood disorder and lack of safety predict reduced physical activity among urban children and adolescents. *American Journal of Health Promotion*, 18(5), 378–386.

Morano, M., Colella, D., Caroli, M. (2011). Gross motor skill performance in a sample of overweigh and no-overweigh preschool children. *International Journal of Pediatric Obesity*, 6(Suppl 2), 42–46.

Murray, R., Ramstetter, C., Council on School Health Executive Committee. (2013). The crucial role of recess in school. *American Academy of Pediatrics*, 131(1), 183–188.

Nassis, G. P., Papantakou, K., Skenderi, K., Triandafillopoulou, M., Kavouras, S. A., Yannakoulia, M., et al. (2005). Aerobic exercise training improves insulin sensitivity without changes in body weight, body fat, adiponectin, and inflammatory markers in overweight and obese girls. *Metabolism*, 54(11), 14721479.

Nemet, D., Wang, P., Funahashi, T., Matsuzawa, Y., Tanaka, S., Engelman, L., Cooper, D. M. (2003). Adipocytokines, body composition, and fitness in children. *Pediatric Research*, 53(1), 148–152.

Norman, A. C., Drinkard, B., McDuffie, J. R., Ghorbani, S., Yanoff, L. B., Yanovski, J. A. (2005). Influence of excess adiposity on exercise fitness and performance in overweight children and adolescents. *Pediatrics*, 115(6), e690–e696.

Okely, A. D., Booth, M. L., Chey, T. (2004). Relationships between body composition and fundamental movement skills among children and adolescents. *Research Quarterly for Exercise and Sport*, 75(3), 238–247.

Pedersen, B., Saltin, B. (2006). Evidence for prescribing exercise as therapy in chronic disease. *Scandinavian Journal of Medicine and Science in Sports*, 16(1), 3–63.

Pescatello, L. S., Franklin, B. A., Fagard, R., Farquhar, W. B., Kelley, G. A., Ray, C. A. (2004). American College of Sports Medicine position stand: Exercise and hypertension. *Medicine and Science in Sports and Exercise*, 36(3), 533–553.

Petty, K. H., Davis, C. L., Tkacz, J., Young-Hyman, D., Waller, J. L. (2009). Exercise effects on depressive symptoms and self-worth in overweight children: A randomized controlled trial. *Journal of Pediatric Psychology*, 34(9), 929–939.

Rahman, T., Cushing, R. A., Jackson, R. J. (2011). Contributions of built environment to childhood obesity. *Mount Sinai Journal of Medicine*, 78(1), 49–57.

Riddell, M. C., Iscoe, K. E. (2006). Physical activity, sport, and pediatric diabetes. *Pediatric Diabetes*, 7(1), 60–70.

Riddiford-Harland, D. L., Steele, J. R., Baur, L. A. (2006). Upper and lower limb functionality: Are these compromised in obese children? *International Journal of Pediatric Obesity*, 1(1), 42–49.

Ruzic, L., Sporis, G., Matkovic, B. R. (2008). High volume-low intensity exercise cAMP and glycemic control in diabetic children. *Journal of Pediatrics and Child Health*, 44(3), 122–128.

Salbe, A. D., Weyer, C., Harper, I., Lindsay, R. S., Ravussin, E., Tataranni, P. A. (2002). Assessing risk factors for obesity between childhood and adolescence: II. Energy metabolism and physical activity. *Pediatrics*, 110(2 Pt 1), 307–314.

Salvadori, A., Fanari, P,. Fontana, M., Buontempi, L., Saezza, A., Baudo, S., Miserocchi, G., Longhini, E. (1999). Oxygen uptake and cardiac performance in obese and normal subjects during exercise. *Respiration*, 66(1), 25–33.

Salvy, S. J., Bowker, J. C., Germeroth, L., Barkley, J. (2012). Influence of peers and friends on overweight/obese youths' physical activity. *Exercise and Sport Sciences Review,* 40(3), 127–132.

Schultz, S., Browning, R., Schutz, Y., Maffeis, C., Hills, A. (2011). Childhood obesity and walking guidelines and challenges. *International Journal of Pediatric Obesity*, 6, 332–341.

Schultz, S., Hills, A., Sitler, M., Hillstrom, H. (2010). Body size and walking cadence affect hip power in children's gait. *Gait Posture*, 32, 248–252.

Schultz, S., Sitler, M., Tierney, R., Hillstrom, H., Song, J. (2009). Effects of pediatric obesity on joint kinematic and kinetics during two walking cadences. *Archives of Physical Medicine and Rehabilitation*, 90(2146), 2146–2154.

Schwimmer, J. (2006). Psychosocial considerations during treatment. In M. Sothern, T. K. von Almen, S. Gordon (Eds.), *Handbook of Pediatric Obesity: Clinical Management* (pp. 55–65). Boca Raton, FL: Taylor & Francis.

Schwimmer, J. B., Burwinkle, T. M., Varni, J. W. (2003). Health-related quality of life of severely obese children and adolescents. *JAMA*, 289(14), 1813–1819.

Siedentop, D. L. (2009). National plan for physical activity: education sector. *Journal of Physical Activity and Health*, 6(Suppl 2), S168–S180.

Singh, G. K., Siahpush, M., Hiatt, R. A., Timsina, L. R. (2011). Dramatic increases in obesity and overweight prevalence and body mass index among ethnic-immigrant and social class groups in the United States, 1976–2008. *Journal of Community Health*, 36(1), 94–110.

Sloan, R. E., Keatinge, W. R. (1973). Cooling rates of young people swimming in cold water. *Journal of Applied Physiology*, 35(3), 371–375.

Sothern, M. S. (2001). Exercise as a modality in the treatment of childhood obesity. *Pediatric Clinics of North America*, 48(4), 995–1015.

Sothern, M. (2002). Encouraging outdoor physical activity in overweight elementary school children. In K. Wellhousen, (Ed.), *Outdoor Play Every Day: Innovative Play Concepts for Early Childhood*. Albany, NY: Delmar.

Sothern, M. (2004). Obesity prevention in children: Physical activity and nutrition. *Nutrition*, 20(7–8), 704–708.

Sothern, M., Caprio, S., Daniels, S., Gordon, S., Ludwig, D. (2010). New ways to overcome old barriers: Engaging pediatricians and primary care physicians in obesity prevention and intervention. *Childhood Obesity*, 6(5), 240–246.

Sothern, M., Gordon, S. (2005). Family-based weight management in the pediatric health care setting. *Obesity Management*, 1(5), 197–202.

Sothern, M., Hunter, S., Suskind, R., Brown, R., Udall, J., Blecker, U. (1999). Motivating the obese child to move: The role of structured exercise in pediatric weight management. *Southern Medical Journal*, 92(6), 577–584.

Sothern, M., Loftin, J., Ewing, T., Tang, S., Suskind, R., Blecker, U. (1999). The inclusion of resistance exercise in a multi-disciplinary obesity treatment program for preadolescent children. *Southern Medical Journal*, 92(6), 585–592.

Sothern, M. S., Loftin, M., Suskind, R. M., Udall, J. N., Blecker, U. (1999a). The health benefits of physical activity in children and adolescents: Implications for chronic disease prevention. *European Journal of Pediatrics*, 158(4), 271–274.

Sothern, M., Loftin, M., Suskind, R., Udall, J., Blecker, U. (1999b). Physiologic function and childhood obesity. *International Journal of Pediatrics*, 14, 135–139.

Sothern, M. S., Loftin, J. M., Udall, J. N., Suskind, R. M., Ewing, T. L., Tang, S. C., Blecker, U. (2000). Safety, feasibility, and efficacy of a resistance training program in preadolescent obese children. *American Journal of the Medical Sciences*, 319(6), 370–375.

Sothern, M., VanVrancken-Tompkins, C., Brooks, C., Thélin, C. (2006). Increasing physical activity in overweight youth in clinical settings. In M. Sothern, T. K. von Almen, S. Gordon (Eds.), *Handbook of Pediatric Obesity: Clinical Management* (pp. 173–188). Boca Raton, FL: Taylor & Francis.

Strong, W. B., Malina, R. M., Blimkie, C. J., Daniels, S. R., Dishman, R. K., Gutin, B., Hergenroeder, A. C., Must, A., Nixon, P. A., Pivarnk, J. M., Rowland, T., Trost, S., Trudeau, F. (2005). Evidence based physical activity for school-aged youth. *Journal of Pediatrics*, 146(6), 732–737.

Stucky-Ropp, R. C., DiLorenzo, T. M. (1993). Determinants of exercise in children. *Preventive Medicine*, 22(6), 880–889.

Tinggaard, J., Mieritz, M. G., Sørensen, K., Mouritsen, A., Hagen, C. P., Aksglaede, L., Wohlfahrt-Veje, C., Juul, A. (2012). The physiology and timing of male puberty. *Current Opinion in Endocrinology, Diabetes and Obesity*, 19(3), 197–203.

Tomaszewski, P., Zmijewski, P., Gajewski, J., Milde, K., Szczepanska, B. (2011). Somatic characteristics of 9-year-old boys with different levels of physical fitness. *Pediatric Endocrinology, Diabetes and Metabolism*, 17(3), 129–133.

Tomporowski, P. D., Lambourne, K., Okumura, M. S. (2011). Physical activity interventions and children's mental function: an introduction overview. *Preventive Medicine*, 52(Suppl 1), S3–S9.

Ullrich-French, S., McDonough, M. H., Smith, A. L. (2012). Social connection and psychological outcomes in a physical activity-based youth development setting. *Research Quarterly for Exercise and Sport*, 83(3), 431–441.

U.S. Centers for Disease Control and Prevention. (2012). Overweight and obesity: consequences. Retrieved June 9, 2012, from http://www.cdc.gov/obesity/childhood/basics.html (updated April 27, 2012).

U.S. Department of Health and Human Services. (2008). Physical activity guidelines for Americans. Retrieved June 25, 2009, from http://www.health.gov/paguidelines.

U.S. Preventive Services Task Force. (2010). Screening for obesity in children and adolescents: U.S. Preventive Services Task Force recommendation statement. *Pediatrics*, 125(2), 361–367.

VanVrancken-Tompkins, C. L., Sothern, M. S. (2006). Preventing obesity in children birth to five years. In *Encyclopedia on Early Childhood Development*. Montreal, Quebec, Canada: Centre of Excellence for Early Childhood Development. Retrieved from http://www.excellenceearlychildhood.ca/liste_theme.asp?lang=EN&act=32.

VanVrancken-Tompkins, C., Sothern, M., Bar-Or, O. (2006). Weaknesses and strengths in the response of the obese child to exercise. In M. Sothern, T. K. von Almen, S. Gordon (Eds.), *Handbook of Pediatric Obesity: Clinical Management* (pp. 67–75). Boca Raton, FL: Taylor & Francis.

Volpe Ayub, B., Bar-Or, O. (2003). Energy cost of walking in boys who differ in adiposity but are matched for body mass. *Medicine and Science in Sports and Exercise,* 35(4), 669–674.

Washington, R. L., Bernhardt, D. T., Gomez, J., Johnson, M. D., Martin, T. J., Rowland, T. W., Small, E., LeBlanc, C., Krein, C., Malina, R., Young, J. C., Reed, F. E., Anderson, S., Bolduc, S., Bar-Or, O., Newland, H., Taras, H. L., Cimino, D. A., McGrath, J. W., Murray, R. D., Yankus, W. A., Young, T. L., Fleming, M., Glendon, M., Harrison-Jones, L., Newberry, J. L., Pattishall, E., Vernon, M., Wolfe, L., Li, S., Committee on Sports Medicine and Fitness and Committee on School Health. (2001). Organized sports for children and preadolescents. *Pediatrics,* 107(6), 1459–1462.

Washington, R., Bernhardt, D., Gomez, J., Johnson, M., Martin, T., Rowland, T., Committee on Sports Medicine and Fitness. (2001). Strength training by children and adolescents. *Pediatrics,* 107(6), 1470–1472.

Zanconato, S., Baraldi, E., Santuz, P., Rigon, F., Vido, L., Da Dalt, L., Zacchello, F. (1989). Gas exchange during exercise in obese children. *European Journal of Pediatrics,* 148(7), 614–617.

Zorba, E., Cengiz, T., Karacabey, K. (2011). Exercise training improves body composition, blood lipid profile and serum insulin levels in obese children. *Journal of Sports Medicine and Physical Fitness,* 51(4), 664–669.

Chapter 2

AEROBIC EXERCISE

Physical fitness, defined as an attribute that includes fitness components such as cardio-respiratory endurance, muscle strength and endurance, flexibility, and body composition (Bovet, Auguste, & Burdette, 2007), is lower in obese versus healthy weight youth. This chapter will focus on the attainment of cardiorespiratory endurance or aerobic fitness through engaging in aerobic exercise.

DEFINING CARDIORESPIRATORY ENDURANCE

Cardiorespiratory endurance is defined as the capacity of an individual to deliver oxygen to the tissues of the body in response to the level of activity (American College of Sports Medicine [ACSM], 2010). The ability of an individual's circulatory and respiratory system to supply fuel and oxygen during sustained physical activity will determine their cardiorespiratory fitness level. Maximal oxygen uptake (VO_2max) is an indicator of cardiorespiratory endurance in both adult and youth populations (Astrand et al., 1986; Casaburi et al., 1989; McArdle & Magel, 1970; Mitchell & Blomqvist, 1971; Rowell, Taylor, & Wang, 1964). The maximal oxygen uptake indicates the functional capacity of the heart, lungs, and skeletal muscle and generally is assumed to be the single-best indicator of physical fitness (ACSM, 2010; Astrand et al., 1986; Ganley et al., 2011). The VO_2max is determined by exercising a subject and determining O_2 intake and O_2 and CO_2 concentrations in expired air. The resulting value is expressed independent of body weight (absolute) in liters per minute (L/min) or relative to body weight (milliliters of oxygen per kilogram of body weight per minute (mL/kg/min). Cardiorespiratory endurance training promotes an enhanced ability to engage in sustained aerobic exercise (ACSM, 2010). Aerobic exercise specifically improves the capacity to uptake, transport, and utilize oxygen. In children and adolescents, the dose of aerobic exercise necessary to achieve improvements in cardiorespiratory fitness requires an intensity greater than 80% of maximal heart rate, a frequency of 3 to 4 days per week and a duration of 30–60 sustained minutes per session. Fitness goals may be seen in as little as 1 month in some children, and after 3 months, most will experience a significant improvement in cardiorespiratory fitness (Baquet, van Praagh, & Berhoin, 2003). In overweight and obese children, an incremental approach to achieving goals necessary for enhanced cardiorespiratory fitness is recommended (Daniels et al., 2009; Sothern, 2001; Strong et al., 2005; U.S. Department of Health and Human Services [U.S. DHHS], 2008).

 Talking Points: Aerobic Exercise (Cardiorespiratory Endurance) (Verbal cues for patients or parents and family members)
Read through the following information with your patient or family member to help him or her to understand the exercise strategy used in the program.

Aerobic exercise is referred to as cardiorespiratory endurance training. This type of workout demands that your large muscles move at moderate or high intensity for long stretches of time. Examples include walking, jogging, dancing, and swimming. Cardiorespiratory training can strengthen your heart and lungs, improve your stamina, keep your body in good, toned shape, and improve your outlook on life. The rule of thumb is that if you can do an activity for longer than 5 minutes without stopping, then you are probably engaging in aerobic exercise.

HEALTH BENEFITS OF AEROBIC EXERCISE IN THE PREVENTION AND MANAGEMENT OF OBESITY AND RELATED COMORBIDITIES IN YOUTH

It is well established that overweight and obese conditions during childhood and adolescence significantly increase the risk for cardiovascular and metabolic disease later in life. In a recent study of 3383 participants ages 12 to 19 years old from the 1999 through 2008

National Health and Nutrition Examination Survey (NHANES), May, Kuklina, and Yoon (2011) found that U.S. adolescents bear a substantial burden of risk factors for cardiovascular disease especially those who are overweight or obese. Adolescents had an overall prevalence for prehypertension and hypertension of 14%, borderline-high to high low-density lipoprotein cholesterol of 22%, high-density lipoprotein cholesterol of 6%, and prediabetes or diabetes of 15%. A consistent dose-response increase in prevalence of each of these risk factors, however, was observed by weight categories: 49% of the overweight and 61% of the obese adolescents had one or more risk factors in addition to their weight status during the 1999–2008 study period, whereas only 37% of normal-weight adolescents had at least one cardiovascular disease risk factor. Regular physical activity is shown to lessen the burden of obesity-related comorbidities, including reductions in blood pressure, increased insulin sensitivity, and decreases in hepatomegaly (Hassink et al., 2008).

The benefits of aerobic exercise to the prevention and management of pediatric obesity and related conditions like hypertension, hypercholesterolemia, asthma, and type 2 diabetes are numerous and cumulative. Over time, aerobic exercise training will result in a multitude of metabolic and physiologic benefits (Daniels et al., 2009; Nassis et al., 2005; Nemet et al., 2003; see Table 2.1). In a recent review, Janssen and LeBlanc (2010) concluded that even small amounts of physical activity over time evoke positive health benefits in children at greater risk of obesity and high blood pressure. In addition to immediate health benefits during childhood, increased physical activity in children and adolescents contributes to the establishment of healthy leisure habits over a lifetime and improved adult cardiovascular and metabolic health.

The achievement of cardiorespiratory (aerobic) fitness in particular may provide protection against developing obesity during childhood, especially in males. Byrd-Williams et al. (2008) performed a study in 160 (53% boys) overweight Hispanic children (mean age at baseline = 11.2) and found that cardiorespiratory fitness at baseline, measured objectively by VO_2max, was protective against increasing adiposity in boys but not in girls. In boys, higher VO_2max at baseline was inversely association with the rate of increase in adiposity ($\beta = -0.001$, p = .03); this effect translated to a 15% higher VO_2max at baseline resulting in a 138 kg lower fat mass gain over the 4-year study period. Among girls, VO_2max was not significantly associated with changes in fat mass ($\beta = 0.0002$, p = .31). The effects of maturation on adiposity, which differ between developing male and female youth, need to be considered when evaluating the obesity preventive value of cardiorespiratory fitness. Likewise, ethnic differences in the response to aerobic training also have been observed. In randomized controlled trial conducted after school, 10 months of exercise improved general and visceral (abdominal) adiposity, bone, and fitness in black girls, 8–12 years of age. The intervention consisted of 80 minutes of physical activity that included 25 minutes of skills instruction, 35 minutes of aerobic physical activity, and 20 minutes of strengthening and stretching. Compared with the control group, the intervention group had a relative decrease in percent body fat (p < .0001), body mass index (BMI; p < .01), and visceral adiposity (p < .01), and a relative increase in bone mineral density (p < .0001) and cardiovascular fitness (p < .05). Higher attendance and heart rate during the exercise sessions were associated with greater increases in bone mineral density (p < .05) and greater decreases in percent body fat (p < .01) (Barbeau et al., 2007).

Steele et al. (2008) reviewed the recent literature (from 2004 onward) that employed objective measures of physical activity to examine the evidence between habitual physical activity, cardiorespiratory (aerobic) fitness, and clustered metabolic risk in youth. On the basis of the limited number of studies available, it was found that both reducing the time spent in sedentary behaviors and increasing overall moderate to vigorous physical activity has beneficial effects on metabolic risk in children and adolescents. Moreover, the studies indicate that habitual physical activity is independently associated with clustered metabolic risk even after adjusting for adiposity. Studies also demonstrate an inverse relationship between cardiorespiratory fitness and clustered metabolic risk. In addition, cardiorespiratory fitness exerts a small to moderate protective effect across all levels of obesity. Overall, studies demonstrate that both habitual physical activity and cardiorespiratory fitness are separately and

Table 2.1 Benefits of Increasing Cardiorespiratory Activities or Improving Cardiorespiratory Fitness

Decreased fatigue in daily activities
Improved work, recreational, and sports performance
Improved cardiorespiratory function Increased maximal oxygen uptake Increased maximal cardiovascular output and stroke volume Increased capillary density in skeletal muscle Increased mitochondrial density Increased lactate threshold Lower heart rate and blood pressure at a fixed submaximal work rate Lower myocardial oxygen demand at a fixed submaximal work rate Lower minute ventilation at a fixed submaximal work rate
Decreased risk of the following: Mortality from all causes Coronary artery disease Cancer (colon, perhaps breast and prostate) Hypertension Non-insulin-dependent diabetes mellitus Osteoporosis Anxiety Depression
Improved blood lipid profile Decreased triglycerides Increased high-density lipoprotein cholesterol Decreased postprandial lipemia
Improved immune function
Improved glucose tolerance and insulin sensitivity
Improved body composition
Enhanced sense of well-being

Source: From Thompson, W., Bushman, B., Desch, J., Kravitz, L., *ACSM's Resources for the Personal Trainer* (3rd ed.), Lippincott Williams & Wilkins, Philadelphia, PA, 2010. With permission.

independently associated with metabolic risk factors in children and adolescents, but possibly through different pathways.

A multitude of studies documented that obese children who are physically fit have similar metabolic risk patterns as healthy weight children with low fitness levels (Dubose, Eisenmann, & Donnelly, 2007; McMurray et al., 2008; Ortega et al., 2008). This confirms that exercise training of sufficient intensity and volume to promote an increase in aerobic fitness has the potential to reduce or prevent pediatric metabolic disease regardless of level of obesity. Specifically, several of the components of the metabolic syndrome are positively altered after aerobic exercise programs in children and adolescents. Mark and Janssen (2008) reported a positive dose-response relationship between increased aerobic activity levels and blood pressure. Moderate aerobic exercise training also was shown to improve overall glucose tolerance in adolescents (Thomas et al., 2009). Recent investigations report significant metabolic benefits of aerobic training in children and adolescents. Zorba, Cengiz, and Karacabey (2011) reported reductions in insulin levels after a 12-week aerobic exercise training program, including walking and jogging exercise in obese children. Aerobic training improved insulin resistance and reduced visceral adiposity in sedentary overweight and obese children participating in an afterschool program (Davis et al., 2012). In addition, a dose-response benefit was identified in those participating in 40 minutes versus 20 minutes of aerobic training daily.

Key Points: Chronic Response of Aerobic Exercise Training

Long-term aerobic exercise training:

- Increases fat free mass and reduces fat mass
- Improves oxidative capacity
- Increases resting metabolism
- Increases fat oxidation
- Improves insulin sensitivity
- Controls low-grade systemic inflammation

Sources: Adapted from Ballor & Keesey, 1991; Bell et al., 2007; Carrel et al., 2005; Carter, Rennie, & Tarnopolsky, 2001; Dao et al., 2004; Gutin et al., 2000; Haddock & Wilkin, 2006; Horowitz, 2001; Hunter et al., 2006; Hurley & Hagberg, 1998; Kanaley et al., 2001; Nassis et al., 2005; Sothern et al., 1999; Stewart et al., 2007; Stiegler & Cunliffe, 2006; Talanian et al., 2007.

Long-term aerobic exercise training in both adults and children is shown in many studies to increase fat-free mass (including skeletal muscle) and reduce fat mass, increase resting metabolism, improve insulin sensitivity, and enhance the ability to use fat as a fuel (oxidative capacity (Ballor & Keesey, 1991; Bell et al., 2007; Carrel et al., 2005; Carter, Rennie, & Tarnopolsky, 2001; Dao et al., 2004; Haddock & Wilkin, 2006; Horowitz, 2001; Hurley & Hagberg, 1998; Hunter et al., 2006; Kanaley et al., 2001; Nassis et al., 2005; Stiegler & Cunliffe, 2006; Talanian et al., 2007; see Table 2.2). It is widely documented that skeletal muscle is the primary site for fat oxidation due to the regulation of mitochondrial activity (Maffeis, 2008). Long-term exercise training stimulates mitochondrial activity, which positively alters skeletal muscle. This further promotes efficiency in synthesizing glycogen, which, in turn, enhances insulin sensitivity. Impaired insulin sensitivity is associated with the accumulation of lipid within skeletal muscle (intramyocellular lipid) (Forouhi et al., 1999; Perseghin et al., 1999; Sinha et al., 2002) and liver (intrahepatic lipid) (Cali et al., 2007; Fabbrini et al., 2009; Larson-Meyer et al., 2006; Perseghin et al., 2006; Ryysy et al., 2000) in adults (Forouhi et al., 1999; Larson-Meyer et al., 2006; Perseghin et al., 1999; Sinha et al., 2002) and adolescents (Cali et al., 2007; Fabbrini et al., 2009; Larson-Meyer et al., 2006; Sinha et al., 2002); and, more recently, it has been associated with intrahepatic lipid accumulation in young, healthy prepubertal children (Bennett et al., 2012; Larsen Meyer et al., 2006). In overweight and obese prepubertal youth, intrahepatic lipid along with subcutaneous fat, but not visceral (abdominal) fat, independently explained the variance in insulin sensitivity (Maffeis et al., 2008). Moreover, in healthy, exclusively prepubertal obese youth, intrahepatic fat accumulation was shown to be more than twice that of nonobese youth (Bennett et al., 2012). Thus, research is clear that aerobically trained skeletal muscle is central to achieving and maintaining a healthy metabolism in overweight and obese children and adolescents (Brambilla, Pozzobon, & Pietrobelli, 2011; Katz et al., 2012; Maffeis, 2008).

 Key Points: Aerobic Exercise Training and Fat Oxidation

Endurance (aerobic) trained muscle stores more glycogen and fat than untrained muscle.

- Oxidative enzyme activity increases
- Free fatty acid levels increase
- Use of fat as an energy source increases
- Muscle and liver glycogen spared
- Lactate threshold increases, reflecting an improved ability to perform exercise aerobically at higher intensities

Sources: Adapted from Byrne & Wilmore, 2001; Hurley & Hagberg, 1998; Kelley et al., 1999; Talanian et al., 2007; Tonkonogi et al., 2000.

Other related emotional health benefits follow interventions that include aerobic exercise training in youth. Students enrolled in kindergarten through third grade with four or more symptoms of hyperactivity and impulsivity disorder participated in an 8-week physical activity program. The intervention, which consisted of 26 minutes of continuous physical activity alternating from moderate to vigorous intensity, produced significant improvements, including in cognitive, motor, social, and behavioral functioning (Smith et al., 2011).

PRESCRIBING AEROBIC EXERCISE TO OVERWEIGHT AND OBESE YOUTH

Current U.S. evidence-based recommendations for physical activity in school-age youth (Strong et al., 2005; U.S. DHHS, 2008) also include specific recommendations for physically inactive youth. They recommend that these youth use an incremental approach to reach the 60-minute-per-day recommendation by increasing physical activity by 10% per week. They further insist that progressing too quickly is counterproductive and may lead to injury. Because overweight and obese youth are shown to have low physical activity levels, these recommendations are applicable. Furthermore, in a recent American Heart Association Childhood Obesity Summit scientists concluded that overweight and obese youth should be given realistic, easily obtainable physical activity goals and should not be compared with normal-weight peers (Daniels et al., 2009). Hassink et al. (2008) also agreed that exercise prescriptions for obese children should involve activities, which are doable, are fun, and develop participatory skills and promote family support.

DANCING

One such entertaining aerobic exercise activity, dancing, was shown in several studies to promote a significant reduction in weight status, especially in girls (Engels et al., 2005; Ildiko et al., 2007; Robinson et al., 2003; Tak et al., 2007). Thus, interventions that include dancing or other types of activities set to music may be useful in the prevention of pediatric obesity (Sothern, 2006). Music, in particular, facilitates increased performance on cardiovascular equipment (Priest, Karageorghis, & Sharp, 2004).

Table 2.2 Physiological Responses to Aerobic Conditioning in Untrained individuals

Variable	Unit of measure	Response
VO_2max	mL/kg/min	↑
Resting heart rate	beats/min	↓
Exercise heart rate	beats/min	↓
Maximum heart rate	beats/min	↔ (or ↓ slight)
a-v O_2 difference	mL O_2/100 mL blood	↑
Maximum minute ventilation	L/min	↑
Stroke volume	mL/beat	↑
Cardiac output	L/min	↑
Blood volume (resting)	L	↑
Systolic blood pressure	mm Hg	↔ (or ↑ slight)
Blood lactate	mL/100 mL blood	
Oxidative capacity of skeletal muscle	Multiple variables	↑

Source: From Thompson, W., Bushman, B., Desch, J., Kravitz, L., *ACSM's Resources for the Personal Trainer* (3rd ed.), Lippincott Williams & Wilkins, Philadelphia, PA, 2010. With permission.

INTERACTIVE COMPUTER GAMES

Interactive computer games (ICG) are similar in intensity to light to moderate traditional physical activities, such as walking, skipping, and jogging (Maddison et al., 2007). Playing If utilized on a regular basis, ICG may have positive effects on children's overall physical activity levels (Ni Mhurchu et al., 2008). Experienced players have higher energy expenditure during varied ICG (Sell, Lillie, & Taylor, 2008).

A study conducted by Bailey and McInnis (2011) evaluated the potential effect of six forms of exergaming (three commercial products and three consumer products) on energy expenditure in children. Results showed that energy expenditure was significantly elevated to a moderate to vigorous intensity level for all forms of interactive gaming. Researchers also found that children in higher BMI percentiles (≥85th percentile) enjoyed the games more than children in lower BMI percentiles. The authors concluded that exergaming may be a potential innovative strategy to reduce sedentary time, increase adherence to exercise programs, and promote enjoyment of physical activity.

Biddiss and Irwin (2010) conducted a systematic review of levels of metabolic expenditure and changes in activity patterns associated with active video game (AVG) play in children to provide a comprehensive synthesis of the current state of knowledge and provide directions for future research and development of AVGs. Play with AVGs was found to increase energy expenditure to light or moderate levels depending on the specific game played. Games that engaged upper- and lower-body movements increased heart rate and energy expenditure significantly compared with games that primarily involved the lower body. Although AVGs can be supported as an enjoyable medium for self-directed physical activity, current evidence yields inconclusive results on the daily use of AVGs to promote physical activity or reduce sedentary behaviors. Therefore, this should not be regarded as a replacement for vigorous exercise. Future research and development should explore long-term use and efficacy of AVGs in promoting physical activity and changing sedentary behaviors.

In a recent study, Graves et al. (2010) compared the physiological cost and enjoyment of exergaming in the Wii Fit with aerobic exercise in adolescents, young adults, and older adults. Results indicated that energy expenditure and heart rate were greater in Wii Fit activities compared with handheld gaming. All three age-groups elicited moderate intensity activity from Wii aerobics, but heart rate fell below the intensity for cardiorespiratory fitness. The authors concluded that the Wii Fit provides enjoyable light- to moderate-intensity activity in adolescents and adults.

 Key Points: What Is "Dance, Dance Revolution"?

"Dance, Dance Revolution" (DDR) is an active screen media device that transforms typical sedentary screen time into physical activity—

- Overweight children expend more energy than normal-weight children during DDR
- DDR is similar to a 12-minute walking treadmill test
- DDR significantly increases energy expenditure when compared with traditional screen time (Unnithan, Houser, & Fernhall, 2006)

In recent studies, DDR was shown to—

- Improve aerobic fitness
- Improve blood pressure
- Elicit higher energy expenditure values compared to similar devices
- Have a broader appeal and greatest ease of use
- Lack sufficient motivation to produce sustained physical activity over time

Sources: Adapted from Lanningham-Foster et al., 2006; Madsen et al., 2007; Murphy et al., 2009.

AEROBIC EXERCISE: INTENSITY, DURATION, AND FREQUENCY

When considering the optimal choice of aerobic exercise in overweight and obese children, it is important to select an activity that the child most likely will perform with a high level of compliance. Instructors should seek to expose overweight and obese children to a variety of physical activities in a nurturing, nonintimidating environment (Sothern, 2001; Sothern, von Almen, & Gordon, 2006; Sothern, von Almen, & Schumacher, 2001). Recommendations for aerobic-type exercise should be individualized according to the child's medical and family history, age, gender and current weight condition, or obesity level (Sothern, 2001, 2004, 2006; Sothern, Hunter, et al., 1999; Sothern, Loftin, et al., 1999). Exercise prescriptions for aerobic activities should include four components: duration, frequency, mode (or type), and intensity (ACSM, 2010).

Key Points: Determining Obesity Level in Overweight and Obese Children and Adolescents

Level I	>120% of 95th BMI or absolute BMI >35 kg/m²	(Severely Obese)
Level II	>95th < 99th% BMI	(Obese)
Level III	>85th < 95th% BMI	(Overweight)
Level IV	≤85th% BMI	(Healthy Weight

Key Points: Determining the Intensity of Aerobic Exercise

- Percent of Maximal Oxygen Uptake (%VO$_2$max mL/kg/min).
- Percent of Heart Rate (%HR max in beats per minute [BPM])
- Speed (miles/kilograms per hour [kg/hr])
- Force (Resistance/Weight in Pounds [lbs]/kilograms [kg])
- Metabolic Equivalent (MET Level) (Ainsworth et al., 2011)

Maffeis (2008) stated that when prescribing the intensity or load to overweight and obese youth, their unique cardiorespiratory capacity must be considered. Because children are more likely to participate in activities that require them to support their excess body weight with their lower extremities, it is important to consider the additional energy expenditure involved. This additional energy expenditure will require more physical effort on the part of the overweight or obese child when compared with a healthy weight child (Loftin et al., 2001, 2003, 2004, 2005; Sothern, 2001). Performance also will be affected negatively (Sothern, 2001; Sothern, Loftin, et al., 1999). In typical school or recreational settings, overweight and obese children are at a disadvantage when participating in physical activities. This may affect

Table 2.3 Suggested Progression for Duration of Exercise (minutes per session) in Overweight and Obese Children and Adolescents

Level	Week 1	Week 5	Week 10
Overweight	30	45	60
Obese	25	40	55
Severely obese	20	35	50

Sources: Adapted from Daniels, S. R., Jacobson, M. S., McCrindle, B. W., Eckel, R. H., Sanner, B. M. *Circulation*, 119(15), 2114–2123, 2009; Sothern, M. *Pediatric Clinics of North America*, 48(4), 995–1015, 2001; Sothern, M., von Almen, T. K., Gordon, S. (Eds.), *Handbook of Pediatric Obesity: Clinical Management*, Taylor & Francis, Boca Raton, FL, 2006; Sothern, M., von Almen, T. K., Schumacher, H., *Trim Kids: The Proven Plan That Has Helped Thousands of Children Achieve a Healthier Weight*, Harper Collins, New York, NY, 2001; Strong, W. B., Malina, R. M., Blimkie, C. J., Daniels, S. R., Dishman, R. K., Gutin, B., et al. *Journal of Pediatrics,* 146(6), 732–737, 2005; U.S. Department of Health Human Services, *Physical Activity Guidelines for Americans*, retrieved June 25, 2009, from http://www.health.gov/paguidelines, 2008.

motivation negatively, which will further decrease physical activity (Sothern, Hunter, et al., 1999; Sothern, von Almen, & Gordon, 2006). Therefore, a gradual increase in exercise intensity, beginning with low to moderate activities, is recommended (Maffeis, 2008; Sothern, 2001; Sothern et al., 2006). Brambilla et al. (2011) agreed but further suggested that activities of low intensity are most appropriate and more numerous. Thus, selecting low-intensity modalities will encourage both overweight and obese children to engage in and sustain physical activity, as well as offer an enormous variety of activities from which to choose. Tables 2.3–2.5 provide appropriate initial recommendations for duration, frequency, and modality for overweight and obese children. Chapter 6 of this textbook provides detailed lesson plans specifically designed to the child's age, weight status, and family and medical history. A sample aerobic training class from Chapter 6 appears at the end of this chapter.

Table 2.4   Suggested Progression for Frequency of Exercise (days per week) in Overweight and Obese Children and Adolescents

Level	Week 1	Week 5	Week 10
Overweight	3	4.5	6
Obese	2	4	5.5
Severely obese	1	3	5

Sources: Adapted from Daniels, S. R., Jacobson, M. S., McCrindle, B. W., Eckel, R. H., Sanner, B. M. Circulation, 119(15), 2114–2123, 2009; Sothern, M. Pediatric Clinics of North America, 48(4), 995–1015, 2001; Sothern, M., von Almen, T. K., Gordon, S. (Eds.), Handbook of Pediatric Obesity: Clinical Management, Taylor & Francis, Boca Raton, FL, 2006; Sothern, M., von Almen, T. K., Schumacher, H., Trim Kids: The Proven Plan That Has Helped Thousands of Children Achieve a Healthier Weight, Harper Collins, New York, NY, 2001; Strong, W. B., Malina, R. M., Blimkie, C. J., Daniels, S. R., Dishman, R. K., Gutin, B., et al. Journal of Pediatrics, 146(6), 732–737, 2005; U.S. Department of Health Human Services, Physical Activity Guidelines for Americans, retrieved June 25, 2009, from http://www.health.gov/paguidelines, 2008.

Table 2.5   Activity Recommendations According to Body Mass Index (BMI) for Overweight, Obese, and Severely Obese Children and Adolescents

Overweight children (>85–95th BMI), 7–18 years	• Limited access to television, video games, computer • Recommended aerobic activities: Weight-bearing activities, such as brisk walking, treadmill, field sports, roller blading, hiking, racquetball, tennis, martial arts, skiing, jump rope, indoor–outdoor tag games • Parent training and fitness education • Pacing skills
Obese children (>95–99th BMI), 7–18 years	• Limited access to television, video games, computer • Recommended aerobic activities: Non-weight-bearing activities, such as swimming, cycling, strength or aerobic circuit training, arm ergometer (crank), recline bike, and interval walking (walking with frequent rests, as necessary) • Parent training and fitness education
Severely obese children (>120% of 95th BMI or absolute BMI >35 kg/m²), 7–18 years	• Limited access to television, video games, computer • Recommended aerobic activities: Non-weight-bearing activities, such as swimming, recline bike, arm ergometer (crank), seated (chair) aerobics, and seated or lying circuit training • Parent training and fitness education • Other emotional and dietary concerns addressed during treatment

Sources: Sothern, M. Pediatric Clinics of North America, 48(4), 995–1015, 2001; Sothern, M., von Almen, T. K., Schumacher, H., Trim Kids: The Proven Plan That Has Helped Thousands of Children Achieve a Healthier Weight, Harper Collins, New York, NY, 2001; U.S. Preventive Services Task Force, Pediatrics, 125(2), 361–367, 2010.

Key Points: Determining the Volume of Physical Activity

- Duration: How long (minutes per session)?
- Frequency: How often (days per week)?

Key Points: Types of Physical Activities

- Aerobic: endurance (longer durations)
- Anaerobic: high-intensity movement, strength (resistance training), power (sprints, jumps)
- Weight bearing: walking, jogging, running, dancing
- Non-weight bearing: cycling, swimming

SAMPLE CLASS

LESSON 2, LEVEL 1: WARMING UP, COOLING DOWN, AND THE METABOLIC ENGINES OF THE BODY

INTRODUCTION

The instructor will discuss the importance of warming up before participating in physical activity. He or she will lead the patients in a 3- to 5-minute warm-up routine to music. The instructor then will lead the students in a 30- to 45-minute low-impact aerobic class while instructing them about the different metabolic engines of the body (e.g., aerobic and anaerobic). He or she will demonstrate the proper way to cool down after exercising.

ACTIVITY I. WARMING UP

The instructor should discuss the importance of warming up before beginning any exercise using the following verbal cues:

Talking Points: Warming Up (Verbal cues for patients or parents and family members)
Read through the following information with your patient to help him or her to understand the exercise strategy used in the program.

You have just tied your sneakers and are about to go for an easy walk or bike ride around the park. Before you do any type of exercise, you will need to warm up for at least 5 minutes before each session. Warming up is simple: Move each part of your body in a slow, controlled manner. When you slowly move an arm, a leg, or a shoulder, your heart sends blood to that body part, delivering fuel to the muscles and tissues that are in motion. Moving your arms and legs helps the heart pump blood throughout your entire body, preparing your body for more movement. Try the suggestions below, or make up your own!
Some Warm-Up Suggestions:

- March in place for 3–5 minutes while moving your arms up and down.
- Do arm circles forward, then back, 20 times.
- Do 10 modified jumping jacks or "side jacks"—instead of jumping, alternate placing each heel out to the side on the floor while the arms go above the head.
- Tap each foot 20 times; then rise on your toes 10 times.

If you do not first warm up before you begin to exercise, you may deprive the arms and legs of essential fuel. Without enough fuel, the muscles cannot perform very well, and they may even become injured. Now let's do some warm-up movements to music.

Table 2.6   Overview: Lesson 2, Level 1 (Red)

Suggested time	Activities	Materials needed
45–60 minutes	Introduction: Warm Up, Metabolic Systems, Cool Down after Exercise	• Parent and patient education materials and books (Sothern et al., 2001) • Exercise attire • CD or digital music player
5–10 minutes	I. Warming Up	
25–35 minutes	II. Activity: The Body's Metabolic Engines	
5–10 minutes	Aerobic and Anaerobic Exercises	
	III. Activity: Cooling Down	
Objectives	After participation in this lesson the student will be able to— 1. Identify safe methods to warm up the body before engaging in an exercise session. 2. Identify differences between aerobic versus anaerobic exercise. 2. Gain knowledge concerning the benefits of aerobic exercise to health. 3. Develop pacing skills to monitor exercise performance to increase duration. 4. Identify movement and exercises that will improve cardiorespiratory (aerobic) endurance. 5. Identify safe methods to cool down the body after engaging in an exercise session.	

The instructor should then play music that has a slow to moderate tempo and lead the students through several warm-up movements for about 3–5 minutes.

Case in Point: Real Words from Real Patients

My mom and dad are divorced. I live with my mom but I see my dad almost every day. My dad is really fit, and he kept bugging me about my weight. He'd make me go jogging with him and he'd get mad if I couldn't keep up. I started my exercise program last week. I was really happy when my teacher said that I didn't have to keep up with my dad anymore. Now my dad and I do fun things like basketball and bike riding. Sometimes I even beat him in bike races—I think he lets me win, but that's ok. I've already lost 12 pounds! Dad is so proud of me.

—Carolyn, age 10 years old

ACTIVITY II. THE BODY'S METABOLIC ENGINES— AEROBIC AND ANAEROBIC ACTIVITIES

During this activity, the instructor will discuss the metabolic system with the children and their families.

Young children are perfectly suited for short bursts of high-energy movement. Any mother of a preschool child knows this first hand. Outdoor tag is a good example (burning about 350–400 calories per hour). Unfortunately, the spontaneous activity of young children decreases as they get older. Scientists do not know whether this is a natural occurrence or whether it is a result of their changing environment. For overweight and obese children and adolescents, activity may be less frequent because they are unable to keep up with the demands of certain sports, dance, or group games. In addition, their metabolic systems— the engines of their bodies—are different. Using a car as a metaphor, overweight and obese children run out of gas sooner because the excess weight makes their engine run harder when they move forward; just as a small car can go farther on the same amount of gas as a large truck.

Regardless of weight, a child's body has three types of engines (or metabolisms), much like a car has three different gears: one for fast takeoffs, one for start-and-stop driving, and one for highway driving:

1. Medium-slow: This engine enables movement for long stretches of time. This is the engine that is fired up for aerobic exercises. It uses a combination of oxygen, fat stored in the body, and sugar (or carbohydrates) for fuel. After about 20 minutes of activity at the same speed, the child's body begins to use more of the stored fat for fuel. If children have not eaten for several hours, their metabolic engines will utilize even more of that stored fat. The longer a child maintains the medium-slow speed, the more calories and fat will be burned.

   Because overweight and obese children have more stored fat than others, they can exercise in the medium-slow engine for hours without running out of gas as long as their pace stays low and consistent. But they must keep it slow and steady for a long period of time. It is all right to move into the fast engine for a moment as long as it is brief and they return to the easier pace.

2. Fast: This engine taps into the body's anaerobic capabilities. "Anaerobic" means "without air"—this engine depends not on oxygen, but primarily on sugar stored in the muscles (glycogen) for its fuel source. Children use this engine whenever the speed of their activity increases to a higher level.

   Overweight and obese children can use the fast engine until the workload becomes too difficult. At this point, a substance called lactic acid will build in his or her muscles. This substance will make his or her muscles burn and feel tired. The breathing rate will increase because he or she is trying to take in more oxygen to shift gears and begin using the medium-slow engine again. Unfortunately, because the fast engine is anaerobic, trying to take in more oxygen by breathing faster will not help. The child's body will not allow him to shift to the medium-slow, aerobic engine unless he or she slows down.

 Key Points: The Engines of the Body

The fast engine has a very small fuel tank. It only takes between 3 and 5 minutes for a child to run out of gas. Unless activity is reduced to a speed or level to allow the child to shift to the medium-slow engine again, he or she will be physically unable to continue.

The fast engine is great for short periods of exercise that promote strength and power. Sprinting is one example. So are stomach crunches.

3. Super Fast: Skilled and powerful athletes such as Olympic weightlifters, jumpers, or sprinters use the super-fast engine. It relies on chemicals made from fuel stored directly in muscle fibers and immediately ready for use. The tank of the super-fast engine is even smaller than the fast engine. When children turn on that engine, they will run out of gas in only 10 seconds.

Children can increase the size of the tanks in each of these engines by engaging in regular exercise training, increasing how often ("frequency") and how long ("duration") he or she spends being physically active during any given week. By doing this, the child eventually will be able to exercise for longer periods of time in all of the metabolic engines.

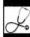

Clinical Reminders for the Health Care Professional: Excess Weight Is Physically Disabling

It is very important to listen to your overweight or obese patient. When they are exercising and say that they are tired, it means that they really are tired. If they say they are hurting, that means they really are hurting. Allow them to slow down or stop to catch their breath. Then, gently encourage them to begin moving again at a pace that is more comfortable. Do not make the mistake of thinking that your patient is faking his or her discomfort, because he or she probably is not. Most important, do not get irritated with your patient's limitations. Remember that his or her excess weight is physically disabling; he or she needs encouragement, not criticism.

It is important not to rush the process. The heavier the overweight or obese child is, the longer it will take for him or her to comfortably use and improve his engines. Obese children take at least 3 months to experience a noticeable change and at least 6 months to 1 year to reach their full potential for improvement. Severely obese children will take longer. Be patient and always refer to the color-coded guidelines in the exercise plan detailed in this book as you gradually add more exercise into his or her routine. Help your patient practice taking his or her heart rate to help him better pace his or her effort. Please refer to the instructions in Lesson 3 (see Chapter 6).

Case in Point: Real Words from Real Patients

My wife and I never realized that just by walking a couple days a week, stretching and flexing with our son, that we would see such dramatic effects. We're all happier, healthier and thinner because of it. Even Sophie, our dog, has started to run in the backyard again!

—Father of 8-year-old boy

Key Points: Exercise Intensity

The body uses different fuel systems for different levels or intensities of work:

Very Vigorous (initiation of movement): When movement is first initiated from a resting position or when activity increases to an extremely vigorous pace for 0–10 seconds, the body uses a fuel called adenosine triphosphate (ATP), which is stored in the muscles.

Vigorous: For 10 seconds to 5 minutes, the body uses a fuel called glycogen, which is also stored in the muscles. After exercising vigorously for about 5 minutes, the muscles produce lactic acid, which causes muscles to feel tired and burn.

Low to Moderate: After 5 minutes—and for hours and hours after as long as the pace is kept to this level—the body uses glycogen plus oxygen in the air plus fat to make fuel and breathe out carbon dioxide.

During this exercise activity, the instructor will demonstrate how the metabolic system works with the children and their families using engines as the metaphor and music as the motivator. He or she will select three different pieces of music with varying tempos: one slow, one medium-fast, and one very fast. After several minutes of playing music with a slower beat, he or she will change it to a song with a faster beat and then one with a very fast tempo. The instructor will vary the pace of movement to match the beat of the music and encourage the children and families to do the same. The instructor will use the following verbal cues:

Talking Points: The Metabolic Engines of the Body (Verbal cues for patients or parents and family members)
Read through the following information with your patient or parent to help him or her to understand the exercise strategy used in the program.

When you exercise, your body depends on three different engines to move. Your body has three engines. Engine 3 is the slowest engine, but, it is the best one for getting rid of fat because you can do it for longer periods of time. Engine 2 is faster than Engine 3, and it works well for becoming stronger and more powerful. Engine 1 is the super-fast engine and is used by very powerful athletes such as Olympic weightlifters and jumpers. I am going to put on some music and you dance around to it.

After several minutes of dancing to one kind of music, the instructor should change it to another, and so on. After moving to each tempo, the instructor should ask the following questions:

- What type of engine are you using now?
- How long do you think you can use this engine?

If you are using Engine 2, the fast engine, you will be able to keep moving only for about 5 minutes. If it is Engine 1, the super-fast engine, you can only keep this up for about 10 seconds. But if you are using Engine 3, the slow engine, you can go on for hours because all this engine needs for fuel is your breathing (oxygen, stored fat, and some of what you have eaten) to make it run. This is the engine you use when exercising at a moderate intensity.

Talking Points: Aerobic Exercise (Verbal cues for patients or parents and family members)
Read through the following information with your patient or parent to help him or her to understand the exercise strategy used in the program.

Explain to your child that when doing aerobic exercises, he should use Engine 3 to burn the most calories. If he kicks into Engine 1 or 2, he is engaging in anaerobic exercise, which will not burn as many calories simply because he will not be able to sustain the pace for long enough time periods.

The instructor should review the following information so patients and families will grasp the difference between the two types of exercises, aerobic and anaerobic (see Table 2.7), using the following cues:

Table 2.7   Examples of Aerobic versus Anaerobic Exercise

Aerobic	Anaerobic
Walking	Running, high speed
Jogging	Body toning (e.g., Pilates)
Cycling	Strength or resistance training
Treadmill or stair climber	Gymnastic stunts
Lap swimming	Interval training
Aerobic dance	Wrestling
Long distance field events	Sprints

Talking Points: Aerobic Versus Anaerobic Exercise (Verbal cues for patients or parents and family members)
Read through the following information with your patient or parent to help him or her to understand the exercise strategy used in the program.

The word "aerobic" means with oxygen. "Anaerobic means" without oxygen. When you do aerobic activities, you send oxygen to the muscles. There, the oxygen mixes with glucose, a sugar that your body produces from carbohydrates and fats. Together, they produce fuel so your body can continue to participate in the aerobic activity. The stronger and better trained your cardiorespiratory system becomes from doing aerobic exercise, the more oxygen is delivered to your exercising muscles, and the more exercise you can do with more ease. The more trained your muscles are, the more they can accept and use that oxygen to make you go.

When you move into Engine 2 or an anaerobic pace, your body only uses the glucose—not oxygen—for fuel. You can do this for only between 3 and 5 minutes because when you burn glucose, a substance called lactic acid builds in your muscles. That is what creates a burning sensation in your muscles and after a short time, depletes your muscles of energy. The more intensely you exercise, the faster the muscle fatigue occurs. At that point, you have to either slow down so that the oxygen demand is lower and the lactic acid is absorbed, or your body will be physically unable to continue.

The point at which your body shifts from aerobic to anaerobic exercise is called the anaerobic threshold. When you exercise hard enough to activate the anaerobic metabolism, your muscles will burn, you will be out of breath, and you will feel tired all over.

This does not mean anaerobic exercise is bad for you. In fact, to become stronger and more fit, you will have to use your anaerobic system to do quite a few activities.

ACTIVITY III. COOLING-DOWN TECHNIQUE

The instructor will provide direction to the children on the techniques for cooling down after exercise. About 5–10 minutes before your patient completes an exercise session—whether it is riding a bike, jogging, swimming, walking, or dancing, he or she will need to start cooling down. The child should do this gradually until he or she is maintaining a slow, easy pace. It is important that children continue at this pace for the last 10 minutes or so of their workout. Cooling down is important because your patient's body needs time to return to its normal heart rate and breathing pattern. Otherwise, the blood traveling to his or her exercising muscles will pool or remain in the muscles. This can make your patient feel dizzy or nauseous, and he or she may experience painful muscle cramps. The instructor should use the following verbal cues:

 Talking Points: Cooling Down (Verbal cues for patients or parents and family members)
Read through the following information with your patient or parent to help him or her to understand the exercise strategy used in the program.

The sign says 2 miles to the end of the park walking track. You are walking at a very brisk pace while swinging your arms vigorously. You are in your target heart rate zone. You know you only have 5–10 minutes left in your training session. What do you do now?

Slow down gradually to a very slow, easy pace for the remaining time. Why do you need to slow down your pace?

Your body needs time to return to its normal heart rate and breathing pattern. If you stop suddenly— that is, just stop in the middle of your training zone—the heart and lungs do not have time to adjust.

Cooling down is just like warming up. You simply move your arms and legs slowly after exercising, and your blood leaves the muscles and returns to the heart and lungs. Your legs even have a built-in pump to help with that process, but you have to keep them moving for the pump to work.

Slowing down before stopping your exercise also helps bring your temperature back to its normal range. That is exactly why it is called cooling down.

No matter what exercise you are doing, always slow the pace for the last 5–10 minutes.

REFERENCES

Ainsworth, B. E., Haskell, W. L., Herrmann, S. D., Meckes, N., Bassett, D. R., Tudor-Locke, C., et al. (2011). 2011 compendium of physical activities. *Medicine and Science in Sports and Exercise*, 43(8), 1575–1581.

American College of Sports Medicine. (2010). *ACSM's Guidelines for Exercise Testing and Prescription* (8th ed.). Philadelphia, PA: Lippincott Williams & Wilkins.

Bailey, B. W., McInnis, K. (2011). Energy cost of exergaming: a comparison of the energy cost of 6 forms of exergaming. *Archives of Pediatric and Adolescent Medicine*, 165(7), 597–602.

Ballor, D. L., Keesey, R. E. (1991). A meta-analysis of the factors affecting exercise-induced changes in body mass, fat mass and fat-free mass in males and females. *International Journal of Obesity*, 15(11), 717–726.

Baquet, G., van Praagh, E., Berhoin, S. (2003). Endurance training and aerobic fitness in young people. *Sports Medicine*, 33(15), 1127–1143.

Barbeau, P., Johnson, M. H., Howe, C. A., Allison, J., Davis, C. L., Gutin, B., et al. (2007). Ten months of exercise improves general and visceral adiposity, bone, and fitness in black girls. *Obesity (Silver Spring, Md.)*, 15(8), 2077–2085.

Barlow, S. (2007). Expert Committee recommendations regarding the prevention, assessment and treatment of child and adolescent overweight and obesity: Summary report. *Pediatrics*, 120(Suppl 4), S164–S192.

Bell, L. M., Watts, K., Siafarikas, A., Thompson, A., Ratnam, N., Bulsara, M., et al. (2007). Exercise alone reduces insulin resistance in obese children independently of changes in body composition. *Journal of Clinical Endocrinology and Metabolism*, 92(11), 4230–4235.

Bennett, B., Larson-Meyer, E., Ravussin, R., Volaufova, J., Soros, A., Cefalu, W., Chalew, S., Gordon, S., Smith, S., Newcomer, B., Goran, M., Sothern, M. (2012). Impaired insulin sensitivity and elevated ectopic and visceral fat in obese versus non-obese healthy prepubertal children. *Obesity*, 20(2), 371–375.

Biddiss, E., Irwin, J. (2010). Active video games to promote physical activity in children and youth: A systematic review. *Archives of Pediatric and Adolescent Medicine*, 164(7), 664–668.

Bovet, P., Auguste, R., Burdette, H. (2007). Strong inverse association between physical fitness and overweight in adolescents: A large school-based survey. *International Journal of Behavioral Nutrition and Physical Activity*, 4(1), 24.

Brambilla, P., Pozzobon, G., Pietrobelli, A. (2011). Physical activity as the main therapeutic tool for metabolic syndrome in childhood. *International Journal of Obesity*, 35(1), 16–28.

Byrd-Williams, C., Shaibi, G., Sun, P., Lane, C., Ventura, E., Davis, J., Kelly, L., Goran, M. (2008). Cardiorespiratory fitness predicts changes in adiposity in overweight Hispanic boys. *Obesity*, 16(5), 1072–1077.

Cali, A. M., Zern, T. L., Taksali, S. E., De Oliveira, A. M., Dufour, S., Otvos, J. D., Caprio, S. (2007). Intrahepatic fat accumulation and alterations in lipoprotein composition in obese adolescents: A perfect proatherogenic state. *Diabetes Care*, 30(12), 3093–3098.

Carrel, A. L., Clark, R. R., Peterson, S. E., Nemeth, B. A., Sullivan, J., Allen, D. B. (2005). Improvement of fitness, body composition, and insulin sensitivity in overweight children in a school-based exercise program: A randomized, controlled study. *Archives of Pediatrics and Adolescent Medicine*, 159(10), 963–968.

Carter, S. L., Rennie, C., Tarnopolsky, M. A. (2001). Substrate utilization during endurance exercise in men and women after endurance training. *American Journal of Physiology, Endocrinology and Metabolism*, 280(6), E898–E907.

Daniels, S. R., Jacobson, M. S., McCrindle, B. W., Eckel, R. H., Sanner, B. M. (2009). American heart association childhood obesity research summit: Executive summary. *Circulation*, 119(15), 2114–2123.

Dao, H. H., Frelut, M. L., Peres, G., Bourgeois, P., Navarro, J. (2004). Effects of a multi-disciplinary weight loss intervention on anaerobic and aerobic aptitudes in severely obese adolescents. *International Journal of Obesity and Related Metabolic Disorders*, 28(7), 870–878.

Davis, C., Pollock, N., Waller, J., Allison, J., Dennis, B., Bassali, R., Melendez, A., Boyle, C., Gower, B. (2012). Exercise dose and diabetes risk in overweight and obese children. *JAMA*, 308(11), 1103–1112.

Dubose, K. D., Eisenmann, J. C., Donnelly, J. E. (2007). Aerobic fitness attenuates the metabolic syndrome score in normal-weight, at-risk-for-overweight, and overweight children. *Pediatrics*, 120, e1262–e1268.

Engels, H. J., Gretebeck, R. J., Gretebeck, K. A., Jimenez, L. (2005). Promoting healthful diets and exercise: Efficacy of a 12-week after-school program in urban African Americans. *Journal of the American Dietetic Association*, 105(3), 455–459.

Fabbrini, E., deHaseth, D., Deivanayagam, S., Mohammed, B. S., Vitola, B. E., Klein, S. (2009). Alterations in fatty acid kinetics in obese adolescents with increased intrahepatic triglyceride content. *Obesity (Silver Spring, Md.)*, 17(1), 25–29.

Forouhi, N. G., Jenkinson, G., Thomas, E. L., Mullick, S., Mierisova, S., Bhonsle, U., McKeigue, P. M., Bell, J. D. (1999). Relation of triglyceride stores in skeletal muscle cells to central obesity and insulin sensitivity in European and South Asian men. *Diabetologia* 42(8), 932–935.

Ganley, K., Paterno, M., Miles, C., Stout, J., Brawner, P., Girolami, G., Warran, M. (2011). Health-related fitness in children and adolescents. *Pediatric Physical Therapy*, 23(3), 208–220.

Graves, L. E., Ridgers, N. D., Williams, K., Strattin, G., Atkinson, G., Cable, N. T. (2010). The physiological cost and enjoyment of Wii Fit in adolescents, young adults, and older adults. *Journal of Physical Activity and Health*, 7(3), 393–401.

Haddock, B. L., Wilkin, L. D. (2006). Resistance training volume and post exercise energy expenditure. *International Journal of Sports Medicine*, 27(2), 143–148.

Hassink, S. G., Zapalla, F., Falini, L., Datto, G. (2008). Exercise and the obese child. *Progress in Pediatric Cardiology*, 25(2), 153–157.

Horowitz, J. F. (2001). Regulation of lipid mobilization and oxidation during exercise in obesity. *Exercise and Sport Sciences Reviews*, 29(1), 42–46.

Hunter, G. R., Byrne, N. M., Gower, B. A., Sirikul, B., Hills, A. P. (2006). Increased resting energy expenditure after 40 minutes of aerobic but not resistance exercise. *Obesity (Silver Spring, Md.)*, 14(11), 2018–2025.

Hurley, B. F., Hagberg, J. M. (1998). Optimizing health in older persons: Aerobic or strength training? *Exercise and Sport Sciences Reviews*, 26, 61–89.

Ildiko, V., Zsofia, M., Janos, M., Andreas, P., Dora, N. E., Andras, P., et al. (2007). Activity-related changes of body fat and motor performance in obese seven-year-old boys. *Journal of Physiological Anthropology, 26*(3), 333–337.

Jacobson, M. (2006). Medical complications and comorbidities of pediatric obesity. In M. Sothern, T. K. von Almen, S. Gordon (Eds.), *Handbook of Pediatric Obesity: Clinical Management* (pp. 31–39). Boca Raton, FL: Taylor & Francis.

Janssen, J., LeBlanc, A. G. (2010). Systematic review of the health benefits of physical activity and fitness in school-aged children and youth. *International Journal of Behavioral Nutrition and Physical Activity, 7*, 40.

Kanaley, J. A., Weatherup-Dentes, M. M., Alvarado, C. R., Whitehead, G. (2001). Substrate oxidation during acute exercise and with exercise training in lean and obese women. *European Journal of Applied Physiology, 85*(1–2), 68–73.

Katz, D., Daniels, S., Gardner, C., Goodman, E., Hassink, S., Sothern, M. (2012). What we don't know: Unanswered questions about childhood obesity. *Childhood Obesity, 8*(1), 7–12.

Larson-Meyer, D. E., Heilbronn, L. K., Redman, L. M., Newcomer, B. R., Frisard, M. I., Anton, S., Smith, S. R., Alfonso, A., Ravussin, E. (2006). Effect of calorie restriction with or without exercise on insulin sensitivity, beta-cell function, fat cell size, and ectopic lipid in overweight subjects. *Diabetes Care, 29*, 1337–1344.

Loftin, M., Heusel, L., Bonis, M., Sothern, M. (2005). Oxygen uptake kinetics and oxygen deficit in obese and normal weight adolescent females. *Journal of Sports Science and Medicine, 4*, 430–436.

Loftin, M., Sothern, M., Trosclair, L., O'Hanlon, A., Miller, J., Udall, J. (2001). Scaling VO_2 peak in obese and nonobese girls. *Obesity Research, 9*(5), 290–296.

Loftin, M., Sothern, M., VanVrancken, C., Udall, J. (2003). Low heart rate peak in obese female youth. *Clinical Pediatrics, 42*(6), 505–510.

Loftin, M., Sothern, M., Warren, B., Udall, J. (2004). Comparison of VO_2 peak during tread-mill and bicycle ergometry in severely overweight youth. *Journal of Sports Science and Medicine, 3*, 254–260.

Maddison, R., Mhurchu, C. N., Jull, A., Jiang, Y., Prapavessis, H., Rodgers, A. (2007). Energy expended playing video console games: An opportunity to increase children's physical activity? *Pediatric Exercise Science, 19*(3), 334–343.

Maffeis, C. (2008). Physical activity in the prevention and treatment of childhood obesity: physio-patholic evidence and promising experiences. *International Journal of Pediatric Obesity, 3*(Suppl 2), S29–S32.

Maffeis, C., Manfredi, R., Trombetta, M., Sordelli, S., Storti, M., Benuzzi, T., Bonadonaa, R. C. (2008). Insulin sensitivity is correlated with subcutaneous but not visceral fat in over-weight and obese prepubertal children. *Journal of Clinical Endocrinology and Metabolism, 93*(6), 2122–2128.

Mark, A. E., Janssen, I., (2008). Dose-response relation between physical activity and blood pressure in youth. *Medicine and Science in Sports and Exercise, 40*, 1007–1012.

May, A., Kuklina, E., Yoon, P. (2011). Prevalence of cardiovascular disease risk factors among us adolescents, 1999-2008. *Pediatrics, 129*(6), 1035–1041.

McMurray, R. G., Bangdiwala, S. I., Harrell, J. S., Amorim, L. D. (2008). Adolescents with meta-bolic syndrome have a history of low aerobic fitness and physical activity levels. *Dynamic Medicine, 7*, 5.

Nassis, G. P., Papantakou, K., Skenderi, K., Triandafillopoulou, M., Kavouras, S. A., Yannakoulia, M., Chrousos, G. P., Sidossis, L. S. (2005). Aerobic exercise training improves insulin sensitivity without changes in body weight, body fat, adiponectin and inflammatory markers in overweight and obese girls. *Metabolism, 54*, 1472–1479.

Nemet, D., Wang, P., Funahashi, T., Matsuzawa, Y., Tanaka, S., Engelman, L., Cooper, D. M. (2003). Adipocytokines, body composition, and fitness in children. *Pediatric Research,* 53, 148–152.

Ni Mhurchu, C., Maddison, R., Jiang, Y., Jull, A., Prapavessis, H., Rodgers, A. (2008). Couch potatoes to jumping beans: A pilot study of the effect of active video games on physical activity in children. *International Journal of Behavioral Nutrition and Physical Activity,* 5, 8.

Ortega, F. B., Ruiz, J. R., Castillo, M. J., Sjostrom, M. (2008). Physical fitness in childhood and adolescence: a powerful marker of health. *International Journal of Obesity,* 32, 1–11.

Perseghin, G., Bonfanti, R., Magni, S., Lattuada, G., De Cobelli, F., Canu, T., et al. (2006). Insulin resistance and whole body energy homeostasis in obese adolescents with fatty liver disease. *American Journal of Physiology, Endocrinology and Metabolism,* 291(4), E697–E703.

Perseghin, G., Scifo, P., De Cobelli, F., Pagliato, E., Battezzati, A., Arcelloni, C., et al. (1999). Intramyocellular triglyceride content is a determinant of *in vivo* insulin resistance in humans: a 1H-13C nuclear magnetic resonance spectroscopy assessment in offspring of type 2 diabetic parents. *Diabetes,* 48(8), 1600–1606.

Priest, D. L., Karageorghis, C. I., Sharp, N. C. (2004). The characteristics and effects of motivational music in exercise settings: the possible influence of gender, age, frequency of attendance, and time of attendance. *Journal of Sports Medicine and Physical Fitness,* 44(1), 77–86.

Robinson, T. N., Killen, J. D., Kraemer, H. C., Wilson, D. M., Matheson, D. M., Haskell, W. L., et al. (2003). Dance and reducing television viewing to prevent weight gain in African-American girls: the Stanford GEMS pilot study. *Ethnicity and Disease,* 13(1 Suppl 1), S65–S77.

Ryysy, L., Hakkinen, A. M., Goto, T., Vehkavaara, S., Westerbacka, J., Halavaara, J., Yki-Jarvinen, H. (2000). Hepatic fat content and insulin action on free fatty acids and glucose metabolism rather than insulin absorption are associated with insulin requirements during insulin therapy in type 2 diabetic patients. *Diabetes,* 49, 749–758.

Sell, K., Lillie, T., Taylor, J. (2008). Energy expenditure during physically interactive video game playing in male college students with different playing experience. *Journal of American College Health,* 56(5), 505–511.

Sinha, R., Dufour, S., Petersen, K. F., LeBon, V., Enoksson, S., Ma, Y. Z., Savoye, M., Rothman, D. L., Shulman, G. I., Caprio, S. (2002). Assessment of skeletal muscle triglyceride content by (1)H nuclear magnetic resonance spectroscopy in lean and obese adolescents: relationships to insulin sensitivity, total body fat, and central adiposity. *Diabetes,* 51(4), 1022–1027.

Smith, A. L., Hoza, B., Linnea, K., McQuade, J. D., Tomb, M., Vaughn, A. J., et al. (2011). Pilot physical activity intervention reduces severity of ADHD symptoms in young children. *Journal of Attention Disorders,* 17(1), 70–82.

Sothern, M. (2001). Exercise as a modality in the treatment of childhood obesity. *Pediatric Clinics of North America,* 48(4), 995–1015.

Sothern, M. (2004). Obesity prevention in children: Physical activity and nutrition. *Nutrition,* 20(7–8), 704–708.

Sothern, M. (2006). The business of pediatric weight management. In M. Sothern, T. K. von Almen, S. Gordon (Eds.), *Handbook of Pediatric Obesity: Clinical Management* (pp. 9–28). Boca Raton, FL: Taylor & Francis.

Sothern, M., Hunter, S., Suskind, R., Brown, R., Udall, J., Blecker, U. (1999). Motivating the obese child to move: The role of structured exercise in pediatric weight management. *Southern Medical Journal,* 92(6), 577–584.

Sothern, M., Loftin, M., Blecker, M., Suskind R., Udall, J. (1999). Physiologic function and childhood obesity. *International Journal of Pediatrics*, 14(3), 1–5.

Sothern, M., VanVrancken-Tompkins, C., Brooks, C., Thélin, C. (2006). Increasing physical activity in overweight youth in clinical settings. In M. Sothern, S. Gordon, T. K. von Almen (Eds.), *Handbook of Pediatric Obesity: Clinical Management* (pp. 173–188). Boca Raton, FL: Taylor & Francis.

Sothern, M., von Almen, T. K., Gordon, S. (Eds.). (2006). *Handbook of Pediatric Obesity: Clinical Management*. Boca Raton, FL: Taylor & Francis.

Sothern, M., von Almen, T. K., Schumacher, H. (2001). *Trim Kids: The Proven Plan That Has Helped Thousands of Children Achieve a Healthier Weight*. New York, NY: Harper Collins.

Steele, R., Brage, S., Corder, K., Wareham, N., Ekelund, U. (2008). Physical activity, cardiorespiratory fitness, and the metabolic syndrome in youth. *Journal of Applied Physiology*, 105(1), 342–351.

Stiegler, P., Cunliffe, A. (2006). The role of diet and exercise for the maintenance of fat-free mass and resting metabolic rate during weight loss. *Sports Medicine (Auckland, N.Z.)*, 36(3), 239–262.

Strong, W. B., Malina, R. M., Blimkie, C. J., Daniels, S. R., Dishman, R. K., Gutin, B., et al. (2005). Evidence based physical activity for school-age youth. *Journal of Pediatrics*, 146(6), 732–737.

Tak, Y. R., An, J. Y., Kim, Y. A., Woo, H. Y. (2007). The effects of a physical activity-behavior modification combined intervention (PABM-intervention) on metabolic risk factors in overweight and obese elementary school children. *Taehan Kanho Hakhoe Chi*, 37(6), 902–913.

Talanian, J. L., Galloway, S. D., Heigenhauser, G. J., Bonen, A., Spriet, L. L. (2007). Two weeks of high-intensity aerobic interval training increases the capacity for fat oxidation during exercise in women. *Journal of Applied Physiology*, 102(4), 1439–1447.

Thomas, A. S., Greene, L. F., Ard, J. D., Oster, R. A., Darnell, B. E., Gower, B. A. (2009). Physical activity may facilitate diabetes prevention in adolescents. *Diabetes Care*, 32, 9–13.

Thompson, W., Bushman, B., Desch, J., Kravitz, L. (2010). *ACSM's Resources for the Personal Trainer* (3rd ed.). Philadelphia, PA: Lippincott Williams & Wilkins.

U.S. Department of Health Human Services. (2008). Physical activity guidelines for Americans. Retrieved June 25, 2009, from http://www.health.gov/paguidelines.

U.S. Preventive Services Task Force. (2010). Screening for obesity in children and adolescents: U.S. Preventive Services Task Force recommendation statement. *Pediatrics*, 125(2), 361–367.

Zorba, E., Cengiz, T., Karacabey, K. (2011). Exercise training improves body composition, blood lipid profile and serum insulin levels in obese children. *Journal of Sports Medicine and Physical Fitness*, 51(4), 664–669.

Chapter 3

STRENGTH (RESISTANCE) TRAINING

Muscular fitness includes parameters of strength, endurance, and power (American College of Sports Medicine [ACSM], 2011) and is one of the four components of fitness (ACSM, 2010). Muscle strength may be defined as the maximum mechanical torque or force generated by skeletal muscle or muscle groups (Stiff, 2001); muscular endurance indicates an ability to maintain force for longer durations (Alberga, Sigal, & Kenny, 2011; Bar-Or & Rowland, 2004; Heyward, 2002) and an ability to perform repeated muscular contractions using high resistance (Pate, 1991). The number of motor units activated over a specific time and the cross-sectional area of the contracting muscle(s) determine the potential for increasing muscular strength and endurance (Bar-Or & Rowland, 2004). Explosive strength or power is defined as performance of work expressed per unit of time or the maximum amount of force produced in the shortest time frame (Bar-Or & Rowland, 2004; Hakkinen et al., 1985). Programs to improve muscular power must include a rapid speed component specific to the desired goals, which typically are related to the improvement of sports performance (Ratamess et al., 2009; Thompson et al., 2010).

It is essential that children, and in particular, overweight and obese children, participate in exercise activities that promote the attainment of muscular strength and endurance (U.S. Department of Health and Human Services [U.S. DHHS], 2008). The ability to participate in daily physical activities is limited in children with weak muscles. Research supports the concept that, if properly administered, strength or resistance-training programs not only may be safe in youth but also may promote enhanced motor performance (Behringer et al., 2011) and help reduce the risk of injury during other physical activities (Faigenbaum & Myer, 2010); however, these benefits are realized only if close supervision is provided by trained, qualified instructors (Ganley et al., 2011). The ACSM (2010, 2011), the National Strength and Conditioning Association (Faigenbaum et al., 2009), and the American Academy of Pediatrics (AAP, Committee on Sports Medicine, 1990; Washington et al., 2001) have all published statements in support of properly administered and supervised, developmentally appropriate muscular strength and endurance training in children and adolescents. It is suggested that a child be of a sufficient age to participate in sports activities before engaging in structured exercise to specifically improve muscular strength and endurance, which is typically 7–8 years of age (Faigenbaum et al., 2009).

Resistance training provides the optimal method of developing the components of muscular strength and endurance in children and adolescents. Resistance training is defined as a type of physical conditioning using varied types of training apparatus, including free weights, weight machines, medicine balls, elastic bands, or one's own body weight as resistance (Alberga et al., 2011), which provides progressively increasing resistive loads and differing movement velocities (Faigenbaum & Myer, 2010). The term "resistance exercise" often is used interchangeably with the terms "strength training" or "weight training" (Alberga et al., 2011). It is important, however, that resistance training not be confused with the sports of body-building, weightlifting, and power lifting, as the goals of these activities are to increase muscle size or improve the amount of maximal weight that can be lifted during a competition. The two types of resistance training are (1) traditional weight training and (2) plyometric exercise.

Talking Points: Resistance Training (Verbal cues for patients or parents and family members)
Read through the following information with your patient or family members to help them to understand the exercise strategy used in the program.

Resistance training comes with a lot of different names and forms (weight training, strength training, circuit weight training, isometrics, and isokinetics). Generally it means that you exercise your muscles against moderate to heavy loads, with few repetitions. Depending on what you do, this is the method for building muscle size, increasing lean body mass, and increasing your strength and power.

Traditional weight training is designed to improve muscular strength through a series of prescribed isoinertial exercise movements (e.g., bench press, squat), utilizing some type of weight (e.g., body weight, dumbbells [free weights], weight machines, exercise bands, and others (ACSM, 2011; de Villarreal, Izquierdo, & Gonzalez-Badillo, 2011; Thompson et al., 2010). This type of training promotes greater force generation through numerous neuromuscular mechanisms, including increased motor unit recruitment and enhanced neural function, alterations in muscle architecture, and others (Ratamess et al., 2009). Results of this type of training are specific to the type of program utilized, intensity, volume, order and type of exercises used, rest periods between sets, and frequency of training bouts (ACSM, 2011; Kraemer & Ratamess, 2004). The individual's training status and genetic predisposition further defines the magnitude of strength improvement (Ratamess et al., 2009).

Plyometric exercise utilizes the elastic properties of the muscles to create greater force and includes jumping movements or motions (Thompson et al., 2010; Trzascoma, Tihanyi, & Trzascoma, 2010). This type of training also is referred to as stretch-shortening cycle exercise, as the muscle is stretched immediately before the muscle shortening or action phase (Faigenbaum et al., 2009; Malisoux et al., 2007). Examples of this type of exercise include skipping, jumping rope, hopping, and trampoline. Research consistently supports the concept that this method of resistance training should be reserved for well-conditioned individuals engaged in sports-specific activities. The selection of the exercise to be used during plyometric training should be specific to the sport of interest to maximize improvements in speed, strength, power, endurance, and flexibility (Arabatzi, Kellis, & de Villarreal, 2010). In a recent position statement from the National Strength and Conditioning Association, the results of numerous studies agreed that if properly designed and supervised, plyometric exercise is a safe and effective modality, which enhances functional abilities and movement biomechanics in young athletes (Faigenbaum et al., 2009). More important, the natural movement patterns of boys and girls during outdoor play typically include plyometric type activities, which may promote an improvement in speed and power. Despite these observations, plyometric exercise poses an inherent risk of injury should training intensity, duration, or frequency exceed the abilities of the developing child (Faigenbaum et al., 2009; Thompson et al., 2010). Particularly in overweight and obese children, plyometric exercise should not be an initial choice for developing muscular strength and endurance as, unlike healthy weight children, they are physically compromised during weight-bearing aerobic exercise (Daniels et al., 2009; Norman et al., 2005; Sothern, 2001; Van Vrancken-Tompkins, Sothern, & Bar-Or, 2006) and have reduced gross motor coordination as well as a biomechanical disadvantage during walking and running (Cliff, Okely, & Morgan, 2011; D'Hondt, Deforche, & Gentier, 2013; Morano, Collella, & Caroli, 2011; Riddiford-Harland, Steele, & Baur, 2006).

MUSCULAR STRENGTH AND ENDURANCE

The muscles of a child's body make movement possible, while bones provide support (Thompson et al., 2010). Skeletal muscle is just one type of muscle and may be controlled voluntarily. The other types of muscles are cardiac and smooth muscle, which are involuntary muscles. There are 100 primary movement muscles and more than 600 total muscles, some of which are responsible for stabilizing the body (Baldwin, 2003). The primary action of skeletal muscles is to produce force that promotes the movement of a joint (Thompson et al., 2010). The primary responsibility of skeletal muscles during joint movement is to pull the bones. To better facilitate this action, the skeletal muscles primarily are arranged in opposing pairs. This arrangement allows one muscle to contract and pull the body part, which is referred to as the **agonist**, while the opposing muscle relaxes to allow the movement, called the **antagonist**. The remaining muscles in proximity to the movement assist by preventing unwanted movement. These muscles, in this context, are classified as **synergists** (Thompson & Floyd, 2001).

Glossary of Terms: (Terms are boldface in text)

Agonist: the prime mover—the muscle directly engaged in muscle action; the muscle whose fibers are shortening or contracting to make the movement possible.

Antagonist: a muscle than has an action opposite to the agonist; the muscle that relaxes to allow the movement to take place

Synergist: muscles located in proximity to the movement that prevent unwanted motion during the exercise

Range of motion (ROM): the distance from start to finish that a body part can move

Multiplanar: an activity that is possible across all possible planes, for example, front and back (anterior/posterior), up and down (vertical), and side to side (mediolateral)

It is important to understand the types of movement that are possible for the major upper and lower extremity joints before prescribing strength training for children. Table 3.1 details this information, identifies the major agonist muscles associated with each movement, and provides examples of strength (resistance) exercise for each movement.

Isotonic strength training is preferred over isometric training (ACSM, 2010). Isotonic training also is called dynamic strength training because the limbs of the body move through a **range of motion (ROM)** during isotonic training. The two parts of an isotonic training movement are concentric and eccentric.

Muscles produce force in three different ways:

1. When the muscle shortens and sufficient force is produced to overcome the amount of weight (external load), it is considered a contraction or concentric muscle action.

2. If there is no change in the length of the muscle, but force is generated, this results in and isometric action.

3. When the muscle is generating force while lengthening and resisting movement from the external load, this is considered eccentric muscle action (Thompson et al., 2010).

According to the ACSM, the most effective training programs utilize concentric–eccentric repetitions and isometric muscle actions, and employ bilateral and unilateral single- and multiple-joint exercise (ACSM, 2011; Dudley et al., 1991; Ratamess et al., 2009). In more recent investigations, however, eccentric training was shown to promote improved functional capacity (Raj et al., 2012), and with the exception of its muscle-damaging nature, it can induce health-promoting effects that may improve quality of life (Vassilis et al., 2010).

Vassilis and colleagues (2010) investigated the influence of chronic weekly bouts of eccentric-only versus concentric-only exercise on muscle physiology and blood chemistry related to specific health-related parameters in adult women. Eccentric training increased muscle strength and performance, improved resting energy expenditure and lipid oxidation, as well as decreased insulin resistance and improved blood lipid profile. Both acute and chronic eccentric exercise, but not concentric exercise, favorably modified the levels of lipids and lipoproteins. Collectively, the type of muscle action (eccentric), intensity of muscle action (maximal), and the number of muscle actions contributed to the effect of training. For the first time, it was reported that only 30 minutes of eccentric exercise over 8 weeks was sufficient to improve health risk factors (Vassilis et al., 2010).

Raj and colleagues (2012) determined the effects of eccentrically biased and conventional resistance training on muscle architecture, one-repetition maximum (1RM), isometric strength, isokinetic force-velocity characteristics, functional capacity, and pulse-wave velocity in older men and women. Both eccentrically biased and conventional resistance training improved 1RM. Significant improvements using eccentrically biased exercise were noted for isometric and concentric torque, vastus lateralis, thickness, and stair climb. Timed up and go, stair descent, and vertical jump improved during conventional resistance training. Pulse-wave

Table 3.1 Major Spine and Lower Extremity Joints, Movements, Range of Motion, Muscles, and Example Resistance Exercises

Joint	Movement	Range of motion	Major agonist muscles	Examples of resistance exercise
Cervical spine	Flexion	50	Strernocleidomastoid, anterior scalene, longus capitis/colli	Machine neck flexion
	Extension	60	Suboccipitals, splenius capitus/cervicus, erector spinae	Machine neck extension
	Lateral flexion	45	Unilateral contraction of flexor-extensor muscles above	Machine neck lateral flexion
	Rotation	80	Unilateral contraction of flexor-extensor muscles above	Machine neck rotation
Lumbar spine	Flexion	60	Rectus abdominis, internal/external oblique abdominus	Crunch, leg raise, machine crunch, high pulley crunch
	Extension	25	Erector spinae, multifidus	Roman chair, machine trunk extension, dead lift, squat
	Lateral flexion	25	Quadratus lumborum, internal/external oblique abdominals, unilateral erector spinae	Roman chair side bend, dumbbell side bend, hanging leg raise
	Rotation		Internal/external oblique abdominals, intrinsic spinal rotators, multifidus	Broomstick twist, machine trunk rotation
Hip	Flexion	120	Iliopsoas, rectus femoris, sartorius, pectineus, tensor fascia latae	Leg raise, sit-up, machine crunch
	Extension	30	Gluteus maximus, hamstrings	Squat, leg press, lunge, machine leg extension
	Abduction	35	Tensor fascia latae, sartorius, gluteus medius and minimus	Cable or machine hip abduction
	Adduction	30	Adductor longus, brevis, and magnus, gracillis, and pectineus	Power squats, cable or machine hip adduction, lunge
	Internal rotation	45	Semitendinous, semimembranosus, gluteus medius and minimus, tensor fascia latae	

continued

Table 3.1 Major Spine and Lower Extremity Joints, Movements, Range of Motion, Muscles, and Example Resistance Exercises (Continued)

Joint	Movement	Range of motion	Major agonist muscles	Examples of resistance exercise
	External rotation	50	Biceps femoris, Sartorius, gluteus maximus, deep rotators (piriformis, superior and inferior gernelli, internal and external obturators, quadrates femoris)	
Knee	Flexion	140	Hamstrings, gracilis, Sartorius, popliteus, gastrocnemius	Leg curl (standing, seated, prone)
	Extension	0–10	Quadriceps femoris	Lunge, squats, machine leg extension
	Internal rotation	30	Gracilis, semimembranosus, Semitendinosus	
	External rotation	45	Biceps femoris	
Ankle: talocrural	Dorsiflexion	15–20	Tibialis anterior, extensor digitorum longus, extensor halluces longus	Ankle dorsiflexion resistance band
	Plantarflexion	50	Gastrocnemius, soleus, tibialis posterior, flexor digitorum longus, flexor hallucis longus	Standing/seated calf raise, donkey calf raise
Ankle: subtalar	Eversion	5–15	Peroneus longus and brevis	Elastic band eversion
	Inversion	20–30	Tibialis anterior and posterior	Elastic band inversion
Scapulothoracic	Fixation		Serratus anterior, pectoralis minor, trapezius, levator scapulae, rhomboids	Push-up, parallel bar dip
	Upward rotation		Trapezius, rhomboids, pectoralis minor, levator scapulae	Upright row, shoulder shrug, seated row
	Downward rotation		Rhomboids, levator scapulae, trapezius	Shoulder shrug
	Elevation Depression		Pectoralis minor, trapezius Serratus anterior, pectoralis minor	Supine dumbbell serratus press, push-up
	Protraction		Rhomboids, trapezius	Seated row
	Retraction			
Glenohumeral (shoulder)	Flexion	90–100	Anterior deltoid, pectoralis major (clavicular head), biceps brachii (long head)	Dumbbell front raise, incline bench press

Table 3.1 Major Spine and Lower Extremity Joints, Movements, Range of Motion, Muscles, and Example Resistance Exercises (Continued)

Joint	Movement	Range of motion	Major agonist muscles	Examples of resistance exercise
	Extension	40–60	Latissimus dorsi, teres major, pectoralis major (strenocostal head)	Dumbbell pullover, chin-up
	Abduction	90–95	Middle deltoid, suprapinatus	Dumbbell lateral raise, dumbbell press
	Adduction	0	Latissimus dorsi, teres major, pectoralis major	Lat pull-down, seated row, cable crossover, flat bench dumbbell fly
	Horizontal abduction	45	Posterior deltoid, teres major, latissimus dorsi	Prone reverse dumbbell fly, reverse cable fly
	Horizontal adduction	135	Pectoralis major, pectoralis minor, anterior deltoid	Flat bench chest fly, pec dec, cable crossover
	Internal rotation	70–90	Latissimus dorsi, teres major, subscapularis, pectoralis major, anterior deltoid	Lat pull-down, bent over row, dumbbell row, rotator cuff exercises, dumbbell press, parallel bar dip, front raises
	External rotation	70–90	Infraspinatus, teres minor, posterior deltoid	External rotator cuff exercises—dumbbell side-lying, cable in, rotator cuff exercises—dumbbell side-lying, cable
Elbow	Flexion	145–150	Bicep brachii, brachialis, brachioradialis	Dumbbell curl, preacher curl, hammer curl, dip, pulley triceps extension, close grip bench
	Extension	0	Tricep brachii, anconeus	Press, push-downs, dumbbell
Radioulnar	Supination	80–90	Biceps brachii, supinator	Dumbbell curl (with supination)
	Pronation	70–90	Pronator quadratus, pronator teres	Dumbbell pronation
Wrist	Flexion	70–90	Flexor carpi radialis and ulnaris, palmaris longus, flexor digitorum superficialis	Dumbbell wrist curl
	Extension	65–85	Extensor carpi radialis longus, brevis, and ulnaris, extensor digitorum longus	Dumbbell reverse wrist curl

continued

Table 3.1 Major Spine and Lower Extremity Joints, Movements, Range of Motion, Muscles, and Example Resistance Exercises (Continued)

Joint	Movement	Range of motion	Major agonist muscles	Examples of resistance exercise
	Adduction	25–40	Flexor and extensor carpi ulnaris	Wrist curl, reverse wrist curl
	Abduction	15–25	Extensor carpi radialis longus and brevis, flexor carpi radialis	Wrist curl, reverse wrist curl

Source: From Thompson, W., Bushman, B., Desch, J., Kravitz, L., *ACSM's Resources for the Personal Trainer* (3rd ed.), Lippincott Williams & Wilkins, Philadelphia, PA, 2010. With permission.

velocity, pennation angle, and fascicle length remained unchanged in both training groups. Eccentrically biased training was shown to be superior to conventional resistance training at increasing torque at high contraction velocities, whereas conventional resistance training was more effective at improving some functional performance measures and vertical jump. These results indicate that eccentrically biased resistance training is a viable alternative to conventional resistance training for older adults and can be performed successfully without assistance using widely available resistance training machines (Raj et al., 2012). Conversely, current recommendations do not encourage the exclusive use of eccentric contractions in a strength training program because of the possibility of severe muscle damage and soreness and other serious related complications (ACSM, 2011). Moreover, its use in developing children has not been explored. Therefore, traditional approaches to strength training that follow ACSM guidelines are recommended for youth (ACSM, 2010; Faigenbaum et al., 2009; Washington et al., 2001).

Key Points: Muscles Are the Engines of the Body

The performance of muscles is improved when stress is applied in excess of their present capacity. Your patient will experience strength gains when sufficient tension is applied to the muscle fibers and associated contractile proteins. This usually occurs between 60% and 80% of the muscle's possible maximum force. Strength training ultimately changes the muscle fibers, which in turn may increase muscle size (hypertrophy). This produces muscles that are more metabolically active, so they are denser and more toned. This is due to three factors:

1. The muscle fibers lengthen and widen, and more fibers may be produced.
2. The muscle undergoes increased vascularization or blood flow and capillary development.
3. Fluid retention or edema can occur in the muscle area (usually happens during protein rebuilding). This is normal and temporary.

THE OVERLOAD PRINCIPLE

The body responds to stress in one or two ways: adaption or breakdown (Ratamess et al., 2009). In muscle adaption, this may be referred to as training effect, such as an increase in strength, power, endurance, or speed. Breakdowns, however, also can result in overuse syndromes and other injuries. It is imperative that strength training workouts be designed in such a way that the body adapts to the challenge of the exercise. This may be achieved only if strength training is dosed carefully so as not to promote the use of excessive force, which may result in injury (ACSM, 2010; Faigenbaum et al., 2009; Ratamess et al., 2009).

 Talking Points: Strength Training (Verbal cues for patients or parents and family members) *Read through the following information with your patient or family members to help them to understand the exercise strategy used in the program.*

Muscles pull bones to make movement possible. If muscles are not strong, then movement will be difficult and you are more likely to have injuries. Also, muscles help to keep your joints stable and keep you upright. Strength exercise will help you to exercise and play better and longer. You will be much less likely to have an injury when you exercise or play. Once you strength train for several weeks, your joints will become more stable and your posture will improve.

Dosing strength training may be challenging because the amount that the muscle is exerted must be greater than its existing potential for strength to improve (Ganley et al., 2011; Sothern, 2001). This concept is based on the overload principle (ACSM, 2010, 2011; Ratamess et al., 2009; Sothern, von Almen, & Schumacher, 2001; Thompson et al., 2010), which results in a training effect specific to the exercise. If stress is excessive, however, the body's response is a stress injury or overuse syndromes. This may occur as a result of improper technique, too much force, inadequate rest, poor nutrition, or dehydration. The goal of training programs is to obtain as much training effect as possible without sustaining stress injury. In weight training, more demanding workouts require more recovery time. Research supports 2–3 nonconsecutive exercise sessions per week with adequate rest in between for novice and intermediate-level participants (Ratamess et al., 2009).

PERIODIZATION TRAINING

Greater increases in muscle performance, quality, and characteristics may be achieved if muscles are exposed to a variety of stimuli, which encourages adaptation (ACSM, 2010; Thompson et al., 2010). When the intensity and volume of strength training is varied systematically during a specific phase of a program, it is referred to as periodization training (Ratamess et al., 2009; Thompson et al., 2010). Periodization schedules can be linear or nonlinear. The specific goals of the individual will determine the type of periodization schedule used. Traditional linear periodization often is used if the goal is to gain maximum power and strength. There are four phases or microcycles, which are designed to promote the following: (1) hypotrophy, (2) strength or power, (3) peak performance, and (4) recovery (Thompson et al., 2010). During the hypotrophy phase, high-volume exercise is recommended to promote muscle size increases. This may be achieved by using a low load with approximately three to five sets of 12–15 repetitions. This is followed by the strength–power phase using slightly increased sets (approximately four to five sets) but reduced repetitions (approximately 8–10) and a moderate load. The peak performance phase uses a very high load, but sets are reduced (approximately three to five sets) and repetitions are low (approximately 1–6). Using these phases, the progression will promote a steady increase in the intensity of the strength training session over several weeks, which then is followed by an active rest or recovery period for approximately 2 weeks (Ratamess et al., 2009; Thompson et al., 2010).

Nonlinear periodization programs allow for variation within each week of a phase (typically 7–14 days) of the program. This type of program is best for individuals with diverse schedules, work or school commitments, or other competitive demands (Sothern, 2001; Sothern et al., 2001). Nonlinear approaches to periodization will contain varied intensities or loads and volumes on each day of training within a phase or microcycle. For example, if the cycle is 10 days, then on the first 1–2 days the training sessions will include exercise to promote increased muscle size (hypotrophy) using decreased loads and sets, but increased repetitions. During the next training day, strength or power gains are the goal, and the load increases as the sets and repetitions decrease. This may be followed by a similar training day 1–2 days later. The phase ends on the 10th day with a peak performance session utilizing power exercises, such as plyometrics, or high load, increased sets and low repetitions. It is possible to apply periodization within a single workout session by varying the intensity or load and number of repetitions during each set. For example, moderate load and high repetitions could be utilized in the first set, which is followed by a higher load with lower repetitions. Regardless of the type of periodization training style utilized, an individual can expect to have strength and power gains that are superior to those achieved during constant-intensity training programs (ACSM, 2011; Ratamess et al., 2009; Thompson et al., 2010).

BENEFITS OF STRENGTH TRAINING IN YOUTH

Aerobic exercise (i.e., swimming and biking) and resistance training offer benefits not only for growth and development but also for reduced risk of chronic disease later in life. Youth resistance training, in particular, has unique positive health outcomes, such as improved cardiovascular risk profile, weight control, strengthened bone, enhanced psychosocial well- being, and improved motor performance skills (Behringer et al., 2011), as well as an increase in young athletes' resistance to sports-related injuries (Faigenbaum et al., 2009). Resistance training has the ability to increase an adolescent's or a child's strength beyond growth and maturation and has been shown to benefit children as young as 5 and 6 years old. The goal of strength or resistance training in children should include the improvement of functional strength (Faigenbaum et al., 2009).

Regular resistance training increases muscular strength and power, and it has a favorable influence on body composition, bone health, and the reduction of sports-related injuries (Faigenbaum & Myer, 2010a; Ratamess et al., 2009; Trzascoma, Tihanyi, & Trzascoma, 2010). Resistance training also improves speed and agility, balance, coordination, jumping ability, flexibility, and gross motor skills (ACSM, 2011; Ratamess et al., 2009). Observations suggest that overweight and obese youth enjoy resistance training because it is not aerobically taxing and provides an opportunity to enhance fitness while gaining confidence in the ability to be physically active (Tompkins et al., 2009). Multifaceted programs, which will increase muscle strength, enhance movement mechanisms, and improve functional abilities, appear to be the most effective strategy for reducing sports-related injury in young athletes. Resistance training targeted to improve low fitness levels, poor trunk strength, and deficits in movement mechanics can offer observable health and fitness benefits to young children (Behringer et al., 2011; Faigenbaum & Myer, 2010a).

Resistance training may increase skeletal muscle mass, therefore increasing whole-body glucose disposal capacity (Corcoran, Lamon-Fava, & Fielding, 2007; Van der Heijden et al., 2010). Research indicates that strength training promotes decreased abdominal fat and improves insulin sensitivity in overweight youth (Davis et al., 2011, Shaibi et al., 2006; Suh et al., 2011). The AAP consistently has supported properly supervised strength and resistance training as a safe method for strength development in preadolescent children (AAP, Committee on Sports Medicine, 1990; Washington et al., 2001). More research is needed; however, it appears that strength and resistance training may be used safely to enhance the efforts to prevent and reverse childhood obesity (Ganley et al., 2011; Shaibi et al., 2006; Sothern, 2001). Young children, in particular, should be provided opportunities to safely climb, run, and jump to encourage the development of muscular strength and endurance (Daniels et al., 2009; Ganley et al., 2011; Sothern et al., 2001). The health benefits of strength training in children include the following: (1) improved strength, (2) increased power, (3) improved muscular endurance, (4) increased bone density and tendon–bone interface strength, (5) improved motor performance (Behringer et al., 2011), (6) enhanced self-satisfaction, (7) increased self-esteem, and (8) positive body image (Sothern, 2001; Sothern et al., 2001; Van Vrancken-Tompkins et al., 2006). The results of strength training provide additional resistance to sports injury in the prepubescent child and reduce the incidence of overuse injury.

Muscular strength also is shown to be an independent predictor of lower insulin resistance in children. In 10- to 15-year-olds (N = 126) upper body strength and waist circumference were the only independent predictors of insulin resistance, accounting for 39% of the variance (p < .001). Children in the highest and middle tertiles of absolute upper body strength were 98% less likely to have high insulin resistance than those with the lowest strength, adjusted for maturation and central adiposity, body mass (odds ratio = .019; p = .003; Benson, Torode, & Singh, 2007).

Several recent experimental studies demonstrate metabolic benefits in children and adoles-cents following strength training (Fedewa et al., 2013). Suh et al. (2011) directly compared the effects of 12 weeks of dietary restriction only, resistance training, and aerobic exercise on insulin sensitivity in overweight South Korean adolescents. Both aerobic and resistance groups significantly improved their insulin sensitivity, while the diet-only group showed no significant changes. (Suh et al., 2011). In another study, a 12-week resistance exercise pro-gram was shown to promote a significant improvement in upper and lower body strength, increased lean muscle mass, and improved hepatic insulin sensitivity without weight loss in obese adolescents. These changes also occurred without concomitant changes in visceral, hepatic, and intramyocellular fat content (Van der Heijden et al., 2010). Likewise, in a simi-lar study, a 16-week strength training program was shown to significantly increase insulin sensitivity in overweight Latino adolescent males at risk for type 2 diabetes. Twenty-two overweight Latino adolescent males were randomly assigned to 2-week resistance training or a nonexercising control (C = 11) for 16 weeks. Strength was measured by 1RM, lean and fat mass by dual-energy x-ray absorptiometry, and insulin sensitivity by the frequently sampled intravenous glucose tolerance test with minimal modeling. Significant increases in strength (p < .05) and insulin sensitivity in the strength training compared with the control group (45.1 ± 7.3% in the RT group versus −0.9 ± 12.9% in controls [p < .01]). Remarkably, results remained significant after adjusting for fat and lean mass (p < .05) (Shaibi et al., 2006).

More recently, Davis et al. (2011) examined the effects of a 16-week circuit training interven-tion, with and without motivational interviewing sessions, on reducing adiposity (visceral adipose tissue [VAT] and hepatic fat) and other type 2 diabetes risk factors in Latina ado-lescent girls who were overweight or obese. Both circuit training and circuit training plus motivational interviewing intervention groups significantly increased fitness and leg press. Compared with controls, circuit training participants decreased waist circumference sub-cutaneous adipose tissue, VAT, fasting insulin, and insulin resistance (HOMA-IR). Circuit training, with or without additional nutritional or behavioral therapy sessions, may reduce adiposity and improve metabolic parameters in overweight and obese Latina adolescent girls (Davis et al., 2011).

Strength training also was shown to improve lean muscle and bone mineral content in obese, prepubertal children ~10 years old who participate in 75-minute strength exercise 3 times/ week plus diet when compared with those on diet alone (Yu et al., 2005). After 6 weeks, the children in the strength exercise plus diet group showed significantly larger increases in lean body mass and total bone mineral content (p < .05).

Conversely, in a recent review article, Alberga et al. (2011) examined the role of resistance exercise in modifying traditional risk factors for cardiovascular disease in obese youth. The authors included controlled studies incorporating a resistance training-only group in adoles-cents with obesity, as well as studies that combined resistance training with aerobic exercise. Resistance training resulted in increased lean body mass and muscular strength and modestly decreased percent body fat. Effects of resistance training on abdominal adiposity, flexibility, muscular power, glycemic control, blood pressure, and lipid profile were inconclusive. The authors concluded that future research should avoid barriers to participation and increase commitment and continuation. Moreover, future research should examine the effects of resistance training alone and in combination with aerobic training on abdominal adiposity, cardiorespiratory fitness, musculoskeletal fitness, and metabolic profile (Alberga et al., 2011).

In adults, progressive resistance training and aerobic exercise elucidate similar reductions in VAT (Ismail et al., 2011). In a recent systematic review and meta-analysis of randomized controlled trials, significant differences in VAT reduction were observed between aerobic exercise therapy and control, but not between progressive resistance training therapy and control. When directly comparing aerobic exercise to progressive resistance training, however, no significant differences in VAT reductions were noted. The authors suggested that in adults aerobic exercise is central for exercise programs aimed at reducing VAT but noted that further investigation is needed regarding the efficacy of combined aerobic exercise and progressive resistance training modalities. Furthermore, combined programs should not sacrifice adequate aerobic training for the inclusion of progressive resistance training (Ismail et al., 2011). This meta-analysis focused only on adult studies; therefore, research studies determining the optimal modality for reducing VAT in youth still are lacking. Nevertheless, in the pediatric scientific literature, it is clear that both aerobic and strength training are essential to maintaining metabolic health and preventing and managing obesity in youth (Faigenbaum et al., 2009).

With the increase in resistance training in schools, health clubs, and sport training centers, it is important to establish safe and effective guidelines by which resistance exercise can improve the health, fitness, and sports performance of younger populations (Faigenbaum & Myer, 2010b). A recent review evaluated the current epidemiology of injury related to the safety and efficacy of youth resistance training and provided age-appropriate training recommendations (Faigenbaum & Myer, 2010b). Several studies reported the incidence of injury in youth from resistance training, weightlifting, and powerlifting, many of which were classified as accidental. Lack of qualified instruction that underlies poor exercise technique and inappropriate training loads could partially explain some of the reported injuries.

Recently, Myer et al. (2009) evaluated resistance training–related injuries presenting to U.S. emergency rooms by subject age and type and mechanism of injury. Two-thirds of injuries sustained in the younger age-group (8–13 years of age) were to the hand and foot and most often were related to "dropping" and "pinching" in the injury descriptions. The older age-groups (19–22 and 23–30 years old) demonstrated a greater percentage of injuries categorized as sprains and strains. The oldest age-group (23–30 years old) demonstrated the greatest percentage of trunk-related injuries. When comparing type of injury, an increased percentage of injuries were classified as a fracture in the 8- to 13-year-old age-group. It appears that children have a lower risk of resistance training–related joint sprains and muscle strains than adults. The majority of youth resistance training injuries were accidents that potentially could have been prevented with increased supervision and stricter safety guidelines. To reduce the occurrence of nonaccidental injuries, an emphasis should be placed on safe equipment and perfecting proper techniques in children and adolescents (Myer et al., 2009).

The risk of musculoskeletal injury resulting from age-appropriate resistance training, weightlifting, and plyometrics does not appear to be any greater than other sports and recreational activities. Resistance training is safe and effective exercise for youth provided that qualified professionals supervise all training sessions and provide age-appropriate instruction on proper lifting procedures and safe training guidelines. Further research should determine the effects of injury prevention strategies on acute and overuse injuries in young athletes. Resistance training protocols then may be developed to aid in the implementation of prevention measures in schools, fitness centers, and sports training facilities catering to youth (Faigenbaum & Myer, 2010b).

Research supports incorporating resistance training into a health-oriented approach to lifelong physical activity for adolescents and children (Faigenbaum et al., 2009). Additional studies are needed, however, to explain the mechanisms responsible for the health-related benefits associated with youth resistance training. There is also a need to establish optimal combinations that will produce long-term training adaptions and increased exercise adherence among youth and explore the potential benefits of resistance training on various medical conditions. Thus, future research should aim to elucidate the mechanisms responsible for the performance enhancement and injury reduction benefits associated with pediatric resistance training to establish the combination of program variables that may optimize long-term training adaptations and exercise adherence (Faigenbaum & Myer, 2010a).

DEVELOPING STRENGTH TRAINING PROGRAMS FOR YOUTH

It is recommended that school-age children should participate in 60 minutes or more of moderate to vigorous physical activity daily that is developmentally appropriate, enjoyable, and involves a variety of activities (Strong et al., 2005; U.S. DHHS, 2008). This recommendation also includes a statement that youth should participate in activities that strengthen the muscles 3 days per week. Resistance training, including weightlifting and plyometric training, has a low risk of injury, no more than any other sport or recreational activity, for children and adolescents if proper age-appropriate training guidelines are followed and appropriately supervised (Faigenbaum et al., 2009). Adverse effects are more likely to occur from at-home use of exercise equipment and less likely to occur with proper supervision, appropriate training design, sensible progression, and careful selection of equipment (Faigenbaum & Myer, 2010b). Youth resistance training guidelines require supervision, enhanced by qualified and enthusiastic instruction, and basic education on weight-room etiquette, proper exercise technique, individual goals, and realistic outcomes (Myer et al., 2009). Resistance training programs should be based in science and should include instruction on proper lifting techniques, safety procedures, and specific methods. Pediatric resistance training programs need to be well designed and supervised by qualified professionals who understand the physical and psychosocial uniqueness of children and adolescents (Faigenbaum et al., 2009). Qualitative recommendations for resistance training in children and adolescents are outlined in Table 3.2.

 Talking Points: Resistance Training Guidelines (Verbal cues for patients or parents and family members)
Read through the following information with your patient or family members to help them to understand the exercise strategy used in the program.

Research shows a significant improvement in body composition and strength performance in everyone—even kids—who engage(s) in this type of exercise. Here are some guidelines for planning your resistance weight training program:

- Allow enough time to adequately warm up and cool down before and after strength training.
- Start with your large muscle groups, preferably your leg muscles.
- Next, work your upper body muscles in unison.
- Now, exercise another large muscle group, such as abdominals or oblique (waistline) muscles. Abdominals typically are performed near the end of the routine.
- Finally, exercise the calf muscles.
- If you feel pain during any of the strengthening exercises, stop them immediately. The pain may indicate an existing injury, a structural problem, or an improper technique.
- Be sure to monitor your results. Use the Strength and Flexibility Workout Chart (Table 3.9) to track how much weight you lift, how many times, and how often you do your strength exercises. This is the only way to determine whether the duration and intensity of each exercise are right for you.
- Genetic factors come into play, and they will affect your results. Respect your own limitations and avoid comparing yourself to others.

Table 3.2 Qualitative Recommendations for Resistance Training in Children and Adolescents

	Not recommended	Recommended
Warm-up	Only static stretching	Involve dynamic movement and movement-based exercises designed to elevate core body temperature, enhance motor unit excitability, improve kinesthetic awareness, and maximize active ranges of motion; 5–10 minutes
Choice and order of exercise		Appropriate for a child's body size, fitness level, and exercise technique experience; the choice of exercises should promote muscle balance across joints and between opposing muscle groups; start with simple exercises and gradually progress to more advanced multijoint movements; large muscle group exercises should be performed before smaller muscle group exercises, and multijoint exercises should be performed before single-joint exercises; perform more challenging exercises earlier in the workout
Training intensity and volume	All exercises need to be performed for the same number of sets and repetitions	First learn how to perform each exercise correctly with a light load; for power exercises, fewer than 6–8 repetitions per set typically are recommended for youth; use child-specific perceived exertion rating scales to assess the exertional perceptions of children during resistance exercise
Rest intervals between sets and exercises	Assume children and adults are the same; it appears that children and adolescents can resist fatigue to a greater extent than adults during several repeated sets of resistance exercise	1 minute; this varies due to training intensity, training volume, exercise choice, and fitness level
Repetition velocity		Resistance train in a controlled manner at a moderate velocity; however, different velocities may be used depending on the exercise
Training frequency	1 day a week	2–3 times per week on nonconsecutive days
Program variation		Periodic variation of the training intensity, training volume, rest interval length, and exercise choice; all youth should begin with a light load and progress gradually to learn proper exercise technique and become skilled in various exercise procedures; 2 loading strategies are required; a power component for novice and

Table 3.2   Qualitative Recommendations for Resistance Training in Children and Adolescents (Continued)

	Not recommended	Recommended
		intermediate lifters consisting of 1 to 3 sets of 3 to 6 repetitions performed not to failure should be integrated into the resistance training program; repetition should be initiated from the proper starting position; should include periods of active rest

Source: From Faigenbaum, A., Kraemer, W., Blimkie, C., Jeffreys, I., Micheli, L., Nitka, M., Rowland, T., *Journal of Strength and Conditioning*, 23(Suppl 5), 60–79, 2009. With permission.

NUMBER OF SETS

Goals determine the number of sets. No studies have determined that single sets are superior to multiple sets in trained or untrained individuals for strength, power, and high-intensity improvements, and hypertrophy of the muscle tissue (Thompson et al., 2010). In adults, multiple sets promote a higher training stimulus, which is required to support the improvement of performance or physical adaption (ACSM, 2011; Kraemer et al., 2002). The goal of strength training in children, however, should focus on the improvement of functional strength and metabolism (Daniels et al., 2009; Egger et al., 2012; Faigenbaum et al., 2009; Ganley et al., 2011; Shaibi et al., 2006; Sothern, 2001; Sothern et al., 1999, 2000, 2001; Suh et al., 2011). In both adults and children, to promote metabolic benefits one to two sets of each of the major muscle groups generally are recommended. When engaging in multiple sets, the duration of the rest period between sets must be considered. Rest time modifies the cardiovascular, hormonal, and metabolic response to the bout of the exercise. Duration of rest also determines the ability and response of the remaining sets of exercise (Thompson et al., 2010). In both adults and children, it generally is recommended that rest intervals be approximately 1-minute duration (Faigenbaum et al., 2009).

VELOCITY—SPEED OF MOVEMENT

In general, moderate velocity is preferred if the goal is to produce the largest strength gains across all testing velocities (Kanehisa & Miyashita, 1983). Recent recommendations suggest that for beginners, slow and moderate velocities may be used safely and effectively (Ratamess et al., 2009). In children, it is recommended that the resistance exercise should be executed in a controlled manner at a moderate velocity (ACSM, 2010; Faigenbaum et al., 2009; Sothern, 2001; Sothern et al., 1999, 2000, 2001). It is acceptable to vary velocities as may be necessitated by the a specific exercise (Faigenbaum et al., 2009)

LOAD: AMOUNT OF RESISTANCE, NUMBER OF REPETITIONS PER SET

In adults, it generally is assumed that high resistance loads (60–80% of 1RM) yield the greatest improvements in strength (ACSM, 2011), especially if the goal is to increase maximal strength. In novice and intermediate participants, moderate loads (60–70% of 1RM) are recommended, whereas heavy loads (>80% of 1RM) should be reserved for experienced individuals (ACSM, 2011). Improved glycemic control, however, has been observed in individuals with type 2 diabetes regardless of whether they participated in moderate-intensity, high-repetition, or high-intensity, low-repetition strength training (Egger et al., 2012). In children, in particular, a light load initially should be utilized while the individual is learning how to perform the exercise correctly (Faigenbaum et al., 2009). After about 2 months of training, the intensity may be increased to a moderate load. Children should not utilize loads >80% unless they have participated in consistent training for more than 12 months. Specific recommendations for children and adolescents are more conservative and novices should begin strength training with a light load (50–70% of 1RM), intermediate

Table 3.3 Recommendations for Progression during Resistance Training for Strength

	Novice	Intermediate	Advanced
Muscle action	ECC and CON	ECC and CON	ECC and CON
Exercise choice	SJ and MJ	SJ and MJ	SJ and MJ
Intensity	50–70% 1RM	60–80% 1RM	70–85% 1RM
Volume	1–2 sets × 10–15 reps	2–3 sets × 8–15 reps	≥3 sets × 6–10 reps
Rest intervals (minutes)	1	1–2	2–3
Velocity	Moderate	Moderate	Moderate
Frequency (d × wk^{-1})	2–3	2–3	3–4

Note: ECC = eccentric; CON = concentric; SJ = single joint; MJ = multiple joint; 1RM = one-repetition maximum; rep = repetition.

participants should begin with moderate loads (60–80% of 1RM), and in youth with training experience exceeding 1 year, heavier loads (70–85% of 1RM) may be utilized (ACSM, 2010; Faigenbaum et al., 2009).

Recommendations for improving muscular strength for novice to intermediate individuals include 8–15 repetitions per set with loads corresponding to 60–70% of 1RM (Ratamess et al., 2009) or the number needed to fatigue the muscle but not to complete exhaustion (ACSM, 2011). Increasing the number of repetitions to 15–25 with a lower intensity (light <50% of 1RM) and a maximum number of two sets will promote increased muscular endurance (ACSM, 2011). According to the National Strength and Conditioning Association (Faigenbaum et al., 2009), children initially should perform 10–15 repetitions with a load of 50–70% of 1RM. After consistent training for 3–12 months, repetitions can be reduced to 8–15 and the load increased to 60–80% of 1RM. If the goal is the improvement of muscular power, fewer than 6–8 repetitions per set typically are used for youth (Faigenbaum et al., 2009).

Strength training ultimately changes the muscle fibers as follows:

1. The muscle fibers lengthen and widen, and more fibers may be produced.

2. The muscle undergoes increased vascularization or blood flow and capillary development.

3. Fluid retention or edema can occur in the muscle area (usually happens during protein rebuilding). This is normal and temporary.

4. These changes may increase muscle size (hypertrophy). It results in muscles that are more metabolically active, so they are denser and more toned.

Table 3.4 Recommendations for Progression during Resistance Training for Power

	Novice	Intermediate	Advanced
Muscle action	ECC and CON	ECC and CON	ECC and CON
Exercise choice	MJ	MJ	MJ
Intensity	30–60% 1RM VEL	30–60% 1RM VEL	30–60% 1RM VEL
Volume	1–2 sets × 3–6 reps	2–3 sets × 3–6 reps	≥3 sets × 1–6 reps
Rest intervals (minutes)	1	1–2	2–3
Velocity	Moderate/fast	Fast	Fast
Frequency (d × wk^{-1})	2	2–3	2–3

Source: From Faigenbaum, A., Kraemer, W., Blimkie, C., Jeffreys, I., Micheli, L., Nitka, M., Rowland, T., *Journal of Strength and Conditioning*, 23(Suppl 5), 60–79, 2009. With permission.
Note: ECC = eccentric; CON = concentric; SJ = single joint; MJ = multiple joint; 1RM = one-repetition maximum; VEL = velocity; STR = strength; rep = repetition.

Talking Points: Growing Healthy Muscles (Verbal cues for patients or parents and family members)
Read through the following information with your patient or family members to help them to understand the exercise strategy used in the program.

Review the following information with your child so he knows what to expect from his strength training exercises.

When you first begin strength training, your body will experience a learning effect due to adaptations that your nervous system undergoes as a result of the training. At this stage, your brain actually is doing most of the work, because it must learn to communicate with your muscles more effectively. As your muscles learn new movements and you become stronger, your brain, essentially, has to record it all. During these initial stages of training, you will notice substantial strength gains from your workout. But those gains will level out, or plateau, once your body is accustomed to the training, and you will have to use different methods to develop more muscles. The key to greater muscle development during a plateau is to—

- Change your training exercises
- Change your training frequency
- Change the relationship between resistance and repetitions

Increase either your training intensity or the amount of weight you are lifting. Make sure you can do the exercise in perfect form for at least 12–15 repetitions before you increase the weight. Increase by 1–2 pounds at a time.

If you remain in the plateau even after taking these steps, make sure you are getting enough sleep (between 9 and 11 hours per night), drinking enough water (muscles are 75% water), and eating a nutritious, well-balanced diet.

Keep in mind that your muscles get stronger after your workout, during the rebuilding period. This is when proteins are resynthesized and connective tissue is rebuilt. You may need to rest more between workout days.

Your goal is to exercise the greatest number of muscle fibers per movement and to exercise those fibers in different movement patterns. Remember to always breathe normally throughout your strength training.

Strength training may provide additional benefits and advantages to overweight and obese children. Because of advanced muscle development and bone age, obese child can perform well in strength training (Bar-Or & Rowland, 2004; Sothern, von Almen, & Gordon, 2006; Sothern, von Almen, & Schumacher, 2001). In addition, many strength exercises require the body to assume positions in which overall body weight is supported. In this case, obese children will perform equally well as if not superior to normal-weight peers (Van Vrancken-Tompkins et al., 2006). Moreover, in especially severely overweight youth, this may enhance performance: Although the excess fat weight is supported, the accompanying increased muscle and bone weight will enable more force to be generated (Sothern, 2001). As such, care should be taken to properly adapt developmentally appropriate strength training sessions to the specific needs of the overweight and obese child and adolescent.

ADAPTING STRENGTH TRAINING TO OVERWEIGHT
AND OBESE CHILDREN

The goal of safe and effective strength training in overweight and obese children is to improve overall health through the attainment of muscular strength, power, and endurance and to improve metabolic function (Davis et al., 2011; Ganley et al., 2011; Shaibi et al., 2006; Sothern, 2001; Van Vrancken-Tompkins et al., 2006). Specifically, the strength training sessions should be designed to ensure functional gains, which include balance, coordination,

Table 3.5   Sequence of Exercises

Order	Muscle group	Type	Intensity	Areas
First	Large	Multijoint exercise	Plyometric or power	Weak
Second	Small	Single-joint exercise	Basic strength	

Source: From American College of Sports Medicine, *ACSM's Guidelines for Exercise Testing and Prescription* (8th ed.), Lippincott Williams & Wilkins, Philadelphia, PA, 2010.

and agility, and to increase the strength and function of tissue so that it resists injury when engaging in physical activities (Bar-Or & Rowland, 2004; Thompson et al., 2010; Van Vrancken-Tompkins et al., 2006). Furthermore, strength training should be of adequate intensity to positively affect the metabolic function of the skeletal muscle cells (Steene-Johannessen et al., 2009), so as to promote an improvement in insulin sensitivity (Davis et al., 2011; Egger et al., 2012; Shaibi, 2006; Suh et al., 2011) and fat oxidation (Tompkins et al., 2009) and a reduction in blood pressure (Daniels et al., 2009), cholesterol (Sung et al., 2002), and abdominal fat (Benson et al., 2007; Davis et al., 2011; Thompson et al., 2010). These specific goals can be attained if the resistance training sessions are designed to gradually increase in intensity over time (ACSM, 2010, 2011; Ratamess et al., 2009).

Joint stability is an important component of safe and effective strength training, and this is even more relevant in overweight children with musculoskeletal problems (Jacobson, 2006). A joint is considered more stable if it is resistant to displacement (Thompson et al., 2010). In contrast to stability is the ROM of a joint; the greater the ROM, the lower the stability of a joint (Baldwin, 2003). Other structures also complement a joint's stability. These include ligaments, which connect bone to bone and help to resist excessive movement; tendons, which link bones to muscles; and muscle fascia, which cover the muscles. The type of equipment that you select for your patient to utilize when participating in training that promotes strength depends on several factors: (1) the condition of your patient (e.g., fitness level, joint stability, age, musculoskeletal problems), (2) the age or maturation level, and (3) the goals of the strength training session (e.g., improve overall strength of the lower or upper extremities, improve stability in a specific joint, improve performance in a specific activity; ACSM, 2010; Ganley et al., 2011; Thompson et al., 2010).

In children younger than 12 years of age, strength may be obtained by engaging in activities that require the child to lift his or her body weight, such as lifting and pulling on playground equipment (Sothern, von Almen, & Schumacher, 2001; Tompkins et al., 2009). Strength training using free weights or weight machines may be safely employed in children as young as 8 years of age, however, if there is interest and motivation (Faigenbaum et al., 2009; Van Vrancken-Tompkins et al., 2006). Free weights may be more advantageous if the child is healthy with no musculoskeletal problems and the goal is to improve overall strength for peak performance. When using free weights, movement is possible in three different planes: anterior–posterior, mediolateral, and vertical (Ratamess et al., 2009; Thompson et al., 2010). Human movement during most exercise or physical activities is **multiplanar**. Thus, free weights provide resistance during movements, which are more likely to be similar to actual sports activities. In contrast, however, correctly performing strength exercise is more difficult with free weights because of the wide range of possible movement across these planes (Ratamess et al., 2009). Therefore, free weights should never be used by children, and in particular overweight children, without adult supervision to ensure correct movement (Myer et al., 2009).

Weight machines, especially those designed specifically for youth, may be more advantageous in overweight children who are unfit or have musculoskeletal problems and poor joint stability, because the direction of the strength training moves are controlled by levers, cams, gears, and pulleys, thus limiting movement across the planes, and reducing the risk for injury (Ratamess et al., 2009). It is important, however, to recognize that weight machines may limit the overall potential of the strength training session because movement is not possible across all possible planes (Ratamess et al., 2009; Thompson et al., 2010). In addition, weight machines are designed to fit most individuals of healthy weight and typical height (Thompson et al., 2010). Severely obese individuals may have a problem fitting comfortably in some of the weight machines. Likewise, very tall or very short individuals may experience discomfort, as well. More important, when engaging a young child in strength training using weight machines, it is essential that the selection of the type of equipment consider their small size. Currently, many manufacturers offer child-size weight machines. For small children, especially those of short stature, and younger children, developmentally appropriate strength training machines are recommended. Under no circumstances should a young or small child engage in strength training using an adult-size weight machine.

Resistance training should be considered an important adjunct to aerobic-based physical activity for overweight and obese children (Sothern et al., 2000). Young children should be provided safe opportunities to climb, run, and jump to encourage development of muscular strength and endurance (Daniels et al., 2009; Ganley et al., 2011; Sothern, von Almen, & Schumacher, 2001). Strength training suggestions for prepubescent children are included in Table 3.6 (Faigenbaum et al., 2009; Ganley et al., 2011; Sothern et al., 2001).

Key Points: Strength Training and Children

The prepubescent child is at an increased risk of injury due to a reduction in joint flexibility caused by rapid growth in the long bones. The results of strength training provide additional resistance to sports injury in the prepubescent child and reduce the incidence of overuse injury.

Sources: Adapted from Sothern, M. S., *Pediatric Clinics of North America*, 48(4), 995–1015, 2001; Sothern, M. S., von Almen, T. K., Schumacher, H., *Trim Kids: The Proven Plan That Has Helped Thousands of Children Achieve a Healthier Weight*, HarperCollins, New York, NY, 2001.

Pediatric health care providers should be careful when recommending strength training to overweight and obese children, especially those with comorbidities such as type 2 diabetes, hypertension, and musculoskeletal disorders (Sothern, von Almen, & Gordon, 2006). More than two decades ago, the AAP separated the terms "resistance training" and "strength training" from the terms "weightlifting," "power lifting," and "bodybuilding" and supported properly supervised strength and resistance training programs as safe methods for strength development in preadolescent children and adolescents (AAP, Committee on Sports Medicine, 1990). More recently, several national medical and scientific organizations (ACSM, 2010; Daniels et al., 2009; Faigenbaum et al., 2009; Washington et al., 2001) unanimously supported properly administered and supervised, developmentally appropriate muscular strength and endurance training in children and adolescents. To date, however, there are still no specific guidelines for strength or resistance training in overweight and obese children (Daniels et al.,

Table 3.6 Strength Training Suggestions for Prepubescent Children

Climbing trees
Swinging on monkey bars
Supervised jumping activities
Swinging on a swing set
Skipping rope
Playing hopscotch
Climbing into and out of a swimming pool
Participating in gymnastics
Dancing
Learning a martial art

2009; Ganley et al., 2011; Sothern, 2001). Because typically overweight and obese children seeking assistance to achieve a healthy weight have low levels of physical activity and fitness, it is best that initial recommendations be based on those specific for novice students (Faigenbaum et al., 2009; Faigenbaum & Myer, 2010a; Ganley et al., 2011). Thus, intensity (load), sets and repetitions, frequency (times per week), speed of movement, and modality (choice of exercise movement) should be modified to reduce the risk of injury and enhance the opportunity for successful completion of the strength exercise bout (Daniels et al., 2009; Hassink et al., 2008; Sothern, 2001; Sothern et al., 2006; Tompkins et al., 2009). In addition, overweight and obese children and adolescents with metabolic disease may experience improved glycemic control when using moderate loads and higher repetitions (Egger et al., 2012).

STRENGTH TRAINING GUIDELINES

The strength training guidelines for overweight and obese children and adolescents in Table 3.7 are recommended to ensure that patients will experience initial success (Sothern, 2001; Sothern et al., 1999; Sothern et al., 2000; Tompkins et al., 2009) and may safely participate in exercises to promote improved muscular strength and endurance. These recommendations are conservative, and where applicable, technique and body positioning are modified to ensure that overweight and obese youth, who are biomechanically (Cliff et al., 2011; D'Hondt et al., 2013; Morano et al., 2011; Riddiford-Harland, Steele, & Baur, 2006) and physically compromised during weight-bearing exercise (Daniels et al., 2009; Jacobson, 2006; McCrindle, Eckel, & Sanner, 2009; Norman et al., 2005; Sothern, 2001; Van Vrancken-Tompkins et al., 2006), are

Table 3.7 Initial Muscular Strength and Endurance Exercise Guidelines for Overweight and Obese Children and Adolescents

Strength training:
2–3 days per week at 50–70% of 1RM.
1–2 sets per exercise.
1 exercise for each major muscle group.
Begin the program using a light load, which is easy for you to lift, until you learn how to do the movement. Then increase to a moderate load or weight at about 60% of what you can lift in one try (this baseline is called the one-repetition maximum [1RM]).
Lift the same amount of weight at each workout until you can perform 12–15 repetitions in perfect form, with little effort.
When you are able to do a strength exercise perfectly 12–15 times, increase the weight by 1–2 pounds.
Use a 2- to 4-second count to lift and lower the weight.
Begin doing strength exercises once per week, gradually working up to twice per week. Never do strength exercises more than three times per week. Always rest at least 1 day between strength workouts.
Rest 1–2 minutes after each set of 8–15 repetitions. One set of each strength exercise is for children under age 14 years. One or two sets are recommended for older children.
Isolate and focus on the muscles you are working by keeping all the other parts of the body stationary and relaxed (abdominals always should be pulled in, also glutes for standing exercises).
Fully extend and contract the muscles without locking the joints when you are performing each strength exercise.
Grip the weight handles lightly to prevent an increase in blood pressure.
Breathe normally throughout the exercises.

Sources: Adapted from American College of Sports Medicine, *ACSM's Guidelines for Exercise Testing and Prescription* (8th ed.), Lippincott Williams & Wilkins, Philadelphia, PA, 2010; Faigenbaum, A., Kraemer, W., Blimkie, C., Jeffreys, I., Micheli, L., Nitka, M., Rowland, T., *Journal of Strength and Conditioning*, 23(Suppl 5), 60–79, 2009; Sothern, M. S., *Pediatric Clinics of North America*, 48(4), 995–1015, 2001; Sothern, M. S., von Almen, T. K., Schumacher, H., *Trim Kids: The Proven Plan That Has Helped Thousands of Children Achieve a Healthier Weight*, HarperCollins, New York, NY, 2001.

provided with the opportunity to increase muscular strength and endurance safely without the additional risk of injury (Sothern, 2001; Sothern et al., 1999, 2000; Sothern, von Almen, & Schumacher, 2001). Also, the recommendations include additional modifications for each specific exercise for children with more severe overweight conditions to further enhance safety and efficacy. The strength training intervention was shown in clinical observational studies to be feasible, safe, and effective in children, 7–17 years of age with mild, moderate, and severe overweight conditions (Sothern et al., 1999, 2000). Once your pediatric patients achieve a healthy weight, guidelines for resistance training outlined in Table 3.2 may be followed.

Talking Points: Strength Training (Verbal cues for patients or parents and family members)
Read through the following information with your patient or family members to help them to understand the exercise strategy used in the program.

Running around the yard and burning calories aerobically is an important component of your child's fitness program—but not the only one. It is now time to focus on strength training.

- If you exercise muscles with some kind of weight (either a hand weight or your own body weight) at least twice a week, they become and stay toned or trained.
- Working with weights forces resistance against the muscle, which trains and strengthens the muscle.
- Trained muscles are metabolically active and actually burn more calories than before they are trained.
- Fat just hangs around, only burning three calories per hour.
- Strength training has many other health benefits: It may enhance motor performance, prevent bone fractures and arthritis, and prevent diseases like osteoporosis, diabetes, and heart disease. It will make your child look better: Strong muscles under her skin will make her look toned and fit.

Key Points: A Few of the Many Benefits of Strength Training
- Improves strength and endurance
- Helps people with cardiac or hypertensive conditions
- Decreases blood pressure
- Increases lean muscles
- Prevents musculoskeletal disorders (especially back problems)
- Improves self-image

Talking Points: Physiologic Feedback (Verbal cues for patients or parents and family members)
Read through the following information with your patient or family members to help them to understand the exercise strategy used in the program.

You can help improve your child's self-concept and his belief in his ability to perform exercise by explaining what happens when muscles are worked. By using a technique called physiologic feedback, you demonstrate how the muscles move the limbs while the child feels, sees, and hears what you are doing. Simply tell your child to make a muscle in his arm. He probably will bend his elbow and try to get his upper arm muscle (bicep) to bulge. Show him how the muscle changes from long (when the arm is straight) to short (when it is bent) to move the lower arm up and down. Ask him to place the hand of the other arm on the muscle so he can feel the muscle shortening as he bends his elbow. This technique will help your child remember the concept of a muscle "contracting."

If these recommendations are followed, by the end of this 12-week program, your patient will have learned a total of 12 strength exercises. The combination of these exercises will provide your patient with a well-balanced workout that targets all of the major muscle groups. It is extremely important that your patient perform all of the exercises each week so that she does not develop strength imbalances that can lead to injury. Spot training is strictly prohibited. One of the greatest predictors of back pain later in life is unbalanced workouts attempted early in childhood or adolescence. It is especially common to see adolescent males performing strength exercises only for the chest (typically bench press) because they equate strength with how much they can "press." If the chest is the only area trained, however, the back will become more vulnerable, especially later in life. Also, refer to the lists in Chapters 5 and 6 of activities and classes that promote strength gains—like martial arts, gymnastics, and monkey bars—especially for younger children.

Talking Points: Strength Training Improves Metabolism (Verbal cues for patients or parents and family members)
Read through the following information with your patient or family members to help them to understand the exercise strategy used in the program.

Aerobic exercise is great for healthy hearts and lungs. But if your child only engages in aerobic exercise, she will be missing a critical component: strength. What good is a car with a great engine but that has no tires, hood, top, or doors? Muscles provide the framework for your child's engine and must be strong to protect him or her from injury. A bone is only as strong as the muscle attached to it.

Muscles must be exercised with some kind of weight at least once or twice a week to keep them tight or toned. This happens through the force of resistance, or strength training. Children can strengthen their muscles through lifting weights (soup cans will do) or simply by lifting a limb or part of their own body (as in modified wall push-ups). Strength training should become a regular part of your child's exercise routine.

Strengthening exercises result in toned muscles. Toned muscles are metabolically active tissues: They burn more calories than fat even when the child is not moving. In fact, a toned muscle burns about 33 calories per hour to maintain itself compared with fat tissue, which burns only two to three calories. Strong muscles are a lot like furnaces. The stronger the muscle, the more intensely the furnace burns. This furnace is called the metabolic rate.

The growing bones and developing joints of overweight and obese children may be at risk for injury if the child engages in strenuous lifting, pushing, jarring, or pulling. Even jumping could cause harm. Severely obese children, in particular, should participate only in strength exercises that offer good support for their joints. The exercises outlined in this chapter were designed especially for overweight and obese children.

Talking Points: Strength Training—Great for Mom and Dad, Too! (Verbal cues for patients or parents and family members)
Read through the following information with your patient or family members to help them to understand the exercise strategy used in the program.

Muscular strength and endurance is defined as the maximum force that a muscle or group of muscles can generate (strength), or the ability of that muscle or group of muscles to repeat contractions over time (endurance). Strength training, sometimes called weightlifting, increases both muscular strength and endurance. Strength training can improve blood pressure and body composition and promote strong bones.

Blood Pressure Responses: Sensible strength training does not produce adverse blood pressure responses. Arm exercise increases systolic blood pressure by approximately 50%. Anyone with high blood pressure should begin at 40–50% of maximum strength.

Heart Rate Response: Heart rate may double during a set of strength exercises. Heart rate returns to normal shortly after resting.

Body Composition Response: Body composition improves as a result of strength training. Research indicates that untrained men and women typically add 3 pounds of muscle after 2 months of strength exercise. At the same time, they may lose from 1–2 pounds of fat, depending on their diets.

With consistent resistance training, overweight and obese children will experience a steady improvement in muscular fitness. Within the first 2–3 months, muscular strength and endurance will improve rapidly as the child's body adapts to the training stimulus. Improvements in muscular fitness of 50% or more may occur after only 6 months of resistance training.

Talking Points: Avoiding Injury (Verbal cues for patients or parents and family members)
Read through the following information with your patient or family members to help them to understand the exercise strategy used in the program.

Listen to your body. If you feel pain in a joint, muscle, or muscle group, this is a good indication that these areas are in recovery. The pain may be due to the accumulation of fluid in and around the area (swelling), which acts as a protective cushion against further damage. Exercising these areas at this point is counterproductive and may lead to overuse injuries. Remember that your muscles, joints, and bones become stronger after your workout when the body is in the process of recruiting satellite cells to promote increased density and strength of the muscles.

STRENGTH TRAINING INSTRUCTIONS AND ILLUSTRATIONS

Instruct your patients to perform these new strength exercises at least once, but preferably twice, this week. Ask them to record their progress on the Strength and Flexibility Workout Chart (Table 3.9). Refer to Table 4.2 to determine the appropriate color-coded training level; each exercise is modified according to the obesity, physical activity, fitness level, and medical condition of the participant. Every week, you will add an additional exercise to their program as follows:

- Light to moderate intensity (50–70% of 1RM)
- A balanced routine of 8–15 exercises specifically designed for overweight children

Your patient should begin performing the exercises as instructed in the illustrations that follow without weight or resistance for a 4-week period. During the fourth week, the exercise trainer should instruct the children on the proper technique during the scheduled weekly session. During the session, parents are enlisted as spotters to ensure safety. The children are instructed to perform the exercise routine according to the exercise illustrations and instruction and as indicated on the exercise record cards, twice per week with at least 1 day of rest between sessions.

Follow these specific instructions and illustrations to safely and effectively prescribe developmentally appropriate strength training activity to your overweight or obese patient. Read the instructions aloud to your patient as he does these exercises, until he no longer needs your assistance.

Table 3.8 Consistent Training for the Sedentary Individual

In formerly sedentary individuals, with *consistent* training, the following improvements in fitness may be expected:	
Training duration (weeks)	Percent improvement in fitness
6–12	~ 25%
12–24	~ 50%
24–36	~ 75%
36–52	~ 100%

Note: After 1 year of consistent training, untrained individuals may reach their individual genetic potential.

Your patient initially should use no weight for the first 4 weeks and then 1-pound weights in each hand and 1- to 3-pound weights on each ankle to perform the exercises after this time. He or she will use this amount of weight until 12–15 repetitions are achieved easily. These weights are inexpensive and can be purchased at most department stores. Your patient also will need a resistance or "stretchy" band, which also is available at most local department or athletic equipment stores. He or she initially will perform eight repetitions per exercise, with an emphasis on proper technique. When eight repetitions are performed in perfect form with ease, the exercises are then increased to nine repetitions. This pattern continues until 12–15 repetitions can be done in perfect form. The amount of weight to be lifted is then increased to 3 pounds for each hand and 5 pounds for each ankle and the repetitions are reduced to eight per exercise. This progression then is repeated. Exercises for the upper- and middle-back muscles use an exercise band. Children use the band with lowest resistance initially and then progress through the same pattern of increased repetitions and intensity. The complete resistance training circuit, consisting of 8–15 different exercises, easily can be performed in 20–30 minutes.

Special Instructions: Parents can be recruited as spotters for the children, or the children can be paired as buddies. As one child is executing the exercise the buddy or parent spots, and then they change places.

PRE-SET WARM-UP

Before engaging in a resistance training routine, the individual should warm up for 3–5 minutes. As an added precaution to help ensure safety and to help prepare the muscles for the initial resistance training set, the exercise instructions include a pre-set warm-up before the initial set of each exercise. Ask your patient to perform 16 unloaded repetitions before the initiation of the first repetition of the initial set using the prescribed weight (force).

POST-SET STRETCH

After engaging in a resistance training routine, the individual should cool down for 3–5 minutes and then participate in a stretching routine for all of the major muscle groups (see Chapter 4). As an added precaution to ensure safety, the exercise instructions include a post-set stretch. Following the final set of resistance exercise, your patient should participate in a stretch or flexibility exercise. Select a flexibility exercise that targets the specific muscle or muscle group utilized during the strength training set(s). See Chapter 4 for specific descriptions and instructions of flexibility exercises for each muscle group.

LEG EXTENSION, SITTING

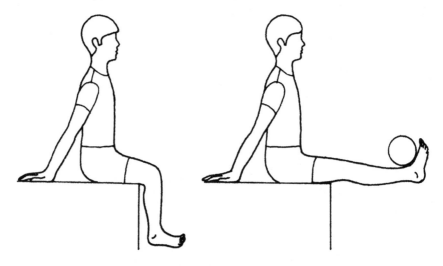

Figure 3.1 Strength exercise 1: Leg extension, sitting

This exercise is appropriate for these levels:	Level 1 Red	Level 2 Yellow	Level 3 Green	Level 4 Blue

Sit in a chair with your arms at your sides. Bend your knees at a 90-degree angle with your feet flat on the floor. Gently flatten your lower back. Perform the pre-set warm-up by following the instructions below without weight for 16 repetitions. Then perform the exercise with the prescribed weight (remember that in the first 4 weeks, you will not use weight).

Slowly extend both your legs from the knee while keeping your upper legs stationary over 2–4 seconds. Do not lift your hips. Extend your legs fully until your upper front thigh muscle is completely contracted, but do not lock your knees. Keep your ankles and feet relaxed. Now take about 2–4 seconds to return to the starting position. Do 8–15 repetitions of these. This exercise strengthens your front thigh muscles (quadriceps).

Perform the postset stretch. Select a flexibility exercise that targets the front thigh (quadriceps) muscles. See Chapter 4 for specific descriptions and instructions of flexibility exercises for each muscle or muscle group.

Take Caution

Remember to breathe normally throughout the exercise. Common errors include lifting the hips; rapidly lifting the weight into an overextended (locked) position; tensing the feet or ankles. Be sure to keep the hips and upper thighs stationary and the feet and ankles relaxed. Do not lock your knees.

LEG CURL, STANDING

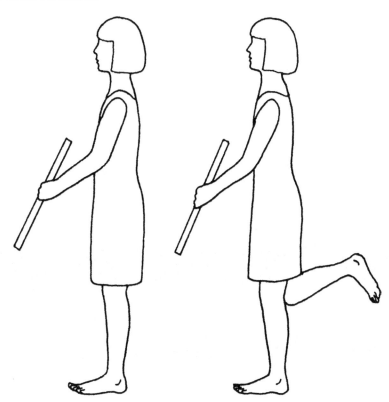

Figure 3.2   Strength exercise 2: Leg curl, standing

This exercise is appropriate for these levels:	Level 1 Red	Level 2 Yellow	Level 3 Green	Level 4 Blue

Stand up straight and tall with your stomach muscles tight, your hips tilted slightly forward, and your knees slightly bent. Hold onto a bar or another stationary object for support. Keep your knees slightly bent. Perform the pre-set warm-up by following the instructions below without weight for 16 repetitions (remember that in the first 4 weeks, you will not use weight).

Slowly raise the heel of one leg upward toward the back of your hip over a 2- to 4-second count. Keep your upper leg and knee stationary.

Now, gently squeeze your heel into the back of your upper leg, fully contracting the upper back thigh muscles.

Slowly (over about 2–4 seconds) return to the starting position. Be sure not to lock your knees. Do 8–15 repetitions of these. This exercise strengthens your back thigh muscles (hamstrings).

Perform the postset stretch. Select a flexibility exercise that targets the hamstring muscles. See Chapter 4 for specific descriptions and instructions of flexibility exercises for each muscle or muscle group.

 Take Caution

Remember to breathe normally throughout the exercise. Common errors include moving the upper leg, tensing the upper body, leaning forward onto the hands, and tightening the feet. Be sure to stand erect, keep the upper leg stationary and feet relaxed.

ROWING, LOW

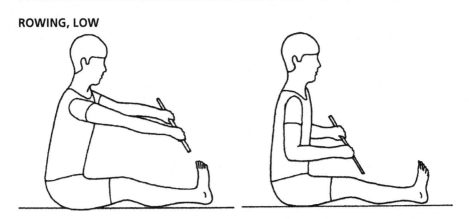

Figure 3.3   Strength exercise 3: Rowing, low

This exercise is appropriate for these levels:	Level 1 Red	Level 2 Yellow	Level 3 Green	Level 4 Blue

Sit upright, leaning slightly forward from your hips. Keep your back straight and your shoulders down. Pull your shoulders back. Perform the pre-set warm-up by following the instructions below without weight for 16 repetitions.

If you are exercising on a machine or are using an exercise band, pull the handles or end of the band back to your upper abdomen over a 2- to 4-second period (remember, in the first 4 weeks, you will not use resistance).

Gently squeeze your shoulder blades together. Now, take about 2–4 seconds, return to the starting position, keeping your back stationary.

Do 8–15 repetitions of this exercise. Be sure to pull back for a full 2–4 seconds. Then, take another 2–4 seconds to return to the starting position. This exercise works your upper back muscle (rhomboid) and your middle back muscle (latissimus dorsi).

Perform the postset stretch. Select a flexibility exercise that targets the upper (rhomboid) and middle back (latissimus dorsi) muscles. See Chapter 4 for specific descriptions and instructions of flexibility exercises for each muscle or muscle group.

 Take Caution

Remember to breathe normally throughout the exercise. Common errors include arching the back and improper position of thumbs, gripping the weights too tightly, and holding your breath. Make sure you keep your back straight, stomach tight, and lightly grip the weights.

OVERHEAD PRESS

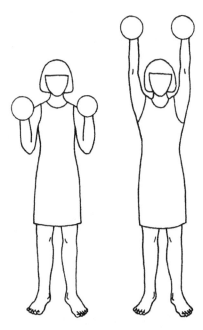

Figure 3.4   Strength exercise 4: Overhead press

This exercise is appropriate for these levels:	Level 3 Green	Level 4 Blue
Please refer to modifications at the end of the instructions for Level 1 (Red) and Level 2 (Yellow)		

Stand tall and erect with your stomach and hips tight. Make a fist with both hands and hold them at shoulder level with your thumbs turned slightly backwards. Perform the pre-set warm-up by following the instructions below without weight for 16 repetitions.

Hold the prescribed weight in each hand (remember that in the first 4 weeks, you will not use weight). Slowly, over 2–4 seconds, raise the weights over your head just in front of your ears, extending your arms fully. Then stretch up and lift your shoulders. Lower your shoulders then bend your elbows out to the side and slowly lower to the starting position over 2–4 seconds. It is very important to keep your back straight and tummy tight throughout this entire movement.

Do 8–15 repetitions of this exercise. As you do them, be sure to lift for 2–4 seconds, and lower for 2–4 seconds. This exercise works your shoulder muscles (deltoids) and the backs of your arms (triceps).

Perform the postset stretch. Select a flexibility exercise that targets the shoulder (deltoid) and rear upper arm (tricep) muscles. See Chapter 4 for specific descriptions and instructions of flexibility exercises for each muscle or muscle group.

> **! Take Caution**
>
> Remember to breathe normally throughout the exercise. Common errors include arching the back and improper position of thumbs, gripping the weights too tightly, and holding your breath. Make sure you keep your back straight, stomach tight, and lightly grip the weights.

Modifications	Level 1 (Red)	Level 2 (Yellow)	Perform the exercise while seated in a sturdy chair. Bend your knees at a 90-degree angle with your feet flat on the floor. Gently flatten your lower back.

SITTING BICEP CURL

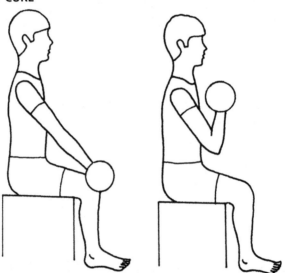

Figure 3.5   Strength exercise 5: Sitting bicep curl

This exercise is appropriate for these levels:	Level 1 Red	Level 2 Yellow	Level 3 Green	Level 4 Blue

Sit upright in a stable chair and clench your fists with your arms extended toward the ground, wrists facing outward. Your elbows should be at the side of your ribs. Perform the pre-set warm-up by following the instructions below without weight for 16 repetitions.

Hold the prescribed weight in each hand (remember that in the first 4 weeks, you will not use weight). Slowly bend your elbows, bringing the weights up to your chest over 2–4 seconds.

Now, slowly return to the starting position over a count of 2–4 seconds, making sure to extend your arms completely.

Do 8–15 repetitions of this exercise. Be sure to lift for 2–4 seconds and lower for 2–4 seconds. This exercise strengthens the front upper arm muscles (biceps).

Perform the postset stretch. Select a flexibility exercise that targets the front upper arm (biceps) muscles. See Chapter 4 for specific descriptions and instructions of flexibility exercises for each muscle or muscle group.

Take Caution

Remember to breathe normally throughout the exercise. Common errors include moving the upper arm or gripping the weight too tightly. Be sure to keep the upper arm stationary and lightly grip the weights.

TRICEP EXTENSION

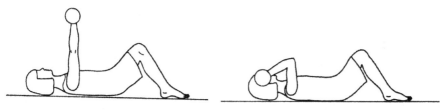

Figure 3.6   Strength exercise 6: Tricep extension

This exercise is appropriate for these levels:	Level 1 Red	Level 2 Yellow	Level 3 Green	Level 4 Blue

Lie on the floor with your knees bent and your stomach muscles tight. Perform the pre-set warm-up by following the instructions below without weight for 16 repetitions. Holding your hand weights, extend your arms straight above your body (remember that in the first 4 weeks, you will not use weight). Keep your thumbs turned back.

Keeping your upper arms still, on a count of 2–4 seconds, slowly bend your elbows and bring your hands down toward your head. Keep your upper arms still, and slowly extend your arms on a count of 2–4 seconds until they are, once again, straight above your body.

Do 8–15 repetitions of this move. Be sure to lower for 2–4 seconds, and lift for 2–4 seconds. This exercise trains and tones the rear upper arm muscles (triceps).

Perform the postset stretch. Select a flexibility exercise that targets the rear upper arm (triceps) muscles. See Chapter 4 for specific descriptions and instructions of flexibility exercises for each muscle or muscle group.

Take Caution

Remember to breathe normally throughout the exercise. Common errors include moving the upper arm and failing to fully extend (straighten) the elbow. Make sure you keep the upper arm stationary and fully straighten the arms at the end of the upward lift.

PELVIC TILT

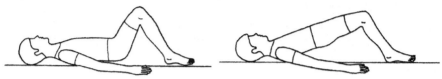

Figure 3.7   Strength exercise 7: Pelvic tilt

This exercise is appropriate for these levels:	Level 1 Red	Level 2 Yellow	Level 3 Green	Level 4 Blue

Lie on the floor with your arms at your sides. Bend your knees at a 90-degree angle to the floor, keeping your feet flat on the floor. Now, press your lower back gently into floor. Keep your upper body relaxed.

Slowly extend your hips upward, raising them off the floor. Tighten your buttock (gluteus) and the back of your thigh muscles (hamstrings) to press your hips upward on the count of 2–4 seconds. Your shoulders and feet will balance you as you raise your hips. Keep raising your hips until your upper body and thighs align. Slowly return to the starting position on a count of 2–4 seconds.

Do 8–15 repetitions of this move. This exercise works your buttock muscles (gluteus) and your hamstrings.

Perform the postset stretch. Select a flexibility exercise that targets the buttock (gluteus) and rear upper leg (hamstrings) muscles. See Chapter 4 for specific descriptions and instructions of flexibility exercises for each muscle or muscle group.

> **!**
> ### Take Caution
> Remember to breathe normally throughout the exercise. Common errors include tensing the upper body and neck. Be sure to keep the back, shoulders, and neck relaxed throughout.

CHEST PRESS

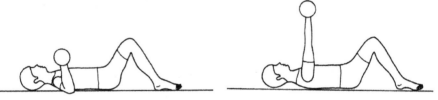

Figure 3.8   Strength exercise 8: Chest press

This exercise is appropriate for these levels:	Level 1 Red	Level 2 Yellow	Level 3 Green	Level 4 Blue

Lie on the floor with your knees bent and your feet flat on the floor. Perform the pre-set warm-up by following the instructions below without weight for 16 repetitions. Then, hold the weights at chest level with your thumbs turned in toward the middle of your body and your elbows bent and out to the side, even with your shoulders (remember that in the first 4 weeks, you will not use weight). Be sure to relax your upper body.

Now, gently press your lower back into floor. To the count of 2–4 seconds, slowly extend the weights upward directly above your chest. Turn the weights inward toward your lower body slightly so your arms are fully extended. Now, lower the weights to a count of 2–4 seconds as you slowly return to the beginning position.

Do 8–15 repetitions of this move. This exercise trains your chest muscles (pectorals).

Perform the postset stretch. Select a flexibility exercise that targets the chest (pectoral) muscles. See Chapter 4 for specific descriptions and instructions of flexibility exercises for each muscle or muscle group.

Take Caution

Remember to breathe normally throughout the exercise. Common errors include moving the weights above the face, rather than above the chest, and arching the back. Make sure to keep the weights in line with the chest and the back flat and pressed against the floor.

LOWER BACK

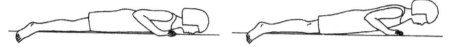

Figure 3.9   Strength exercise 9: Lower back

This exercise is appropriate for these levels:	Level 1 Red	Level 2 Yellow	Level 3 Green	Level 4 Blue

Lie on the floor on your stomach with your legs extended and your hands alongside your chest, palms down. Bend your elbows and spread your fingers on the floor. Keep your head in line with your body, with your face downward.

Using your lower back muscles, slowly and smoothly lift your upper body from the floor as one unit for the count of 2–4 seconds. Use your hands for support but do not push with them. Instead, lift with your back muscles. Keep your head in line with your back.

Now, slowly, to the count of 2–4 seconds, return to the starting position. Do 8–15 repetitions of this move. This exercise trains your lower back muscles.

Perform the postset stretch. Select a flexibility exercise that targets the lower back muscles. See Chapter 4 for specific descriptions and instructions of flexibility exercises for each muscle or muscle group.

Take Caution

Remember to breathe normally throughout the exercise. Common errors include pulling the head back, making jerky movements, and pushing with the hands. Remember to keep the head in line with the upper body and move slowly using your back muscles to lift.

STOMACH CRUNCHES

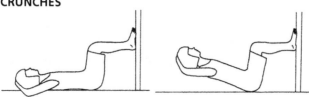

Figure 3.10   Strength exercise 10: Stomach crunches

This exercise is appropriate for these levels:	Level 1 Red	Level 2 Yellow	Level 3 Green	Level 4 Blue

Lie on the floor with your arms behind your head. Interlock your fingers behind the base of your neck and keep the elbows out to the side, in line with your shoulders. Bend your knees at a 90-degree angle and put your feet flat against a wall. Keep your chin tilted slightly back while relaxing your head in your hands throughout the movement.

Press your lower back gently against the floor. Hold in your abdomen while lifting your upper body from the lower trunk on the count of 2–4 seconds. Do not roll your head and shoulders forward. Look up at the ceiling, keeping your head relaxed in your hands throughout the movement.

Now, on the count of 2–4 seconds, return to the starting position. Keep your elbows pointed outward during entire exercise.

Do 10–20 repetitions of this move. This exercise trains your stomach muscles (abdominal).

Perform the postset stretch. Select a flexibility exercise that targets the stomach (abdominal) muscles. See Chapter 4 for specific descriptions and instructions of flexibility exercises for each muscle or muscle group.

! Take Caution

Remember to breathe normally throughout the exercise. Common errors include moving the weights above the face, rather than above the chest, and arching the back. Make sure to keep the weights in line with the chest and the back flat and pressed against the floor.

SQUAT, STANDING

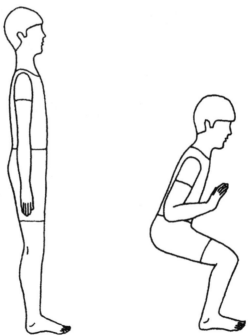

Figure 3.11   Strength exercise 11: Squat, standing

This exercise is appropriate for these levels:	Level 3 Green	Level 4 Blue
Please refer to modifications at the end of the instructions for Level 1 (Red) and Level 2 (Yellow)		

Stand tall and erect with your stomach muscles tight. Do not lock your knees. Your hands may be on your hips, or you can use them to hold onto a support. Keep your knees and feet facing forward with about 18–20 inches between your feet.

Slowly to the count of 2–4 seconds, bend your knees to no more than a 90-degree angle and lean your body slightly forward, bending at the hip while keeping your back straight and your stomach tight. Keep your heels on the ground as you lower your hips. Do not allow your knees to extend past your feet. Again to the count of 2–4 seconds, return to the starting position.

Do 8–15 repetitions of this move. You are training the front thigh muscles (quadriceps), the back thigh muscles (hamstrings), and the buttocks (gluteus).

Perform the postset stretch. Select a flexibility exercise that targets the front thigh (quadriceps), rear thigh (hamstrings), and buttocks (gluteus) muscles. See Chapter 4 for specific descriptions and instructions of flexibility exercises for each muscle or muscle group.

 Take Caution

Remember to breathe normally throughout the exercise. Common errors include bending the knees too much, allowing the knees to move forward of the feet, arching the back, and locking the knees when returning to the starting position. Remember to lower the hips just until the knees are over the feet and keep your stomach tight. Keep the back straight and never lock your knees when returning to the upright position.

Modifications	Level 1 (Red)	Level 2 (Yellow)	Perform the exercise with a sturdy chair behind you. Bend your knees with your feet flat on the floor while you lower your hips toward the chair seat. Once you feel the seat begin to lift upward, return to the original standing position.

STANDING CALVES

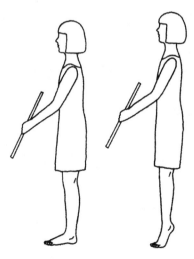

Figure 3.12   Strength exercise 12: Standing calves

Table 3.9   Strength & Flexibility Workout Chart

You'll only need one copy of this form for the entire 12 weeks, but be sure to fill it out carefully – and you will be amazed at your progress.

Strength Training Exercises

Name of Exercise	Muscles working	Sunday		Monday		Tuesday		Wednesday		Thursday		Friday		Saturday	
	Suggested Days: Monday, Wednesday and Friday	Rest at least one day between strength work-outs. Don't do strength exercises more than 3 times per week.													
		#	Lbs	#	Lbs	#	Lbs	#	Lbs	#	Lbs	#	Lbs	#	Lbs
Leg Extension	Quad-driceps														
Leg Curl	Ham strings														
Rowing, Low	Upper Back														
Overhead Press	Shoulders														
Bicep Curl	Biceps														
Tricep Extension	Triceps														
Pelvic Tilt	Gluteals/Abdominal														
Chest Press	Pectorals (Chest)														
Lower Back Extension	Low Back														
Stomach Crunches	Abdominal														
Squat, Standing	Gluteals/Quad-riceps														
Standing Calves	Rear calves														

Table 3.10 Flexibility/Stretching Exercise

Suggested Days: You can do flexibility/stretching exercise every day.

Name of Exercise	Muscles Stretched	Sunday		Monday		Tuesday		Wednesday		Thursday		Friday		Saturday	
		#	Sec	#	Sec	#	Sec	#	Sec	#	Sec	#	Sec	#	Sec
Shoulder Stretch	Shoulders and Back														
Chest Stretch	Pectorals (Chest)														
Upper Back Stretch	Upper Back and Neck														
Single Rear Shoulder Stretch	Shoulders and Back														
Lying Quad Stretch	Quad-riceps														
Seated Ham-string Stretch	Ham-strings														
Relax Your Back	Back, Legs, Arms, Neck, Torso														
Modified Butterfly Stretch	Hips, Ham-strings, Gluteals														
Butterfly Stretch	Hips, Ham-strings, Gluteals														
Straddle Stretch	Hips, Ham-strings, Gluteals, Back														
Flex @ Your Desk	Back, Chest, Shoulders														
Calf Stretch	Rear Calves														

This exercise is appropriate for these levels:	Level 1 Red	Level 2 Yellow	Level 3 Green	Level 4 Blue

Stand erect with your stomach muscles tight and your hips tilted slightly forward. Hold onto a bar or other stationary object for support.

Slowly, over a count of 2–4 seconds, lift your heels and rise on the balls of your feet as high as possible.

Now, again over a count of 2–4 seconds, slowly return to the starting position. Be careful not to lock your knees.

Do 8–15 repetitions of this move. You are training the calf muscles (gastrocnemius).

Perform the postset stretch. Select a flexibility exercise that targets the calf (gastrocnemius) muscles. See Chapter 4 for specific descriptions and instructions of flexibility exercises for each muscle or muscle group.

Take Caution: Common Errors

Remember to breathe normally throughout the exercise. Common errors include hyperextending (locking) the knees and moving too rapidly. Remember to keep your stomach tight and back straight. Never lock your knees while doing this exercise. Don't forget to encourage your patient to record his or her progress on the Strength and Flexibility Workout Chart (Table 3.9).

SAMPLE CLASS

Chapter 6 provides a 40-week exercise curriculum, which includes strength training group classes. Below is a sample class from the Red, Level 1 program, which is designed for children with severe obesity but also may be used safely in healthy, overweight, and obese youth.

Table 3.11 Overview: Lesson 4, Level 1 (Red)

Suggested time (Total: 40–60 minutes)	Activities	Materials needed
5–10 minutes	Introduction: Muscular Strength and Endurance	• Parents and patient education materials and books (Sothern et al., 2001) – Exercise attire

10–15 minutes	I. Activity: Muscle and Fat Weight-Lifting (Resistance Training) Demonstration and Instruction (MPEP PUMP)	– Hand weights and ankle weights
		  – Exercise mats
		  – Resistance bands
		  – Fat and lean weight models

25–35 minutes	II. Activity: Muscular Strength and Endurance Strength Training Circuit	• Staff
		  – Exercise specialist
		  – Exercise assistant

Objectives	After participation in this lesson the student will be able to— 1. Identify safe methods to participate in exercises to improve muscular strength and endurance 2. Gain knowledge concerning the benefits of resistance training to health. 3. Safely participate in a resistance training circuit under the supervision of a parent or other adult. 4. Gain knowledge concerning the specific muscle or muscle group that is responsible for varied types of body movement.	

LESSON 4, LEVEL 1: MODERATE-INTENSITY PROGRESSIVE EXERCISE PROGRAM (MPEP) PUMP—MUSCULAR STRENGTH AND ENDURANCE EXERCISES

INTRODUCTION

The instructor will discuss the benefits of strength training and factors that affect the results. Proper technique and methods will be emphasized. Strength or resistance training may be used safely to enhance the efforts to prevent and reverse childhood obesity and other chronic pediatric diseases in clinic-based interventions (Bar-Or & Rowland, 2004; Faigenbaum & Myer, 2010a, 2010b; Faigenbaum et al., 2009; LeMura & Maziekas, 2002; Metcalf & Roberts, 1993; Stratton et al., 2004).

Key Points: Benefits of Resistance Training

Resistance training is defined as weight training, strength training, circuit weight training, isometrics, and isokinetics. This type of training involves exercising the muscles against moderate to heavy loads, generally with few repetitions, and it results in varying degrees of muscle size increase (hypertrophy), increased lean body mass, and increased strength and power. For many years, resistance weight training evoked a negative image and was avoided by athletic and medical professionals. Recently, however, major research studies determined that this type of training using moderate loads (50–70% of 1RM), and following prescribed regimens, produced the following benefits:

- Improvement in both strength and cardiovascular endurance
- Safe and effective exercise conditioning in cardiac and hypertensive patients when set guidelines are followed
- Significant decreases in resting blood pressure and possibly successful antihypertensive therapy
- Improvement in body composition by increase of lean muscle mass and decrease of fat stores
- Prevention of musculoskeletal disorders, especially in the back area
- Improvement of self-image and self-efficacy (feeling of control over one's situation)
- Acceleration of heart rate and blood pressure responses within clinically acceptable levels during exercise
- Favorable modification of risk factors for coronary artery disease
- Possible provision of up to 15% increase in aerobic endurance (maximum oxygen uptake [VO_2max])
- Possible promotion of the use of glucose and fat by muscles, improving insulin sensitivity, lipoprotein lipid profiles, blood pressure, and increase of high-density lipoprotein cholesterol.

ACTIVITY I. MUSCLE AND FAT

The instructor should pass around models of muscle tissue and fat tissue for the kids to feel and observe using verbal cues.

Talking Points: Muscle and Fat (Verbal cues for patients or parents and family members)
Read through the following information with your patient or family members to help them to understand the exercise strategy used in the program.

This is only one pound of fat. Notice how big it is, but it is very light. This is 2 pounds of muscle. Notice how small it is but that it is much heavier than fat. When you have too much fat it makes you look very large. But, if you have a lot of muscle you will look lean.

> Muscles have very little brains—they remember only after being shown many times. They will stay tight without you telling them to, if you exercise them with weight at least twice a week.
>
> The most important thing is that a muscle that you have exercised becomes a trained muscle. Trained muscles burn calories even when you are not exercising them. Fat tissue just hangs around.
>
> Strength training can improve blood pressure, body composition, and promote strong bones.

ACTIVITY II. DEMONSTRATION AND INSTRUCTION

The instructor reviews the technique for each of the strength exercises using the illustrations, descriptions, and instructions previously detailed in this chapter. Children should begin performing the exercises as instructed in the illustrations in this chapter without weight or resistance for a 4-week period. During the fourth week, the exercise trainer will instruct the children on the proper technique during the scheduled weekly session. During the session, parents are enlisted as spotters to ensure safety. The children are instructed to perform the exercise routine according to the illustrations in this chapter and as indicated on the exercise record cards, twice per week with at least 1 day of rest between sessions.

Clinical Reminders for the Health Care Professional: Exercise Safety

Parents can be recruited as spotters for the kids, or the kids can be paired as buddies. As one child is executing the exercise, the buddy or parent spots, and then they change places.

ACTIVITY III. MUSCULAR STRENGTH AND ENDURANCE— STRENGTH TRAINING CIRCUIT

The children will participate in a circuit strength training session. The strength training stations will follow the exercises illustrated previously detailed in this chapter and on the Strength and Flexibility Workout Chart (Table 3.9). During the circuit, the instructor will discuss facts concerning strength training.

Talking Points: Safe and Effective Resistance Training for Youth (Verbal cues for patients or parents and family members)
Read through the following information with your patient or family members to help them to understand the exercise strategy used in the program.

Resistance training comes with a lot of different names and forms (weight training, strength training, circuit weight training, isometrics, and isokinetics). Generally it means that you exercise your muscles against moderate to heavy loads, with few repetitions. Depending on what you do, this is the method for building muscle size, increasing lean body mass, and increasing your strength and power.

Ask your pediatrician about which kinds of strengthening activities are safe for your overweight child. His growing bones and developing joints may be at risk for injury if he asks too much of his body by strenuous lifting, pushing, jarring, or pulling. Even jumping could cause harm. Severely obese children should participate in only those strength exercises that offer good support for their joints. The exercises outlined in this chapter were designed especially for overweight children. In the fourth week, your child should start the process of exercising with weights. Children under 14 years of age should begin at the lowest intensity. No matter what the child's age, you should focus on the child's technique. Upon getting your pediatrician's approval and ensuring that the equipment is in good condition, encourage your child to strengthen his or her muscles by following the guidelines in this chapter.

As the children move from one station of the circuit to another, strength exercises, specifically designed for overweight children, are performed in one set of 8–12 repetitions. The movement time is 2–4 seconds concentric and 2–4 seconds eccentric through a full ROM. Children under 14 years of age begin at the lowest intensity. Proper technique is emphasized. Participants increase load (weight or resistance) only when the 12th repetition is performed with ease and in perfect form.

 Key Points: Guidelines for Resistance Training

Force and Weight Aspects

Individuals should begin the program at 50–70% of maximum strength threshold. This weight should be maintained until 12–15 repetitions can be performed at specified velocities and in perfect form (technique). At this time an increase in weight of 5–10% is recommended.

Speed of Movement (Velocity)

A 2- to 4-second count for both the lifting and lowering phases with constant movement throughout is recommended. The movement should be performed with no rest and with a slight hold at the highest force resistance. The velocity can be increased slightly when using free weights, and a hold is not necessary.

Frequency

Untrained individuals should begin the program at a frequency of once per week with twice per week the maximum. Trained individuals can begin the program at a frequency of twice per week, with a minimum of once per week to prevent a loss in strength and muscle size. A minimum of 1 day between workouts is necessary to guarantee enough rest to promote strength gains. For individuals working at peak workloads, 2–3 days of rest between workouts is advisable. This will help to prevent overwork and injury. It is inadvisable to work out with weights more frequently than three times per week.

Duration

A period of 1–2 minutes per station is suggested. Each station should consist of one set of between 8 and 15 repetitions performed as specified. This will induce a balanced workout of muscular strength, muscular endurance, and slight VO_2max improvement provided there is a minimum rest period with no more than 1 minute between stations (a rest of 15–30 seconds is recommended).

Technique

Body alignment should follow ACSM guidelines with positioning for maximum isolation of designated muscles or muscle groups. The general technique for all exercises is as follows:

Movement should occur only in the joint adjacent to the muscle(s) being contracted. All other body parts should be stationary and relaxed.
As the movement begins, the individual should focus on the muscle(s) being worked, and fully contract (squeeze and shorten) the muscle into the holding point. When extending the weights, a maximum range of motion should be achieved.
There should be a light grip on the handles unless specifically working the forearm. This prevents an unnecessary elevation in blood pressure.
Techniques specific to each exercise should be illustrated by a weightlifting instructor or trainer.

Breathing should be continuous and at a normal rate throughout with no specific inhalation or exhalation phase. To aid in concentration a quiet, nondistracting atmosphere is recommended. Warm-up should consist of approximately 5 minutes of low-impact jogging moves, range of motion without weight, and gentle stretching. Cooldown should be a similar process with more intense stretching.

Safety

At least one spotter is required on all free-weight stations. A spotter is encouraged on all stations to aid the subject, especially through the latter repetitions of maximum force.

Injury Prevention

It is suggested that exercises be performed as specified only. It is advisable that a spotter be utilized to correct faulty technique as muscle reaches fatigue.

Muscle Soreness

Slight muscle soreness and tightness are normal 1–2 days following weight training. Research suggests that this may be due to the muscle-rebuilding process. Proper cooldown and adequate stretching are encouraged for prevention of soreness. If the soreness is light, gentle stretching and range-of-motion exercise are beneficial, along with elevation and ice for swelling. If there is no swelling then a warm bath and massage are beneficial. For severe soreness, the RICE method (rest, ice, compression, and elevation) is recommended. If pain persists after 3 days, it is recommended that the individual be seen by a physician.

Sources: Adapted from American College of Sports Medicine, *ACSM's Guidelines for Exercise Testing and Prescription* (8th ed.), Lippincott Williams & Wilkins, Philadelphia, PA, 2010; Faigenbaum et al., 2009; Sothern, M. S., *Pediatric Clinics of North America*, 48(4), 995–1015, 2001; Sothern, M. S., von Almen, T. K., Schumacher, H., *Trim Kids: The Proven Plan That Has Helped Thousands of Children Achieve a Healthier Weight*, HarperCollins, New York, NY, 2001.

The children initially use 1-pound weights in each hand and 1- to 3-pound weights on each ankle to perform the exercises. They initially perform eight repetitions per exercise, with emphasis on proper technique. When eight repetitions are performed in perfect form with ease, the exercises are then increased to nine repetitions. This pattern continues until 12 repetitions can be done in perfect form. The amount of weight to be lifted is then increased to 3 pounds for each hand and 5 pounds for each ankle and the repetitions are reduced to eight per exercise. The progression described previously is repeated. Exercises for the upper and middle back muscles use an exercise band. Children use the band with lowest resistance initially and then progress through the same pattern of increased repetitions and intensity. The complete resistance training circuit, consisting of 8–12 different exercises, easily can be performed in 20–30 minutes.

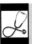

Clinical Reminders for the Health Care Professional: Strength Training for Overweight and Obese Youth

Appropriate strength training for overweight and obese children should include the following: Moderate-high intensity: 50% (beginners) to 70% (intermediate) of 1RM

- A balanced routine of 8–15 exercises specifically designed for overweight and obese children
- One (beginners) to two (intermediate) set(s) of 8–15 repetitions
- Movement time: 2–4 seconds concentric; 2–4 seconds eccentric

Children under 14 years begin at the lowest intensity. Proper technique is emphasized. Participant increases load (weight or resistance) only when the 12–15th repetition is performed with ease and in perfect form.

Glossary

Muscular Strength and Endurance: The maximum force that a muscle or group of muscles can generate (strength), or the ability of that muscle or group of muscles to repeat contractions over time (endurance). Strength training, sometimes called weightlifting, increases both muscular strength and endurance.

Alberga, A. S., Sigal, R. J., Kenny, G. P. (2011). A review of resistance exercise training in obese adolescents. *The Physician and Sports Medicine*, 39(2), 50–63.

American Academy of Pediatrics, Committee on Sports Medicine. (1990). Strength training, weight and power lifting, and body building by children and adolescents. *Pediatrics*, 86(5), 801–803.

American College of Sports Medicine. (2010). *ACSM's Guidelines for Exercise Testing and Prescription* (8th ed.) Philadelphia, PA: Lippincott Williams & Wilkins.

American College of Sports Medicine. (2011). Position stand: Quantity and quality of exercise for developing and maintaining cardiorespiratory, musculoskeletal, and neuromotor fitness in apparently healthy adults: Guidance for prescribing exercise. *Medicine and Science in Sports and Exercise*, 43(7), 1334–1359.

Arabatzi, F., Kellis, E., de Villarreal, E. (2010). Vertical jump biomechanics after plyometric, weight lifting, and combined (weight lifting + plyometric) training. *Journal of Strength and Conditioning Research*, 24(9), 2440–2448.

Baldwin, K. (2003). *Kinesiology for Personal Fitness Trainers*. New York, NY: McGraw-Hill.

Bar-Or, O., Rowland, T. (2004). *Pediatric Exercise Medicine: From Physiologic Principles to Health Care Application*. Chaimpaign, IL: Human Kinetics.

Behringer, M., Vom Heede, A., Matthews, M., Mester, J. (2011). Effects of strength training on motor performance skills in children and adolescents: a meta-analysis. *Pediatric Exercise Science*, 23(2), 186–206.

Benson, A. C., Torode, M. E., Fiatarone Singh, M. A. (2007). A rationale and method for high-intensity progressive resistance training with children and adolescents. *Contemporary Clinical Trials*, 28(4), 442–450.

Cliff, D. P., Okely, A. D., Morgan, P. J. (2011). Movement skills and physical activity in obese children: Randomized controlled trial. *Medicine and Science in Sports and Exercise*, 43(1), 90–100.

Corcoran, M. P., Lamon-Fava, S., Fielding, R. A. (2007). Skeletal muscle lipid deposition and insulin resistance: effect of dietary fatty acids and exercise. *American Journal of Clinical Nutrition*, 85(3), 662–667.

Daniels, S. R., Jacobson, M. S., McCrindle, B. W., Eckel, R. H., Sanner, B. M. (2009). American Heart Association childhood obesity research summit: Executive summary. *Circulation*, 119(15), 2114–2123.

Davis, J. N., Gyllenhammer, L. E., Vanni, A. A., Meija, M., Tung, A., Schroeder, E. T., Spruijt-Metz, D., Goran, M.I. (2011). Startup circuit training program reduces metabolic risk in Latino adolescents. *Medicine and Science in Sports and Exercise*, 43(11), 2195–2203.

de Villarreal, E., Izquierdo, M., Gonzalez-Badillo, J. (2011). Enhancing jump performance after combined vs. maximal power, heavy-resistance, and plyometric training alone. *Journal of Strength and Conditioning Research*, 25(12), 3274–3281.

D'Hondt, E., Deforche, B., Gentier, I., De Bourdeaudhuij, I., Vaeyens, R., Philippaerts, R., Lenoir, M. (2013). A longitudinal analysis of gross motor coordination in overweight and obese children versus normal-weight peers. *International Journal of Obesity*, 237(1), 61–67. doi: 10.1038/ijo.2012.55. Epub 2012 Apr 17.

Dudley, G., Tesch, P., Miller, B., Buchanan, P. (1991). Importance of eccentric actions in performance adaptions to resistance training. *Aviation, Space, and Environmental Medicine*, 62(6), 543–550.

Egger, A., Niederseer, D., Diem, G., Finkenzeller, T., Ledl-Kurkowski, E., Forstner, R., Pirich, C., Patsch, W., Weitgasser, R., Niebauer, J. (2012). Different types of resistance training in patients with type 2 diabetes mellitus: effects on glycemic control, muscle mass and strength. *European Journal of Preventive Cardiology*. [Epub ahead of print].

Faigenbaum, A., Kraemer, W., Blimkie, C., Jeffreys, I., Micheli, L., Nitka, M., Rowland, T. (2009). Youth resistance training: Updated position statement paper from the National Strength and Conditioning Association. *Journal of Strength and Conditioning*, 23(Suppl 5), 60–79.

Faigenbaum, A. D., Myer, G. D. (2010a). Pediatric resistance training: benefits, concerns, and program design considerations. *Current Sports Medicine Reports*, 9(3), 161–168.

Faigenbaum, A. D., Myer, G. D. (2010b). Resistance training among young athletes: safety, efficacy and injury prevention effects. *British Journal of Sports Medicine*, 44(1), 56–63.

Fedewa, M., Gist, N., Evans, E., Dishman, R. (2013). Exercise and insulin resistance in youth: A meta-analysis. *Pediatrics*, 133(1), 1–12.

Ganley, K., Paterno, M., Miles, C., Stout, J., Brawner, P., Girolami, G., Warran, M. (2011). Health-related fitness in children and adolescents. *Pediatric Physical Therapy*, 23(3), 208–220.

Häkkinen, K., Komi, P. V., Alén, M. (1985). Effect of explosive type strength training on isometric force- and relaxation-time, electromyographic and muscle fibre characteristics of leg extensor muscles. *Acta Physiologica Scandinavica*, 125(4), 587–600.

Hassink, S. G., Zapalla, F., Falini, L., Datto, G. (2008). Exercise and the obese child. *Progress in Pediatric Cardiology*, 25(2), 153–157.

Heyward, V. H. (2002). *Advanced Fitness Assessment and Exercise Prescription* (4th ed.). Champaign, IL: Human Kinetics.

Ismail, I., Keating, S. E., Baker, M. K., Johnson, N. A. (2011). A systematic review and meta-analysis of the effect of aerobic vs. resistance exercise training on visceral fat. *Obesity Reviews*, 13(1), 68–91.

Kanehisa, H., Miyashita, M. (1983). Specificity of velocity in strength training. *European Journal of Applied Physiology*, 52, 104–106.

Kraemer, W. J. Adams, K., Cafarelli, E., Dudley, G. A., Dooly, C., Feigenbaum, M. S., Fleck, S. J., Franklin, B., Fry, A. C., Hoffman, J. R., Newton, R. U., Potteiger, J., Stone, M. H., Ratamess, N. A., Triplett-McBride, T., American College of Sports Medicine. (2002). ACSM position stand: Progression models in resistance training for healthy adults. *Medicine and Science in Sports and Exercise*, 34(2), 364–380.

Kraemer, W., Ratamess, N. (2004). Fundamentals of resistance training: Progression and exercise prescription. *Medicine and Science in Sports and Exercise*, 36, 674–678.

LeMura, L. M., Maziekas, M. T. (2002). Factors that alter body fat, body mass, and fat-free mass in pediatric obesity. *Medicine and Science in Sports and Exercise*, 34(3), 487–496.

Malisoux, L. Jamart, C., Delplace, K., Nielens, H., Francaux, M., Theisen, D. (2007). Effect of long-term muscle paralysis on human single fiber mechanics. *Journal of Applied Physiology*, 102, 340–349.

Morano, M., Colella, D., Caroli, M. (2011). Gross motor skill performance in a sample of overweight and non-overweight preschool children. *International Journal of Pediatric Obesity*, 6(Suppl 2), 42–46.

Myer, G. D., Quatman, C. E., Khoury, J., Wall, E. J., Hewett, T. E. (2009). Youth versus adult "weightlifting" injuries presenting to United States emergency rooms: Accidental versus nonaccidental injury mechanisms. *Journal of Strength and Conditioning Research*, 23(7), 2054–2060.

Norman, A. C., Drinkard, B., McDuffie, J. R., Ghorbani, S., Yanoff, L. B., Yanovski, J. A. (2005). Influence of excess adiposity on exercise fitness and performance in overweight children and adolescents. *Pediatrics*, 115(6), e690–e696.

Pate, R. (1991). Health-related measures of children's physical fitness. *Journal of School Health*, 61(5), 231–233.

Raj, I. S., Bird, S. R., Westfold, B. S., Shield, A. J. (2012). Effects of eccentrically biased versus conventional weight training in older adults. *Medicine and Science in Sports and Exercise*, 44(6), 1167–1176.

Ratamess, N., Alvar, B., Evotoch, T., Housh, T., Kibler, B., Kraemer, W., Triplett, T. (2009). Progression models in resistance training for healthy adults. *Medicine and Science in Sports and Exercise*, 687–708. doi:101249/MSS0b013e3181915670.

Riddiford-Harland, D. L., Steele, J. R., Baur, L. A. (2006). Upper and lower limb functionality: Are these compromised in obese children? *International Journal of Pediatric Obesity*, 1(1), 42–49.

Shaibi, G. Q., Cruz, M. L., Ball, G. D., Weigensberg, M. J., Salem, G. J., Crespo, N. C., Goran, M. I. (2006). Effects of resistance training on insulin sensitivity in overweight Latino adolescent males. *Medicine and Science in Sports and Exercise*, 38(7), 1208–1515.

Sothern, M. S. (2001). Exercise as a modality in the treatment of childhood obesity. *Pediatric Clinics of North America*, 48(4), 995–1015.

Sothern, M., von Almen, T., Gordon, S. (Eds.). (2006). *Handbook of Pediatric Obesity: Clinical Management*. Boca Raton, FL: Taylor & Francis.

Sothern, M., Loftin, J., Ewing, T., Tang, S., Suskind, R., Blecker, U. (1999). The inclusion of resistance exercise in a multi-disciplinary obesity treatment program for preadolescent children. *Southern Medical Journal*, 92(6), 585–592.

Sothern, M., Loftin, M., Udall, J., Suskind R., Ewing, T., Tang, S., Blecker, U. (2000). Safety, feasibility and efficacy of a resistance training program in preadolescent obese children. *American Journal of the Medical Sciences*, 319(6), 370–375.

Sothern, M. S., von Almen, T. K., Schumacher, H. (2001). *Trim Kids: The Proven Plan That Has Helped Thousands of Children Achieve a Healthier Weight*. New York, NY: HarperCollins.

Steene-Johannessen, J., Anderssen, S. A., Kolle, E., Andersen, L., (2009). Low muscle fitness is associated with metabolic risk in youth. *Medicine and Science in Sports and Exercise*, 41(7), 1361–1367.

Stiff, M. (2001). Biomechanical Foundation of Strength and Power Training. Biomechanics in sport. In V. Zatsiorsky (Ed.), *Biomechanics in Sport: Performance Enhancement and Injury Prevention* (pp. 103–139). London: Blackwell Scientific.

Strong, W. B., Malina, R. M., Blimkie, C. J., Daniels, S. R., Dishman, R. K., Gutin, B., Hergenroeder, A. C., Must, A., Nixon, P. A., Pivarnk, J. M., Rowland, T., Trost, S., Trudeau, F. (2005). Evidence based physical activity for school-aged youth. *Journal of Pediatrics*, 146(6), 732–737.

Suh, S., Jeong, I. K., Kim, M. Y., Kim, Y. S., Shin, S. S., Kim, J. H. (2011). Effects of resistance training and aerobic exercise on insulin sensitivity in overweight Korean adolescents: A controlled randomized trial. *Diabetes and Metabolism Journal*, 35(4), 418–426.

Sung, R., Yu, C., Chang, S., Mo, S., Woo, K., Lam, C. (2002). Effects of dietary intervention and strength training on blood lipid level in obese children. *Archives of Disease in Childhood*, 86, 407–410.

Thompson, W., Bushman, B., Desch, J., Kravitz, L. (2010). *ACSM's Resources for the Personal Trainer* (3rd ed.). Philadelphia, PA: Lippincott Williams & Wilkins.

Thompson, C., Floyd, R. (Eds.). (2001). *Manual of Structural Kinesiology* (14th ed.). New York, NY: McGraw-Hill.

Tompkins, C., Soros, A., Sothern, M., Vargas, A. (2009). Effects of physical activity on diabetes management and lowering risk for type 2 diabetes. *American Journal of Health Education*, 40(5), 286–290.

Trzaskoma, L., Tihanyi, J., Trzaskoma, Z. (2010). The effect of a short-term combined conditioning training for the development of leg strength and power. *Journal of Strength and Conditioning Research*, 25(9), 2498–2505.

U.S. Department of Health and Human Services. (2008). Physical activity guidelines for Americans. Retrieved from www.health.gov/paguidelines.

Van der Heijden, G., Wang, Z., Chu, Z., Toffolo, G., Manesso, E., Saurer, P., Sunehag, A. (2010). Strength exercise improves muscle mass and hepatic insulin sensitivity in obese youth. *Medicine and Science in Sports and Exercise*, 42(11), 1973–1980.

VanVrancken-Tompkins, C., Sothern, M., Bar-Or, O. (2006). Strengths and weaknesses in the response of the obese child to exercise. In M. Sothern, T. K. von Almen, S. Gordon (Eds.), *Handbook of Pediatric Obesity: Clinical Management* (pp. 67–75). Boca Raton, FL: Taylor & Francis.

Vassilis, P., Nikolaidis, M. G., Theodorou, A. A., Panayiotou, G., Fatouros, I. G., Koutedakis, Y., Jamurtas, A. Z. (2010). A weekly bout of eccentric exercise is sufficient to induce health-promoting effects. *Medicine and Science in Sports and Exercise*, 43(1), 64–73.

Washington, R., Bernhardt, D., Gomez, J., Johnson, M., Martin, T., Rowland, T., Committee on Sports Medicine and Fitness. (2001). Strength training by children and adolescents. *Pediatrics*, 107(6), 1470–1472.

Yu, C. C., Sung, R. Y., So, R. C., Lui, K. C., Lau, W., Lam, P. K., et al. (2005). Effects of strength training on body composition and bone mineral content in children who are obese. *Journal of Strength and Conditioning Research/National Strength and Conditioning Association*, 19(3), 667–672.

Chapter 4

FLEXIBILITY TRAINING

Flexibility is an important health-related dimension of fitness (American College of Sports Medicine [ACSM], 2011) and is defined as the ability of an individual to move a joint through its complete range of motion (ROM; ACSM, 2010) or the ROM that a joint is able to move through without experiencing pain (Thompson et al., 2010). Flexibility also is defined as the total achievable excursion (within the limits of pain) of a body part through its ROM and typically is enhanced by the process of stretching (Jenkins & Beazell, 2010). The ability of a muscle and its related noncontractile tissues, such as ligaments and tendons, to fully extend determines the flexibility of a specific joint (Ganley et al., 2011). The determinants of flexibility also may be divided into static (tissues, stage of collagen subunits in the tissue, inflammation, and temperature of tissue) and dynamic factors (neuromuscular variables, such as voluntary muscle control and the inherent neuromuscular feedback to the musculo-tendinous unit) and external factors (such as pain). Flexibility usually is assessed in terms of ROM measured by one of the following tools: a goniometer, the Leighton flexometer, or the electrogoniometer (Ganley et al., 2011). Field tests, such as the commonly used sit-and-reach test, offer alternatives to such assessments, although normative data for children are lacking.

FLEXIBILITY AND STRETCHING ACTIVITIES

Many factors determine flexibility, including the type of tissue surrounding the joint, the structure and properties of the joint, and the health and temperature of the tissues (Thompson et al., 2010). Joints possess specific structural properties that will determine the ROM possible during flexibility exercise. Individual limitations in ROM are determined by age, gender, physical activity, fitness status, and genetically influenced joint structural factors. Stretching activities are the most common methods to improve joint flexibility. Stretching movements can be active (performed by the individual) or passive (performed by a trainer as an assist to the individual). It is well accepted that well-controlled static stretching movements versus ballistic stretching are most appropriate for developing youth (Santonja et al., 2007).

Talking Points: Exercise Activity Ideas—Flexibility in Motion (Verbal cues for patients or parents and family members)
Read through the following information with your patient or family members to help them to understand the exercise strategy used in the program.

If your child enjoys how flexibility exercises make him feel, consider enrolling him in a class where stretching and flexibility are core to the discipline. These days, schools, academies, and various organizations offer a wide range of kid-friendly karate and dance classes, as well as yoga and gymnastics. Your options include tap, ballet, jazz dancing, rhythm gymnastics, tumbling, cheerleading, dance teams, swimming, synchronized swimming (water ballet), springboard diving, martial arts (karate, judo, self-defense, tai bo), tai chi, and ice skating.

Most classes are structured for fun and to be a challenge—but be certain that the one your child chooses is appropriate for his level of fitness. Talk to the instructor before enrollment to determine whether he will work with you and be responsive to your child's unique needs, while always ensuring his safety.

Before engaging in stretching activities, individuals should engage in a brief, aerobic exercise warm-up. Studies demonstrate that greater ROM during stretching occurs after an active warm-up (Wenos & Konin, 2004). Also, the elastic properties of a muscle are enhanced and the ROM is improved as the temperature of the muscle increases (Gilette & Holland, 1991). Breathing is an important consideration during stretching activities, and proper techniques aid in relaxation and the reduction of stress and muscle tension. Individuals are advised to exhale slowly as the stretch is initiated and the body moves to the end point and exhale as they return to the starting position. Correct posture is essential during stretching activities. Shoulders should remain back and the spine and hips should be held in a neutral position to avoid injury.

There are three types of stretching activities: (1) static, (2) dynamic, and (3) proprioceptive neuromuscular facilitation (PNF) (ACSM, 2010, 2011).

Static stretching consists of a slow controlled movement into a position, which then is held for a predetermined amount of time (ACSM, 2010, 2011; Thompson et al., 2010). Significant gains in flexibility have been reported after participation in static stretching. Recommendations vary from one source to another, but it commonly is assumed that the static stretch should be held for a period of at least 15–30 seconds to gain optimal benefits. There are no additional benefits to holding a static stretch for longer than 30 seconds (ACSM, 2011; see Table 4.1).

Talking Points: Benefits of Stretching (Verbal cues for patients or parents and family members)
Read through the following information with your patient or family members to help them to understand the exercise strategy used in the program.

Ensure that your child always stretches after she participates in aerobic or strengthening exercises. This will prevent soreness and possibly even injury. Stretching is also a great way to unwind at the end of the day.

Dynamic stretching refers to movements across a ROM in a specific direction as to promote increased flexibility (ACSM, 2010, 2011). Sports or recreational warm-up periods typically include dynamic stretching, which are specific to the needs of the athlete movements (Thompson et al., 2010). Dynamic stretching is a valuable tool to improve muscle function, agility, overall posture, and balance, especially in individuals with limited ROM.

Dynamic stretching also includes ballistic stretching, which refers to rapid stretching or short ROM that simulates many movements specific to sports activities (ACSM, 2011). Unlike well-controlled dynamic stretching, ballistic stretching is associated with musculoskeletal injuries, especially in untrained individuals. As the overweight child is at increased risk for these types of injuries, ballistic stretching should be avoided during the initial phases of the exercise program. Ballistic stretching may be employed once there are significant improvements in overall fitness in overweight children when the goal is to improve sports performance, but activities should be supervised by a qualified exercise professional (ACSM, 2011; Jenkins & Beazell, 2010).

Table 4.1 Recommendations for Flexibility Training

Frequency 2–3 days per week, 2–4 stretch repetitions
Intensity Static: Move to a position of mild discomfort prior to holding the stretch; 13–15 range on Borg scale
Duration Static: Less than 30 seconds as no benefit to more than 30 seconds; 10–30 seconds
Mode (type) Involve the major muscle and tendon groups

Source: From Thompson, W., Bushman, B., Desch, J., Kravitz, L., *ACSM's Resources for the Personal Trainer* (3rd ed.), Lippincott Williams & Wilkins, Philadelphia, PA, 2010.

PNF combines passive and isometric stretching techniques (ACSM, 2010; Thompson et al., 2010). Initially, a muscle group is stretched passively and then, while in the stretched position, it contracts isometrically against resistance. This is followed by another passive stretch through the increased ROM. A partner usually provides resistance during the resistance phase of the stretch cycle; thus, PNF should be performed only with an experienced, qualified personal trainer.

BENEFITS OF FLEXIBILITY TRAINING

Flexibility training is shown to improve posture and balance, and regardless of age, joint ROM is improved after participation in stretching exercises (ACSM, 2011). Research indicates that flexibility training not only prevents injury but also improves sport performance; however, static stretching and stretching too vigorously before athletic events has negative implications (Jenkins & Beazell, 2010).

Recently, a randomized controlled clinical trial was used to assess whether the ACSM flexibility training recommendation parameters improved hip flexion ROM in 173 active young adult university students, which included 122 men and 51 women (Sainz de Baranda & Ayala, 2010). Hip flexion passive ROM was determined through a bilateral straight-leg raise test at pre-, 4 weeks, 8 weeks, and post- (12 weeks) intervention. Mean passive ROM was improved for each intervention stretching group, whereas the control group's mean passive ROM decreased. Thus, by following the ACSM flexibility training recommendations, individuals can expect an improvement in hip flexion ROM. These benefits are realized regardless of the type of flexibility activity employed, as no significant differences were found between stretch technique and single stretch duration (Sainz de Baranda & Ayala, 2010).

Talking Points: Benefits of Flexibility Training (Verbal cues for patients or parents and family members)
Read through the following information with your patient or family members to help them to understand the exercise strategy used in the program.

Flexibility training, or stretching, is just as important as aerobics and strength training. Inflexible joints and muscles inhibit your child from participating in activities to her fullest potential. They also can lead to chronic muscle and joint disorders. If you participate in stretching exercises with your child, you will be helping yourself offset chronic pain and disease, too.

Stretching can be done often and almost anywhere. We encourage it during television time. Make sure you arrange the room in which your child watches television so that she can sprawl on the floor and perform her stretches. Also, make sure he or she warms up or moves around for about 3–5 minutes before doing stretches.

Meroni and colleagues (2010) conducted a randomized controlled trial to determine whether passive or active stretching technique produces greater hamstring flexibility and whether the gains are maintained. The 6-week stretching program was composed of one passive and one active stretching group. ROM measurement was implemented at preintervention, 3 and 6 weeks, and again at 4 weeks after the cessation of training to evaluate outcomes. Overall, active stretching, using the active knee extension ROM (AKER) test produced the greater gain in flexibility. These gains were maintained almost completely after 4 weeks. Similar results were not seen in the passive group. Furthermore, active stretching was more time efficient and required lower compliance to generate positive results.

Marangoni (2010) implemented a study of 68 volunteers, all of whom worked at computers for prolonged periods of time and reported pain for at least 3 weeks. The study evaluated the effects of regular stretching exercises on pain associated with working at a computer workstation. A secondary aim sought to determine whether the type of media used (e.g., computer program or print materials) for exercise instruction had an effect on outcomes. A pretest–posttest control group design and ANOVA analysis concluded that the computer-generated stretching program promoted a 72% reduction in pain, the print version contributed to a 64% reduction and the control group experienced an increase in pain of 1%. In conclusion, both software and hard copy stretching interventions contributed to a decrease in pain as there were no significant differences between outcomes of either intervention

In a recent study, Puentedura and colleagues (2011) compared the immediate effects of a hold-relax (HR) PNF stretching technique versus static stretching on hamstring flexibility in 30 healthy, asymptomatic subjects randomly assigned to one of two stretching intervention groups. Each individual's left leg was treated as the control and received no intervention. The right leg was measured for ROM based on the AKE test pre- and postintervention using the Acumar digital inclinometer. Both groups reported significant increases in hamstring flexibility in the intervention leg compared with baseline measurements. There was no significant difference, however, between HR-PNF or static stretching techniques with regard to increasing immediate postintervention hamstring flexibility. Thus, HR-PNF provided no additional benefit to promoting enhanced flexibility over that afforded by traditional static stretching.

A pretest–posttest controlled, experimental study was performed in a clinical research laboratory to compare the acute effect of the contract-relax stretching technique on active-knee ROM using either target muscle contraction or an uninvolved muscle contraction (Azevedo et al., 2010). Sixty healthy men were assigned to one of three groups: the contract-relax group, which performed a traditional hamstring contract-relax stretch; the modified contract-relax group, which performed hamstring contract-relax stretching using contraction of an uninvolved muscle distant from the target muscle; or the control group, which did not stretch. The effects of the various stretching techniques on ROM were measured by the AKER test. Results indicated that ROM gains were similar between both stretching groups. The authors concluded that regardless of whether the target stretching muscle was contracted or the uninvolved muscle was contracted, the ROM gain was the same.

Recently Jenkins and Beazell (2010) developed a program at the Runner's Clinic at the University of Virginia that includes flexibility training targeting hip flexors, hamstrings, quadriceps, rectus femoris, iliotibial band, gastrocnemius, and toe flexors and plantar fascia. Several flexibility exercises utilized in this program were shown in previous studies to improve hamstring flexibility (Fasen et al., 2009) and reduce patellofemoral pain (Peeler & Anderson, 2007). These studies were performed in adults, however; therefore, caution should be used when employing these techniques in children, especially overweight or obese children who have special musculoskeletal needs.

MODIFYING FLEXIBILITY EXERCISE FOR OVERWEIGHT AND OBESE CHILDREN

Flexibility training, or stretching, is just as important as aerobic and strength training. Inflexible joints and muscles can inhibit children from participating in activities to their fullest potential. Inflexibility also can lead to chronic muscle and joint disorders. Stretching should be performed after aerobic or strengthening exercises to help prevent soreness and possible injury (Sothern, von Almen, & Gordon, 2006; Sothern, von Almen, & Schumacher, 2001). The available research clearly supports well-controlled static stretching movements versus ballistic stretching in developing youth (Santonja et al., 2007). These findings are even more relevant in the overweight and obese, prepubertal child who are at an increased risk of injury resulting from a reduction in joint flexibility caused by rapid growth in the long bones. Even in the absence of an injury, musculoskeletal pain may occur in overweight children, especially in the lower extremities (Schultz et al., 2011). This may limit their ability to engage in certain movements designed to increase flexibility. Thus, it is important to tailor specific flexibility exercises to the level of overweight of each individual child. After establishing individualized goals, flexibility exercises will promote improved ROM in major muscle-tendon groups, specific to the muscle groups involved in the stretching motion (ACSM, 2011).

FLEXIBILITY TRAINING IN OVERWEIGHT CHILDREN WITH BONE AND JOINT PROBLEMS

In clinical evaluations, the most common musculoskeletal disorders identified in overweight and obese children and adolescents are Blount disease (tibia vara), genu varum, and slipped capital femoral epiphysis (Krebs et al., 2003; Sothern, von Almen, & Gordon, 2006). In particular, Blount disease and slipped capital femoral epiphysis are of greatest concern (Jacobson, 2006). Blount disease may occur with or without pain and is observed as a lateral outward bowing of the affected lower limbs. Symptoms of slipped capital femoral epiphysis include hip or knee pain, limp, and an externally rotated and abducted leg. Affecting primarily younger children with excessive weight, both of these conditions present a barrier to increasing physical activity as movement worsens the condition. Because of the limited mobility of overweight and obese children with bone and joint problems, it is essential that health care providers consult with an orthopedic specialist before instructing the child to perform stretching exercise (Jacobson, 2006).

FLEXIBILITY TRAINING PROGRAM: INSTRUCTIONS AND ILLUSTRATIONS

Instruct your patients to perform these flexibility exercises at least once, but preferably five times, each week. It is very important that your patient breathe normally throughout the execution of each of the stretching exercises. It is best to perform these flexibility exercises at the end of the aerobic or strength training session after performing a cooldown routine (see Chapters 2, 3, and 6). Instruct your patient to record his or her progress on the Strength and Flexibility Workout Chart (Table 3.9). Use Table 4.2 to determine the appropriate color-coded training level for your patient as each exercise is modified according to the obesity, physical activity, and fitness level, and medical condition of the participant.

Consider the following example: A severely obese (Level 1, Red) football player, with good strength and flexibility, excellent cardiorespiratory endurance, and well-controlled asthma should begin with the Level 3, Green exercise program. On the other hand an overweight (Level 3, Green) sedentary girl with high glucose levels, poor strength, and cardiorespiratory endurance but excellent flexibility should begin the Level 1, Red exercise program. When a patient's condition is identified as "in between" a color-coded level, health care providers always should select the lower of the levels to ensure initial success and reduce the risk of injury and overtraining.

Table 4.2 Select the Level That Best Corresponds to the Greatest Number of Selected Categories

Color code	Weight level	Physical activity level	Cardiorespiratory fitness level	Muscular strength and endurance	Flexibility	Comorbidity, (e.g., asthma, hypertension, diabetes)
Red	Level 1 Severe Obesity >120% of 95th BMI or absolute BMI >35 kg/m²	Sedentary	Unfit	Poor	Poor	Uncontrolled or severe
Yellow	Level 2 Obesity >95–<99th percentile BMI	Moderately active	Moderately fit	Average	Average	Controlled or moderate
Green	Level 3 Overweight >85–<99th percentile BMI	Active	Fit	Good	Good	Well controlled or mild
Blue	Level 4 Healthy Weight >5–<85th percentile BMI	Very active	Very fit	Excellent	Excellent	No comorbidities

SHOULDER STRETCH

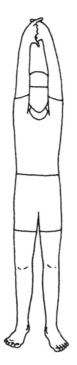

Figure 4.1   Flex exercise 1: Shoulder stretch

This exercise is appropriate for these levels:	Level 3 (Green) Overweight Condition	Level 4 (Blue) Healthy Weight Condition
Please refer to modifications at the end of the instructions for Level 1 (Red) Severe Obese Condition and Level 2 (Yellow) Obese Condition		

Stand with your feet about 18 inches apart. Now, bend your knees slightly. Push your hips forward just a bit. Keep your stomach muscles tight. Inhale as you raise both arms up above your head with your upper arms just ahead of your ears. Interlock your fingers, and turn your hands inside out. Stretch upward at a slight angle forward. Hold this position for 15–30 seconds. Lower arms and relax. Repeat this process one more time, holding this position again for 15–30 seconds.

 Take Caution

Remember to breathe normally throughout this exercise. Common errors include arching the back and locking (hyperextending) the knees. Make sure your back is flat, stomach is tight and contracted, and knees are slightly bent or "soft."

Modifications	Level 1 (Red) Severe Obese Condition	Level 2 (Yellow) Obese Condition	Do not turn the hands inside out during the exercise after interlocking the fingers.

CHEST STRETCH

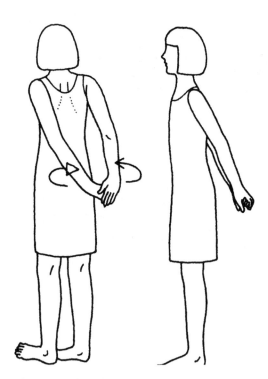

Figure 4.2   Flex exercise 2: Chest stretch

This exercise is appropriate for these levels:	Level 3 (Green) Overweight Condition	Level 4 (Blue) Healthy Weight Condition
Please refer to modifications at the end of the instructions for Level 1 (Red) Severe Obese Condition and Level 2 (Yellow) Obese Condition		

Stand with your feet about 18 inches apart. Slightly bend your knees and push your hips forward as you tighten your stomach. Pull your arms back and interlock your hands as you roll and press your shoulders back and squeeze your shoulder blades together. Keep breathing and keep your head, neck, and shoulders relaxed. Slightly tilt your chin upward. Hold this position for 15–30 seconds. Release, lower arms, and relax. Repeat this process one more time, holding this position again for 15–30 seconds.

> **! Take Caution**
>
> Remember to breathe normally throughout this exercise. Common errors include arching the back, locking (hyperextending) the knees, and tensing the head and neck. Make sure your back is flat, stomach is tight and contracted, and knees are slightly bent or "soft." Make sure your head and neck are relaxed.

Modifications	Level 1 (Red) Severe Obese Condition	Level 2 (Yellow) Obese Condition	Do not interlock your hands behind your back. Open the palm and roll the thumbs out and away from the body when you squeeze your shoulder blades together.

UPPER BACK STRETCH

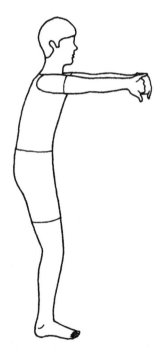

Figure 4.3   Flex exercise 3: Upper back stretch

This exercise is appropriate for these levels:	Level 3 (Green) Overweight Condition	Level 4 (Blue) Healthy Weight Condition
Please refer to modifications at the end of the instructions for Level 1 (Red) Severe Obese Condition and Level 2 (Yellow) Obese Condition		

Stand with your feet about 18 inches apart. Bend your knees slightly and push your hips forward as you tighten your stomach muscles. Bring your arms forward in front of your chest, interlock your fingers, and turn your hands inside out. Round your upper back as you drop your chin down toward your chest. Now, push your hands away from your body, stretching your upper back in between your shoulder blades. Hold this position for 15–30 seconds. Repeat this process one more time, holding this position again for 15–30 seconds.

> **! Take Caution**
>
> Remember to breathe normally throughout this exercise. Common errors include arching the back and locking (hyperextending) the knees. Make sure your back is flat, stomach is tight and contracted, and knees are slightly bent or "soft."

Modifications	Level 1 (Red) Severe Obese Condition	Level 2 (Yellow) Obese Condition	Do not turn your hands inside out during the exercise after interlocking your fingers.

SINGLE REAR-SHOULDER STRETCH

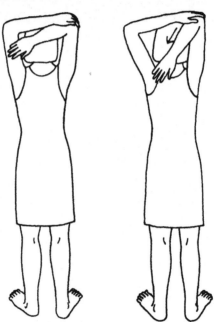

Figure 4.4   Flex exercise 4: Single rear-shoulder stretch

This exercise is appropriate for these levels:	Level 3 (Green) Overweight Condition	Level 4 (Blue) Healthy Weight Condition
Please refer to modifications at the end of the instructions for Level 1 (Red) Severe Obese Condition and Level 2 (Yellow) Obese Condition		

Stand with your feet about 18 inches apart. Tighten your hips and push them slightly forward. Now, tighten your tummy and slightly bend your knees. Raise your right arm straight up above your head just to the side of your right ear. Bend your elbow, and drop your hand down in between your shoulder blades. Now, reach up with your left arm. Bring it over your head to grab your right elbow. Gently pull your right elbow toward your left side. Hold this position for 15–30 seconds. Gently release. Repeat this exercise with your left arm. Repeat this process one more time, holding this position for each arm again for 15–30 seconds.

> **!** **Take Caution**
>
> Remember to breathe normally throughout this exercise. Common errors include arching the back and locking (hyperextending) the knees. Make sure your back is flat, stomach is tight and contracted, and knees are slightly bent or "soft." Be careful not to pull too hard on your elbow. You should feel a gentle nudge but not pain.

Modifications	Level 1 (Red) Severe Obese Condition	Level 2 (Yellow) Obese Condition	Grab the upper arm across the front of the head.

LYING QUAD STRETCH

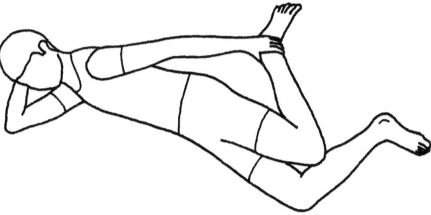

Figure 4.5   Flex exercise 5: Lying quad stretch

This exercise is appropriate for these levels:	Level 3 (Green) Overweight Condition	Level 4 (Blue) Healthy Weight Condition
Please refer to modifications at the end of the instructions for Level 1 (Red) Severe Obese Condition and Level 2 (Yellow) Obese Condition		

Lie on the floor on your right side. Support your head with your right hand. Bend both your knees, but bend your left leg back further and grab the left ankle with your left hand.

Pull your left heel into the back of your left hip as you move your knee back. Hold this stretch for 15–30 seconds. Gently release your ankle. Now, repeat this move while lying on your left side, holding your right ankle. Repeat this process for each leg one more time, holding this position again for 15–30 seconds.

> **Take Caution**
>
> Remember to breathe normally throughout this exercise. Common errors include forgetting to support the head with the hand, allowing the knee to turn upward toward the ceiling, forgetting to bend the opposite leg and grabbing the toes or foot instead of the ankle. Make sure your head is supported and your knee is level with the floor. Do not forget to also bend the opposite leg and grab your ankle, not your feet or toes.

Modifications	Level 1 (Red) Severe Obese Condition	Level 2 (Yellow) Obese Condition	Grab the back bottom of your pants if you cannot reach your ankle.

SEATED HAMSTRING STRETCH

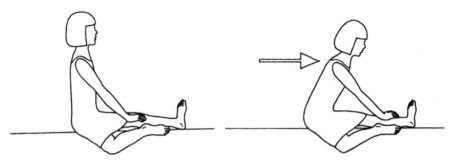

Figure 4.6 Flex exercise 6: Seated hamstring stretch

This exercise is appropriate for these levels:	Level 1 (Red) Severe Obese Condition	Level 2 (Yellow) Obese Condition	Level 3 (Green) Overweight Condition	Level 4 (Blue) Healthy Weight Condition

Sit on the floor with both of your legs extended and your tummy held tight. Relax your head, neck, and shoulders. Now, slightly bend the knee of your left leg out to the side until your left heel rests between the ankle and knee of your right leg. Make sure your right knee and right foot are pointed toward the ceiling. Now, place both of your hands on your right knee. Keeping your upper body straight and your head up, bend forward from the hip as you slide your hands down your right leg. Hold this stretch for 15–30 seconds. Now, repeat this move with the left leg straight and the right leg bent. Repeat this process one more time for each leg, holding this position again for 15–30 seconds.

 Take Caution

Remember to breathe normally throughout this exercise. Common errors include bending the opposite leg too much and rolling the neck and shoulders forward. Remember you need to bend the opposite leg only slightly and you should bend from the hip as you bring your chest down to your leg. Keep your head and shoulders in line as you perform the stretch.

RELAX YOUR BACK

This exercise is appropriate for these levels:	Level 1 (Red) Severe Obese Condition	Level 2 (Yellow) Obese Condition	Level 3 (Green) Overweight Condition	Level 4 (Blue) Healthy Weight Condition

Lie on your back. Relax your head and neck into your hands. Gently press your lower back into the floor. Slowly bring your knees into the chest and squeeze gently. Keep breathing. Keep your upper body relaxed. Drop one foot while bending your knee. Squeeze the other knee gently into your chest. Slowly pull the knee across your body to stretch the outer hip.

Extend the opposite arm, palm down. Turn your head toward the opposite direction. Slowly return the knee to chest. Repeat with other leg. Return both knees, and then the rest of your body, to the starting position.

Slowly slide one arm upward along the floor. Stretch your arm toward your head with your upper arm alongside your ear. Repeat with other arm. Place arms behind your head and relax your head and shoulders. Tilt your hips upward as you gently press your lower back into the floor. Tighten and hold in the lower abdomen. Keeping the same lower body position, again slowly extend arms overhead. Do not lift the shoulder, neck, or head. Keep upper body relaxed. The spine should be aligned completely with the floor and should be relaxed.

Continue to hold the stomach tight and press the spine gently into the floor. Begin to "walk" the feet out until the back begins to rise off the floor. Tilt the hips again and press spine into floor, holding stomach tight. Over time, your stomach muscles will become stronger, enabling you to achieve and maintain this position. Keep your back flat and the spine gently pressed into the floor. Relax your shoulders and head while keeping stomach tight. Release the position, allowing the back to slowly arch. Relax your abdomen.

Slowly and gently, stretch hands away from feet. Let your rib cage expand, arch back, and stretch your stomach. Relax all muscles. Slowly, return knees to the chest and gently squeeze. Slowly return to the original stretch position. Drop feet with knees bent for safety. Relax all muscles. Slowly return knees to the chest and gently squeeze. Return to starting position. Roll onto your stomach. Sit back on your heels while extending arms forward, palms down. Keep your face down, head in line with the back. Gently stretch. Inhale as you return to a standing position.

MODIFIED BUTTERFLY STRETCH

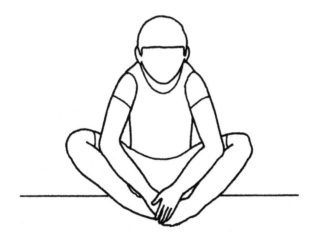

Figure 4.7   Flex exercise 8: Modified butterfly stretch

Sit on the floor and spread your legs out to each side. Make sure your tummy is tight and your head, neck, and shoulders are relaxed. Slowly bring your feet together and grasp your ankles.

Bend forward as you hold your ankles, bringing your chest and chin down toward the floor. Make sure you look straight ahead and do not roll your back or drop your chin. Hold this stretch for 15–30 seconds. Return to the sitting position. Repeat this process one more time, holding this position again for 15–30 seconds.

Take Caution

Remember to breathe normally throughout this exercise. Common errors include rolling the neck and shoulders forward. Remember you should bend from the hip as you bring your chest down toward the floor. Keep your head and shoulders in line as you perform the stretch.

BUTTERFLY STRETCH

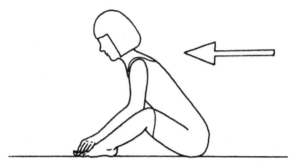

Figure 4.8 Flex exercise 9: Butterfly stretch

This exercise is appropriate for these levels:	Level 3 (Green) Overweight Condition	Level 4 (Blue) Healthy Weight Condition
Please refer to modifications at the end of the instructions for Level 1 (Red) Severe Obese Condition and Level 2 (Yellow) Obese Condition		

Sit on the floor with your legs extended out to each side. Tighten your tummy, and keep your head, neck, and shoulders relaxed. Bring your feet together and grasp your ankles. Pull your feet toward your body until you feel a gentle stretch. Now, place your elbows on your knees as you continue to hold your ankles. Bend forward, looking straight ahead as you bring your chest and chin to the floor. Press your elbows on your knees as you bend forward. Do not roll your shoulders or drop your head. Hold this stretch for 15–30 seconds. Slowly return to starting position. Then repeat this process one more time, holding this position again for 15–30 seconds.

Take Caution

Remember to breathe normally throughout this exercise. Common errors include rolling the neck and shoulders forward. Remember you should bend from the hip as you bring your chest down toward the floor. Keep your head and shoulders in line as you perform the stretch. Be careful not to press too hard on the knees or pull too tightly on the ankles.

Modifications	Level 1 (Red) Severe Obese Condition	Level 2 (Yellow) Obese Condition	This stretch is not appropriate for Level 1 (Red) Severe Obese Condition or 2 (Yellow). Perform the modified butterfly stretch only.

STRADDLE STRETCH

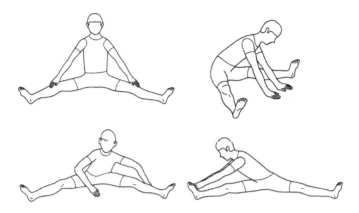

Figure 4.9 Flex exercise 10: Straddle stretch

This exercise is appropriate for these levels:	Level 1 (Red) Severe Obese Condition	Level 2 (Yellow) Obese Condition	Level 3 (Green) Overweight Condition	Level 4 (Blue) Healthy Weight Condition

Sit upright on the floor with your legs extended forward, and your hands alongside your hips. Slowly extend your legs out to each side as far as you comfortably can. Turn your knees and toes up toward the ceiling. Place your hands behind your hips keeping your head, shoulders, and trunk in line. Bend from the hip forward until you feel a gentle stretch on your inner thighs. Do not roll your head and shoulders forward. Bring your hands in between your legs and slowly "walk" them forward and then to each side until you feel a gentle stretch in the inner thigh. Hold each stretch for 15–30 seconds. Gently release and "walk" hands back until you are back in the upright position. Repeat this process one more time, holding each position again for 15–30 seconds.

Take Caution

Remember to breathe normally throughout this exercise. Common errors include rolling the neck and shoulders forward. Remember you should bend from the hip as you bring your chest down toward the floor. Keep your head and shoulders in line as you perform the stretch.

FLEX AT YOUR DESK

If you think you can only stretch at home, think again. Here are some stretches to do at your desk at school. Ask your teacher if the entire class can participate in them. Everyone will feel better for it.

The following exercise is appropriate for these levels:	Level 1 (Red) Severe Obese Condition	Level 2 (Yellow) Obese Condition	Level 3 (Green) Overweight Condition	Level 4 (Blue) Healthy Weight Condition

Turn sideways in your desk or push your chair back. Bend over from the hips and let your chest rest on your thighs. Let your head fall below your knees as your hands fall to the ground. Hold for 15–30 seconds. Inhale as you slowly return to your upright position. Repeat one more time.

Take Caution

Remember to breathe normally throughout this exercise. Make sure you are seated in a sturdy chair (without wheels). Remember to inhale as you lift your head after performing the stretch.

The following exercise is appropriate for these levels:	Level 3 (Green) Overweight Condition	Level 4 (Blue) Healthy Weight Condition
Please refer to modifications at the end of the instructions for Level 1 (Red) Severe Obese Condition and Level 2 (Yellow) Obese Condition		

Sit with your back straight and flat against the back of the chair. Bring your arms up above your head and interlock your fingers. Then turn your hands inside out and keep your arms in front of your ears. Stretch your hands and arms upward toward the ceiling. Hold 15–30 seconds and then repeat.

Take Caution

Remember to breathe normally throughout this exercise. Make sure you are seated in a sturdy chair (without wheels). Common errors include arching the back and tensing the head and neck. Remember to keep the stomach tight and contracted and the back flat against the back of the chair. Make sure your head and neck are relaxed.

Modifications	Level 1 (Red) Severe Obese Condition	Level 2 (Yellow) Obese Condition	Do not turn the hands inside out during the exercise after interlocking the fingers.

The following exercise is appropriate for these levels:	Level 3 (Green) Overweight Condition	Level 4 (Blue) Healthy Weight Condition
Please refer to modifications at the end of the instructions for Level 1 (Red) Severe Obese Condition and Level 2 (Yellow) Obese Condition		

Sit with your back straight and flat against the back of the chair. Raise your right arm straight up above your head just to the side of the right ear. Bend your elbow and drop your hand to the back of your neck. Reach up with the other arm and grasp the elbow. Gently pull. Hold 15–30 seconds. Repeat with the other arm.

Take Caution

Remember to breathe normally throughout this exercise. Make sure you are seated in a sturdy chair (without wheels). Common errors include arching the back, tensing the head and neck, and pulling too hard on the elbow. Remember to keep the stomach tight and contracted and the back flat against the back of the chair. Make sure your head and neck are relaxed. Be careful not to pull too hard on your elbow. You should feel a gentle nudge, but not pain.

Modifications	Level 1 (Red) Severe Obese Condition	Level 2 (Yellow) Obese Condition	Grab the upper arm across the front of the head.

The following exercise is appropriate for these levels:	Level 1 (Red) Severe Obese Condition	Level 2 (Yellow) Obese Condition	Level 3 (Green) Overweight Condition	Level 4 (Blue) Healthy Weight Condition

Sit on the edge of your chair. Pull your arms back and roll your thumbs out to the side while gently pressing your elbows together. Press your shoulders back and squeeze your shoulder blades together, tilt your chin upward, and stretch your chest. Hold 15–30 seconds and then repeat.

 Take Caution

Remember to breathe normally throughout this exercise. Make sure you are seated in a sturdy chair (without wheels). Common errors include tensing the head and neck. Make sure your head and neck are relaxed.

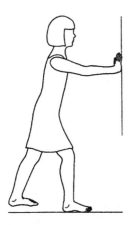 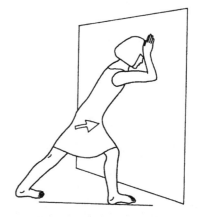

Figure 4.10   Flex exercise 12: Calf stretch

This exercise is appropriate for these levels:	Level 1 (Red) Severe Obese Condition	Level 2 (Yellow) Obese Condition	Level 3 (Green) Overweight Condition	Level 4 (Blue) Healthy Weight Condition

Stand in front of a wall and place your hands on the wall in line with your chest. Move one leg 2–3 feet behind the other. Now, bend your front leg and press the heel of the back leg toward the floor until you feel a gentle stretch in the calf muscle. Push on the wall, bringing your head in between your arms with your face toward the floor, continuing to push the heel backward until you feel a full stretch from your hands down through the heel. Hold this stretch for 15–30 seconds. Now, repeat this move with your other leg. Repeat this process for each leg one more time, holding this position again for 15–30 seconds.

> **! Take Caution**
>
> Remember to breathe normally throughout this exercise. Common errors include failing to place the heel of the back leg on the floor and forgetting to place the head in between the arms with the face down toward the floor. Position your back leg so that you can easily place the heel on the floor and feel the stretch in the back of your calf muscle. Relax your head and neck as you look down with your head in between your upper arms.

SAMPLE CLASS

In this section you will find instructions and illustrations for a lesson—which can be taught in a group, family setting—focusing on flexibility. Additional lessons can be found in Chapter 6.

LESSON 6, LEVEL 1: FLEXIBILITY—THE BODY'S BALANCING ACT AND THE FLEX TEST

INTRODUCTION

The instructor will discuss the importance of flexibility. Flexibility refers to the maximum ability to move a joint through its full ROM. Flexibility keeps your body in balance. Stretching will help you improve and maintain flexibility. If you neglect flexibility in your training, you may acquire muscle or joint injuries or chronic disorders. One of these disorders, pronation distortion syndrome is characterized by knee flexion, internal rotation, and adduction (knock-kneed) and excessive foot pronation (flat feet). Individuals with this condition develop patterns of injury including plantar fasciitis, posterior tibialis tendinitis (shin splints), patellar tendinitis, and low back pain. Obese people are at higher risk (Irving et al., 2007; Kaufman et al., 1999; Moen et al., 2009). Stretching will help you improve and maintain flexibility.

Table 4.3   Overview: Lesson 6, Level 1 (Red)

Suggested time (Total time: 35–45 minutes)	Activities	Materials needed
10–15 minutes	Introduction: Flexibility: Flex Test	Parents and patient education materials and books (Sothern et al., 2001)
25–30 minutes	I. Activity: Flex Test—A Balancing Act	Parents and patient education materials and books (Sothern et al., 2001) Exercise attire Mats
Objectives	After participation in this lesson the student will be able to— 1. Identify movements that will increase muscular flexibility. 2. Gain knowledge concerning the benefits of muscular flexibility to health. 3. Identify imbalances in the posture that lead to bone and joint problems. 4. Identify movement and exercises that will improve posture, muscular flexibility, and reduce the risk of injury.	

ACTIVITY I. FLEX TEST

Students will be guided through the Flex Test sequence in partners. The instructor will emphasize the importance of balance as it relates to flexibility and strength. Students should be shown how to keep the knees slightly bent or "soft" and not overextended during activities. Corrective exercises, designed to improve the imbalanced areas of the body, will be introduced. The program flexibility exercises in this chapter will be reviewed while set to music.

Talking Points: Flexibility and Balance (Verbal cues for patients or parents and family members)
Read through the following information with your patient or family members to help them to understand the exercise strategy used in the program.

Aerobic exercise is great for healthy hearts and lungs. But if your child engages in only aerobic exercise, she will be missing two critical components: strength and flexibility. What good is a car with a great engine but that has no tires, hood, top, or doors? Muscles provide the framework for your child's engine and must be strong to protect her from injury. A car runs more efficiently when it is in alignment. The same holds true for the human body. The function of flexibility is to maintain balance. When your child was born, she was in perfect proportion. She was symmetrical—that is, the left side was identical to the right. The front of the body was in balance with the rear. After years of using one part of the body more than another, imbalances occur. This can result in poor posture, unfit appearance, or injury and pain in a bone or joint.

Stretching and flexibility are important to your patient's exercise routine to maintain good posture and overall balance. Using the car as a metaphor helps children understand the value of good posture and a balanced body. Individuals cannot drive a car that has a flat tire—it is unbalanced. In the same regard, children cannot achieve a healthy lifestyle if they do not have a balanced body. When children are born, their body was a perfectly designed machine—just like a brand new car. It was symmetrical, meaning that the left side was identical to the right, and the front was in balance with the rear. But after years of using one part of the body more than the other parts, the body can get out of balance. Although, children do not have flat tires to show us that they are out of balance, they do have poor posture, or worse, an injury or pain in their bones and joints.

Talking Points: Importance of Balance (Verbal cues for patients or parents and family members)
Read through the following information with your patient or family members to help them to understand the exercise strategy used in the program.

If you overtrain or neglect to stretch your chest muscles or undertrain your back area, you could walk around looking like a gorilla (instructor demonstrates). Moreover, your back could begin to hunch over and you will start to look like a very old outer space alien (instructor demonstrates).
But if your chest is flexible and your back is strong, you will appear taller, thinner, and stronger. This is why you have been doing stretch-and-flex exercises since the first week of the program. Do these exercises whenever and wherever you can. It is easy to do them while you are watching television, playing outside, or relaxing in your room after you warm up for 3–5 minutes.

The Flex Test is a way to check to see whether your patient has any of these imbalances. Flex exercises can help correct those imbalances and prevent others from occurring. Guide the patient and his or her parent through the following Flex Test series. Then continue with the information that follows.

The Flex Test

Examine the figures below and answer the question beneath each. If your answer is "yes," note which side (left or right) is particularly problematic.

Do you look like this?

Then try this:
Chest stretch

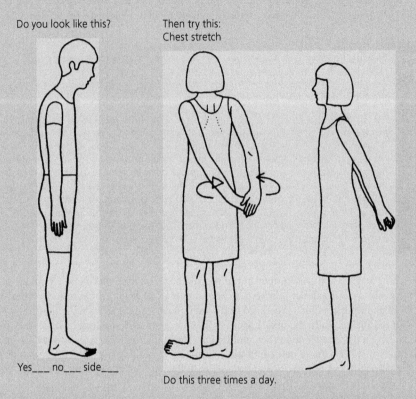

Yes___ no___ side___

Do this three times a day.

Then try this:
Rowing, low

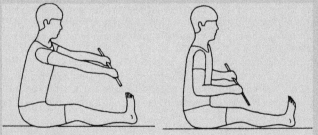

Do 8–12 repetitions two to three times per week.

Do you look like this?

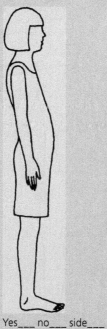

Yes___ no___ side___

Then try this:

Stomach crunch and pelvic tilt

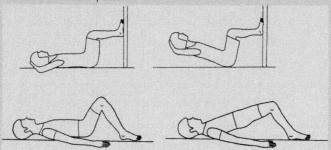

Do 8–20 repetitions two to three times per week.

Do you look like this?

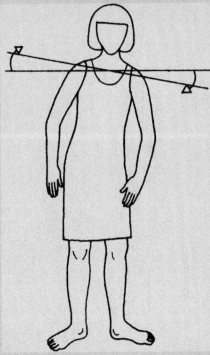

Yes___ no___ side___

Then try this:
Shoulder stretch

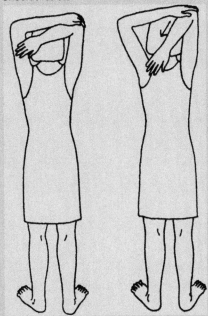

Do this three times a day.

And try this:

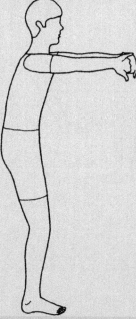

Do this three times a day.

Do you look like this?

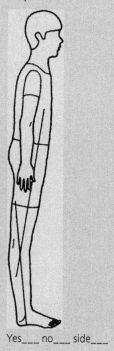

Yes___ no___ side___

Then try this:

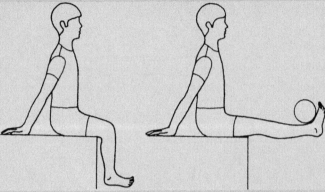

Leg extension, sitting and leg curl, standing

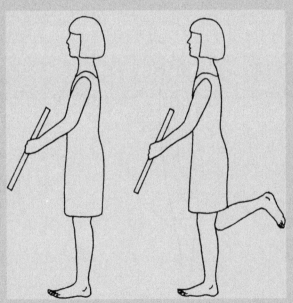

Do these three times per week.

And try this:

Lying quad stretch

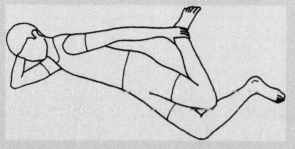

Do this three times a day.

Important: Keep knees "soft" or slightly bent when standing (do not lock or hyperextend the knees). This automatically takes stress off the knee joints and the lower back.

Do you look like this?

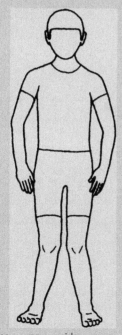

Yes___ no___ side___
or

Do you look like this?

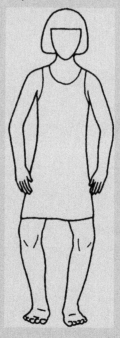

Yes___ no___ side___
or

Do you look like this?

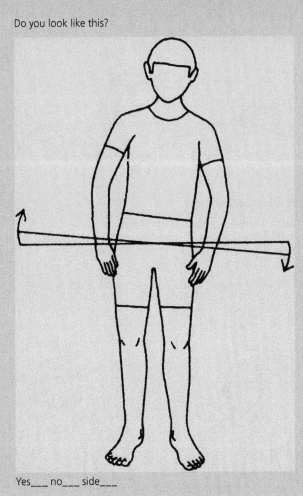

Yes___ no___ side___

Then see your pediatrician or family physician. He or she will likely refer you to an orthopedic specialist.

REFERENCES

American College of Sports Medicine. (2010). *ACSM's Guidelines for Exercise Testing and Prescription* (8th ed.). Philadelphia, PA: Lippincott Williams & Wilkins.

American College of Sports Medicine. (2011). Position stand: Quantity and quality of exercise for developing and maintaining cardiorespiratory, musculoskeletal, and neuromotor fitness in apparently healthy adults: Guidance for prescribing exercise. *Medicine and Science in Sports and Exercise*, 43(7), 1334–1359.

Azevedo, D., Melo, R., Correa, R., Chalmers, G. (2010). Uninvolved versus target muscle contraction during contract-relax proprioceptive neuromuscular facilitation stretching. *Physical Therapy in Sport*, 12(3), 117–121.

Fasen, J., O'Connor, A., Schwartz, S., Watson, J., Plastaras, C., Garvan, C., et al. (2009). A randomized controlled trial of hamstring stretching: Comparison of four techniques. *Journal of Strength and Conditioning Research*, 23(2), 660–667.

Ganley, K., Paterno, M., Miles, C., Stout, J., Brawner, P., Girolami, G., Warran, M. (2011). Health-related fitness in children and adolescents. *Pediatric Physical Therapy*, 23(3), 208–220.

Gilette, T., Holland, G. (1991). Relationship of body core temperature and warm-up to hamstring range of motion. *Journal of Orthopaedic and Sports Physical Therapy*, 13(3), 126–131.

Hammer, W. I. (1999). Muscle imbalance and post-fascilitation stretch. In W. I. Hammer (Ed.), *Functional Soft Tissue Examination and Treatment by Manual Methods* (pp. 415–446). Gaithersburg, MD: Aspen Publishers.

Liebenson, C. (1996). Integrating rehabilitation into chiropractic practice (blending active and passive care). In C. Liebenson (Ed.), *Rehabilitation of the Spine* (pp. 13–44). Baltimore, MD: Williams & Wilkins.

Irving, D., Cook, J., Young, M., Menz, H. (2007). Obesity and pronated foot type may increase the risk of chronic plantar heel pain: a matched case-control study. *BMC Musculoskeletal Disorders*, 8, 41.

Jacobson, M. S. (2006). Medical complications and comorbidities of pediatric obesity. In M. S. Sothern, T. K. von Almen, S. T. Gordon (Eds.), *Handbook of Pediatric Obesity: Clinical Management* (pp. 31–39). Boca Raton, FL: Taylor & Francis.

Janda, V. (1993). Muscle strength in relation to muscle length, pain and muscle imbalance. In K. Harms-Rindahl (Ed.), *Muscle Strength* (pp. 89–91). New York, NY: Churchill Livingstone.

Jenkins, J., Beazell, J. (2010). Flexibility for runners. *Clinical Journal of Sports Medicine*, 29(3), 365–377.

Kaufman, K., Brodine, S., Shaffer, R., Johnson, C. Cullison, T. (1999). The effect of foot structure and range of motion on musculoskeletal overuse injuries. *American Journal of Sports Medicine*, 27, 585–593.

Krebs, N. F., Baker, R. D., Greer, F. R., Heyman, M. B., Jaksic, T., Lifshitz, F. et al.; American Academy of Pediatrics Committee on Nutrition. (2003). Prevention of pediatric overweight and obesity. *Pediatrics*, 112(2), 424–430.

Marangoni, A. (2010). Effects of intermittent stretching exercises at work on musculoskeletal pain associated with the use of a personal computer and the influence of media on outcomes. *Work*, 36(1), 27–37.

Meroni, R., Cerri, C., Lanzarini, C., Barindelli, G., Della Morte, G., Gessaga, V., Cesana, G., De Vito, G. (2010). Comparison of active stretching technique and static stretching technique on hamstring flexibility. *Clinical Journal of Sports Medicine*, 20(1), 8–14.

Moen, M., Tol, J., Weir A., Steunebrink, M., De Winter, T. (2009). Medial tibial stress syndrome: A critical review. *Sports Medicine*, 39, 523–546.

Peeler, J., Anderson, J. E. (2007). Effectiveness of static quadriceps stretching in individuals with patellofemoral joint pain. *Clinical Journal of Sport Medicine*, 17(4), 234–241.

Puentedura, E., Huijbregts, P., Celeste, S., Edwards, D., In, A., Landers, M., Fernandez-de-las-Penas, C. (2011). Immediate effects of quantified hamstring stretching: Hold-relax proprioceptive neuromuscular facilitation versus static stretching. *Physical Therapy in Sport*, 12(3), 122–126.

Sainz de Baranda, P., Ayala, F. (2010). Chronic flexibility improvement after 12 week of stretching program utilizing the ACSM recommendations: hamstring flexibility. *International Journal of Sports Medicine*, 31(6), 389–396.

Santonja Medina, F., Saniz de Baranda Andujar, P., Rodriguez Garcia, P., Lopez Minarro, P., Canteras Jordana, M. (2007). Effects of frequency of static stretching on straight-leg raise in elementary school children. *Journal of Sports Medicine and Physical Fitness*, 47(3), 304–308.

Schultz, S. P., Browning, R. C., Schutz, Y., Maffeis, C., Hills, A. P. (2011). Childhood obesity and walking: Guidelines and challenges. *International Journal of Pediatric Obesity*, 6(5–6), 332–341.

Sothern, M., von Almen, T. K., Schumacher, H. (2001). *Trim Kids: The Proven Plan That Has Helped Thousands of Children Achieve a Healthier Weight*. New York, NY: HarperCollins.

Sothern, M. S., von Almen, T. K., Gordon, S. T. (Eds.). (2006). *Handbook of Pediatric Obesity: Clinical Management*. Boca Raton, FL: Taylor & Francis.

Thompson, W., Bushman, B., Desch, J., Kravitz, L. (2010). *ACSM's Resources for the Personal Trainer* (3rd ed.). Philadelphia, PA: Lippincott Williams & Wilkins.

Wenos, D., Konin, J. (2004). Controlled warm-up intensity enhances hip range of motion. *Journal of Strength and Conditioning Research*, 18(3), 529–533.

Chapter 5

MOTIVATING OVERWEIGHT CHILDREN TO INCREASE PHYSICAL ACTIVITY

More than 11% of United States children ages 6–17 years old are physically inactive (Singh et al., 2008). Inactivity is significantly higher and physical activity is significantly lower among females (Pratt et al., 2008; Seabra et al., 2012), ethnic minority groups, children from non-English-speaking households and socioeconomically disadvantaged backgrounds, and overweight and obese children (Salvy et al., 2012). These children also have lower perceived physical competence, have less parental support for physical activity, and are less attracted to physical activity (Seabra et al., 2012). Research indicates that, in particular, overweight and obese children and adolescents are less physically active, perceive physical activity more negatively, and find sedentary activity more reinforcing than physical activity when compared with normal weight youth (Salvy et al., 2012; Sothern et al., 2006).

Education studies indicate that physical fitness improves students' self-image and promotes a positive school environment. Children's feelings of self-worth and self-esteem begin developing in the early elementary years (O'Brien, 1989). Some types of exercise training may improve self-esteem in prepubescent youth (Metcalf & Roberts, 1993). Furthermore, regular physical training may promote the attainment of self-esteem during the elementary years, which may transfer to improved self-worth in the later, more difficult, pubertal and postpubertal years (Haugen, Ommundsen, & Seiler, 2013). Exercise programs must be goal oriented with easily attainable outcomes to ensure individual student success (Sothern et al., 2006). Exercise techniques must be appropriate to the physical development level of the student (Sothern, 2001; Sothern et al., 2001; Sothern et al., 2006; Strong et al., 2005; U.S. Department of Health and Human Services [U.S. DHHS], 2008). Childhood is a critical time when children's physical activity behaviors are formed and during which they develop healthy attitudes toward physical activity. Physicians and health care professionals can help their overweight and obese pediatric patients adopt a healthier and more physically active lifestyle in several ways (Deforche, Haerens, & de Bourdeauhuij, 2011; McInnis, Franklin, & Rippe, 2003). A thorough understanding of the determinants of exercise initiation and adherence is essential to selecting the best methods to promote physical activity in overweight and obese children and adolescents.

DETERMINANTS TO PHYSICAL ACTIVITY

Many factors are described as determinants to increased physical activity and adherence to exercise programs. Environmental factors, such as a perceived lack of time, have been proposed as primary deterrents to physical activity. Although individuals report a lack of available time for physical activity, other complex issues affect this perception. Poor behavioral skills, that is, limit setting and time management, may contribute more to the lack of opportunity for physical activity, or the individual may lack adequate motivation to be physically active. Lack of time then becomes a perceived determinant as opposed to an environmental one (Chalip et al., 1984; Dishman, 1994; Sonstroem, 1998). Measuring self variables, such as perceived competence, self-efficacy, and self-esteem, may describe the psychological benefits associated with physical activity (Godin & Shephard, 1985; Sonstroem, 1998); however, these do not predict behavior unless incentives are present or past history is considered (Dishman, 1994). Stralen and colleagues (2011) reviewed the literature to identify psychosocial and environmental mediators of energy balance-related behaviors for youth and concluded that self-efficacy and intention are relevant mediators to target in physical activity interventions.

The mother's perception of barriers to exercise and her report of family social support are important predictors as well (Holm et al., 2012). Stucky-Ropp and DiLorenzo (1993) concluded that children are influenced by important socialized family variables. Furthermore, families serve as important learning environments for enhancing health-related behaviors, including physical activity in children. More recently, Holm and colleagues (2012) evaluated the influence of parental participation on change in physical activity in 83 families enrolled in a family-based child weight gain–prevention program. Both maternal and paternal change in physical activity strongly predicted change in physical activity in their children. Week-end activity, in particular, was positively affected. These and other studies confirm that targeting families rather than individuals may provide a more beneficial effect in increasing physical activity. This certainly has been shown to be effective in multidisciplinary weight management research studies (Hassink & Kessler, 2010). More important, encouraging parents to increase physical activity, especially on weekends, represents a highly effective method to engage parental involvement in interventions to promote increased physical activity (Holm et al., 2012; Sothern et al., 2001).

Duncan, Duncan, and Strycker (2005) observed similar findings of social support for youth ages 10–14 years. A positive correlation was observed between physical activity and youth, and parent, sibling, and friend support. In particular, children in this age-group who perceived a greater level of support from friends had the higher levels of physical activity. Another positive correlation was observed between parents, siblings, and friends watching a game and the youth's level of physical activity (Duncan et al., 2005). Recently Knowlden and Sharma (2012) concluded that any effort to prevent childhood obesity should include interventions to increase physical activity where the parents are targeted as the primary agents of change.

Taylor and colleagues (1999) examined the relationship between specific components of physical activity during childhood and adolescence and exercise habits in adulthood. An interesting finding was the inverse relationship between adult physical activity and those who were forced to exercise as preteens and during teen years. Also, an inverse correlation was identified between adult physical activity and those who were encouraged to exercise during preteen years. These results indicate that being forced and encouraged during childhood may facilitate negative attitudes toward physical activity and may extend into adulthood (Taylor et al., 1999).

Child enjoyment of physical activity is the most prominent predictor of exercise behavior (Hassink & Kessler, 2010; Milteer et al., 2011; Sothern, 2006; Sothern et al., 2006; Stucky-Ropp & DiLorenzo, 1993; U.S. DHHS, 2008). Young children are distracted easily and are incapable of focused activity for long periods of time. This contributes to the sporadic nature of their physical activity (Borra et al., 1995; Sothern et al., 2006). Adults can engage in long-duration exercise easily because of their enhanced ability to concentrate. Although most individuals engage in activity because they enjoy the effort, children need activity to be fun for them to continue. Adults are more able to engage in challenging activities that may be slightly painful to reach performance or aesthetic goals. Young children, on the other hand, are not concerned with appearance and are not overly concerned with winning or competition (Borra et al., 1995; French et al., 1994; Moore et al., 1995).

The idea of learned helplessness has been suggested as a probable reason for lack of motivation to participate in healthy behaviors (Hunter et al., 1990). Learned helpless children justify the causes of bad events in their lives as stable in time, global in effect, and internal to themselves. Such children develop a cluster of helplessness deficiencies, such as passivity or nonassertiveness, unaware or unable to see alternatives, sadness, lowered self-esteem, lowered achievement-oriented behaviors, and lacking in initiative and persistence (Nolen-Hoeksema, Girgus, & Seligman, 1986). Both children and adults avoid situations they believe exceed their capabilities and make them feel helpless. They, however, undertake and do develop self-confidence behaviors that they believe they can implement and from which they will derive benefit. Given appropriate skills and incentives, personal efficacy beliefs are some major determinants of children's choice of behaviors. Personal efficacy beliefs can help determine how much effort they will expend, and how long they will sustain effort in dealing with uncomfortable or new situations (Bandura, 1986).

Social influences on youth sport and physical activity remains an understudied area of research. In recent years, however, interest has been growing in the roles that peers and friends play, both in positive and negative ways, to youth physical activity. Recent findings indicate that overweight and obese youth are alone more often, have fewer friendships, and are less likely to have reciprocated or mutual friendships when compared with nonoverweight youth (Salvy et al., 2012). Companionship provided by friends is associated with positive affect during physical activity, a characteristic defined as social facilitation. Unexpectedly, in both overweight and nonoverweight youth, exercise intensity is greater when performed with one or more individuals. It also is suggested that overweight and obese children and adolescents may be motivated to increase physical activity in the presence of other youth to create a favorable impression or in an effort to combat the negative stigma attached to their increased weight status. But, unfortunately, overweight and obese youth often are teased by their peers because of their physical appearances. Likewise, they often are subjected to peer rejection, ostracism, and physical and verbal victimization, which lessen their engagement in physical activity pursuits (Losekam et al., 2010). Regrettably, only peer experiences that are characterized by positive interactions, mutual affection, cooperation, and respect increase the probability of engaging in physical activity through social facilitation. And, it only takes one single episode of ostracism to negatively influence feelings of belonging, self-esteem, cognitions, and mood in overweight and obese youth (Salvy et al., 2012).

Talking Points: Support From Family and Friends (Verbal cues for patients or parents and family members)
Read through the following information with your patient or family members to help them to understand the exercise strategy used in the program.

Previously your child may have shied away from doing any exercise at all, fearing discrimination from lean peers who could accomplish the same activities with relative ease. It is important to find peers that your child feels comfortable with—preferably other active kids who want to stay healthy or maybe lose weight, and who will participate in team sports or other activities at the same pace as your child. Seek out other children in your child's social circles at school, church, scouting, and other clubs or associations. Arrange regular meetings at the park or in someone's backyard where the kids can play and practice the sports and activities they like.

Of greater concern is research indicating that weight criticism during physical activity and manifestations of victimization are predictive of a reduction in perceived ability relative to peers and a decline in overall physical activity (Salvy et al., 2012). Therefore, a vicious cycle is established, for example, increased peer adversity during physical activity pursuits leads to social isolation, which in turn decreases physical activity and increases sedentary behavior. Thus, to achieve meaningful results to physical activity participation, it is necessary to promote the modification of the overweight and obese child's existing social and peer networks and include methods that involve fostering the creation of new positive social networks and experiences (Sothern et al., 2001, 2006).

Case in Point: Real Words from Real Patients and Their Families
Read through the following information with your patient or family members to help them to understand the exercise strategy used in the program.

Austin had always wanted to play football, but, because of his weight, he was never picked at recess games and lacked the confidence to try out for the playground teams—so, he eventually quit trying. After 1 month on the program, however, Austin lost 8 pounds and became more confident about his physical skills. He and his father began passing the football each evening, and the whole family participated in weekend football games. Austin knew his skills were improving, and soon enough, he mustered the confidence to try out for his neighborhood park team. Next thing he knew, Austin was playing tackle for the team, and was being chosen regularly for pick-up games during school recess.

When designing exercise programs for obese children, the instructor should consider activities that are mastered easily. Such activities will ensure that students experience initial success when participating in physical activity if adherence to the program is desired (Sothern, 2001; Sothern et al., 2006).

MOTIVATIONAL THEORIES AND MODELS FOR ENCOURAGING POSITIVE BEHAVIOR CHANGE

Modern strategies for chronic disease prevention and management include a variety of social learning theories and health promotion models (Sothern, 2006; Sothern et al., 2006; Sung-Chan et al., 2012). Many of these theories and models are based on the results of behavioral research. Because diseases related to poor lifestyle choices can be altered by changes in individual behavior patterns, the physician or health care professional should possess a thorough knowledge of these behavioral theories and models (Blair, 1993; Sothern, 2006; Sothern & Gordon, 2005). Over the past few decades, the utilization of behavioral theories has increased in the scientific research literature relating to pediatric weight management (Knowlden & Sharma, 2012). Several theories have been applied; however, the two most widely employed are the theory of planned behavior (Ajzen, 1991; Crawley & Koballa, 1994) and the social cognitive theory (Bandura; 2004; Knowlden & Sharma, 2012; Nixon et al., 2012).

THE THEORY OF PLANNED BEHAVIOR
The theory of planned behavior attempts to clarify many of the issues that surround negative behavior patterns (Ajzen, 1991; Crawley & Koballa, 1994). Because previous research in human behavior patterns failed to provide good predictors for behavior change, this theory was developed to account for many of the variables associated with alterations in behavior. These variables include individual attitude and disposition and specific personality traits (Ajzen, 1991). The theory of planned behavior, using central concepts from the behavioral sciences, provides a framework that allows the understanding and prediction of individual behavior patterns in specific situations and across a wide variety of personality types. This framework moderates the relationship of intention to behavior from perceived behavioral control. For instance, if perceived behavioral control is high, then the intention will convert to behavior. In contrast, if the perceived behavioral control is low, then it is not likely that the intention will convert to behavior (Baranowski et al., 2003).

Mummery, Spence, and Hudec (2000) examined the theory of planned behavior in predicted physical activity in a nationwide sample of Canadian school youth in grades 3, 5, 8, and 11. Measures of the theory of planned behavior included physical activity intention, attitude, subjective norm, and perceived behavioral control. The direct measures of the theory of planned behavior explained 47% of the variability in predicting physical activity intention. In particular, perceived behavioral control made the largest contribution to predicting physical activity intention. Conversely, Trost, Saunders, and Ward (2002) observed that the theory of planned behavior could not account for a substantial portion of the variance in intentions or moderate to vigorous physical activity in sixth-grade youth. Further research is needed with the theory of planned behavior within the context of diet, physical activity, and obesity in children (Baranowski et al., 2003).

TRANSTHEORETICAL MODEL OF BEHAVIOR CHANGE
Although exercise is shown to improve weight status and overall health, it is unknown which individuals are most ready to adhere to an exercise program or to achieve the greatest results from a given program. Few tools have been developed to quickly measure a patient's readiness to participate in an exercise program. It is possible, however, to evaluate a participant's readiness for change using a scale based on the transtheoretical model of behavior change

as developed by Prochaska and DiClemente (1983). This model proposes that individuals must progress through a series of stages of change and engage in specific change processes to achieve behavior change. Within this theory is the concept of stage distribution, which proposes that within any given population, individuals are in various stages related to behavior change. It is believed that clinicians promoting or prescribing behavior change must prescribe therapies based on each individual's stage of change. Use of the transtheoretical model or its clinical modality, motivational interviewing, has been shown to be successful in many settings (Zimmerman et al., 2000).

Talking Points: Social Learning Theories—The Backbone of Behavior Change
(Verbal cues for patients or parents and family members)
Read through the following information with your patient or family members to help them to understand the exercise strategy used in the program.

Social learning theories state that children who can grasp the concepts behind specific behavioral changes and who are physically able to make these changes will do so willingly if they believe they will benefit from the new behaviors. This is why parents must provide positive reinforcement, rewards, and incentives to children who alter negative behaviors and engage in new healthy ones. Additionally, kids will participate in new behavior if they believe they can do it. This is why it is also important to establish easy-to-attain goals—ones kids absolutely will reach. Also, when kids learn to listen to their bodies (e.g., to slow down if they are exercising too hard, speed up if the exercise is not challenging enough), they acquire a new mastery or understanding of their body as well as of how to carry out a healthier lifestyle. These elements, coupled with your positive role modeling, add up to the strongest probability that your child will indeed participate and be successful.

SELF-DETERMINATION THEORY

The scientific literature supports the use of self-determination theory for a variety of life contexts, including education, sport, exercise, and physical education (Rosenkranz et al., 2012). The self-determination theory proposes a similar concept; social-contextual factors (i.e., motivational strategies used by teachers) can influence an individuals' motivation and subsequent behavior by satisfying three basic needs: (1) autonomy, which is the need to experience one's behavior as self-endorsed; (2) competence, which is the need to effectively interact with one's environment and achieve positive outcomes; and (3) relatedness, which is the need to feel supported and connected with others. Strategies based on the self-determination theory model have been shown to satisfy these psychological needs in the physical activity context and are essential to well-being, learning, and the development of autonomous forms of motivation. Self-determination theory has been implemented successfully in programs to promote physical activity in adolescents and adult women (Silva et al., 2010).

SOCIAL COGNITIVE THEORY

Social cognitive theory identifies a core set of determinants, the mechanisms through which they work, and optimal ways of translating this knowledge into effective health practices (Bandura, 1986, 2004). Social cognitive theory recognizes that human behavior is influenced by the dynamic interaction, referred to as reciprocal determinism, between an individual and their environment (Glanz, Rimer, & Viswanath, 2008). This theory acknowledges that behavior is learned through mechanisms of modeling coupled with an individual's self-regulation toward adopting and maintaining behaviors (Bandura, 2004). Ultimately, social cognitive theory postulates that human motivation and action are driven extensively by forethought (Conner & Norman, 2005). This theory suggests that behavior change and maintenance of behavior are a function of one's expectations of their ability to perform the behavior (self-efficacy) and the expectation of the outcome resulting from performing that behavior (outcome expectations) (Bandura, 2004; Glanz et al., 2008; Keller et al., 1999). Sometimes referred to as "mastery," the attainment of the belief that an individual has the ability to perform the desired behavior can be increased through the implementation of specific strategies that endure initial success (Sothern et al., 1999; Sothern et al., 2001; Sothern et al., 2006).

Key Points: Promoting Physical Activity in Overweight Youth Using Social Cognitive Theory

- Mastery Experiences: Set short-term, achievable physical activity goals and provide activity rewards for those achieved.
- Physiologic Feedback: Teach pacing techniques, such as breathing and heart rate monitoring; reevaluate the child's condition every 3–6 months.
- Role Modeling: Parents do not have to be thin, but they must set a good example by participating in physical activities and reducing screen time.
- Knowledge Transfer: Enroll children in structured dance, sport, or movement classes. Make sure the teachers are qualified and understand limitations

Sources: Adapted from Sothern et al., 1999; Sothern et al., 2001, 2006.

Talking Points: Suggestions for Increasing Mastery (Verbal cues for patients or parents and family members)
Read through the following information with your patient or family members to help them to understand the exercise strategy used in the program.

- Expose children to varied activities in a nonintimidating and nurturing environment.
- Encourage participation in aerobic activities appropriate for age and size.
- Realize that young children have immature metabolic systems. Do not impose adult exercise goals.

Source: From Sothern et al., 2001.

According to social cognitive theory, children are motivated to behave a certain way if they believe that the targeted behavior will benefit them and if they believe they can perform the intended behavior. Self-efficacy beliefs influence goals and shape the outcomes individuals expect their efforts to produce. An individual with high self-efficacy usually expects to see favorable results, whereas those with low self-efficacy tend to expect poor outcomes. In addition, those with low self-efficacy tend to give up easily, whereas those with high self-efficacy tend to overcome difficulties that they may encounter. Chronic disease treatment intervention programs for youth may be enhanced through the application of the training concepts of social cognitive theory. Goal setting is a proven strategy to encourage successful behavior change and improved self-efficacy.

Handouts for Patients and Parents

Class 1 _____ (date)
Goal-Setting and Action Planning

My goal for this week is to:

_____

1. Does it say exactly what I plan to *do*?
2. Do I have control over it?
3. Can I tell when I've done it?
4. Does it say what I *will* do instead of what I *won't* do?
5. Is it easy to do?

Source: From Sothern et al., 2001.

Talking Points: Suggestions for Providing Physiologic Feedback (Verbal cues for patients or parents and family members)
Read through the following information with your patient or family members to help them to understand the exercise strategy used in the program.

- Encourage children to self-monitor physical activity and provide activity rewards for goals achieved.
- Do not draw attention to unhealthy activities with negative comments. Instead, praise children when they choose active play instead of television.
- Teach children that all movement is physical activity and will burn calories.

Source: From Sothern et al., 2001.

Bandura (2004) suggested that before individuals alter their current lifestyle to that of a healthy one, they must have the knowledge of health risks associated with their present condition. Because individuals self-evaluate their behavior, they abstain from behaviors that breed self-dissatisfaction. A challenge facing physicians and health care professionals is helping individuals believe they possess the ability to, in fact, adapt a healthier lifestyle and help strengthen their belief in themselves that they do have the power and ability to make these changes.

 Talking Points: Suggestions for Encouraging Knowledge Transfer (Verbal cues for patients or parents and family members)
Read through the following information with your patient or family members to help them to understand the exercise strategy used in the program.

Genetics loads the gun, but environment pulls the trigger. Even if your child is genetically designed to be overweight, his or her environment and behaviors can be adjusted to combat this predisposition. Your child may become chubby even with adjustments. He or she does not have to be doomed to a life of ill health.

Source: From Sothern et al., 2001.

Although individuals may know the health risks associated with negative behaviors, it is self-efficacy that governs whether or not they will translate that knowledge into a more healthful behavior. For instance, those with low self-efficacy, although aware of the health risks, still will not take action, whereas those with high levels of self-efficacy will combine their beliefs with positive outcome expectations. Stated simply, individuals with high levels of self-efficacy believe that the benefits of adapting a healthy lifestyle will outweigh the disadvantages of the lifestyle change. Sonstroem (1998) suggested that no matter what model is utilized to analyze physical activity behaviors, it is vital that it is used repeatedly over time and as a complete and whole intervention.

 Talking Points: Suggestions for Encouraging Positive Parental Role Modeling (Verbal cues for patients or parents and family members)
Read through the following information with your patient or family members to help them to understand the exercise strategy used in the program.

- Families that play together, stay healthy together.
  - Reserve at least half a day of each weekend for family physical fitness.
- Alternate a game of family flag football outdoors with games on television. Play the first and third quarters and watch the second and fourth.
- Create an environment for active play both inside and outside the home.

Source: From Sothern et al., 2001.

Two systematic reviews, Belanger-Gravel et al. (2010) and Nixon et al. (2012), found social cognitive theory to be the most commonly used model for interventions, which reported significant favorable changes in one or more physical outcome measures. In addition, Tierney et al. (2011) recommended interventions that target self-efficacy, consider anticipated outcomes, and provide reinforcement to increase motivation. In addition, individuals should draw support from those around them, including peers, relatives, and health care professionals to overcome difficulties associated with participation in physical activity.

MOTIVATIONAL INTERVIEWING

Motivational interviewing is a patient-centered, directive approach to counseling for behavior change that emphasizes individual autonomy. Motivational interviewing strives to help patients move toward behavior change by assisting them in the process of identifying, articulating, and strengthening personally relevant reasons for change and by addressing ambivalence about the change (DiLillo & West, 2011). Motivational interviewing does not provide advice and information in a prescriptive manner, but rather seeks to promote behavior change using an empathic, interactive style that supports self-determination, enhanced self-efficacy and underscores individual control. Characteristics of motivational interviewing include (1) the collaboration between the provider and patient; (2) the elicitation and reinforcement of change talk, which involves framing the targeting lifestyle behavior changes into the context of broader life goals; and (3) patient's personal values. Motivational interviewing may be an effective approach for the prevention and treatment of pediatric obesity by targeting changes in diet, physical activity and other behaviors contributing to childhood obesity (DiLillo & West, 2011). Numerous randomized trials have demonstrated the efficacy of motivational interviewing for addictive behaviors. There are only a limited number of studies, especially among pediatric populations, of motivational interviewing for weight control, and findings on the effectiveness are inconsistent (DiLillo & West, 2011; Resnicow, Davis, & Rollnick, 2006). Resnicow et al. (2006) identified only two studies in which motivational interviewing was used to intervene on pediatric obesity: (1) the Healthy Lifestyles Pilot Study and (2) the Go Girls study. Future research in the behavioral weight management application of motivational interviewing is needed to determine the feasibility and effectiveness of incorporating this strategy into weight-loss settings. Studies should determine the type and extent of provider training necessary to ensure adequate skill development and the cost-effectiveness of motivational interviewing (DiLillo & West, 2011). Despite inconsistent results, evidence from the implementation of motivational interviewing in interventions that address other health problems supports the concept that this strategy, when delivered in conjunction with behavioral counseling, may enhance weight loss and likely will increase adherence to behavioral recommendations (DiLillo & West, 2011; Resnicow et al., 2006). Additionally, motivational interviewing may be helpful in promoting weight maintenance after an initial loss has been achieved (DiLillo & West, 2011).

MOTIVATIONAL TECHNIQUES AND STRATEGIES TO INCREASE PHYSICAL ACTIVITY IN OVERWEIGHT YOUTH

INITIAL EVALUATION

Before prescribing any type of physical activity program, physicians and health care professionals should evaluate their patient's level of self-efficacy (Sothern et al., 2006). Those individuals with a high level of self-efficacy need minimal guidance and can succeed in changing their behavior in most situations. Those with limited self-efficacy beliefs, however, require more intense, tailored personal guidance and structure. Positive reinforcement and repeated successful experiences will build belief in an individual's ability and help with any difficulties or setbacks they may encounter during the intervention (Sothern, 2006; Sothern et al., 1999).

In addition to evaluating a patient's level of self-efficacy, the individual's readiness to begin a physical activity program should be assessed. Health care professionals should consider whether the patient actually desires help or if he or she recognizes the need for weight loss. The patient's motivation and stress levels should be assessed and discussed along with the subject's relationship with food since because this may warrant the inclusion of other forms of counseling as well. At this point, the health care professional and patient should develop achievable goals together (Kushner & Weinsier, 2000).

To achieve greater physical activity compliance, the physician or health care professional should take the time to understand and discuss any social or physical barriers the patient might encounter associated with them being physically active. These can include an overweight or obese parent, feeling uncomfortable exercising in public or thinking that certain exercises have to be painful or extremely vigorous to be beneficial (Albright et al., 2000). In promoting physical activity with their patients, the physician or health care professional should help establish realistic expectations and correct overly pessimistic or optimistic attitudes (Sothern, 2006; Sothern et al., 2006). Both long- and short-term goals should be established as well as routine times and places for physical activity. The physician or health care professional should relay the benefits of social support and prepare patients for situations that may present challenges to exercising (i.e., holidays). The patient should develop some sort of contract with the health professional and practice self-reinforcement with rewards (Gordon et al., 2000). In addition to a physical activity program, daily lifestyle activities should be emphasized as a way to increase overall physical activity levels and energy expenditure (Gordon et al., 2000; Jakicic et al., 1995).

Talking Points: Guidelines for Parents to Promote Positive Behavior Change (Verbal cues for parents)
Read through the following information with your patient or family members to help them to understand the exercise strategy used in the program.

Anchoring behavioral changes into everyday life takes practice. Research shows that by following these guidelines, your child's behavior will change over time.

Provide positive reinforcement. Kids will do anything for attention, and the type you give (positive or negative) is thought to drive and maintain the child's behavior. So, for example, if you give attention for positive actions, chances are your child will repeat that behavior in the future. Likewise, if you respond to unhealthy action, chances are your child will repeat that behavior in the future. It is essential to focus on positive behaviors that reinforce weight-loss goals while ignoring, redirecting, or consciously problem solving negative behaviors.

Ultimately, the best way to train yourself to develop and maintain new habits (i.e., catching your child at being good and commenting on it) is to practice. When you slip up, take a deep breath, regroup, and direct your attention to the healthy changes your child has been making. Recommit to the program as many times as it takes.

Be a strong and consistent role model. Children—especially young children— emulate behavior of the significant role models in their lives. As such, children look primarily to their parents as role models for their behavior. Studies show that groups in which both parents and children participated in weight-loss programs had significantly better long-term maintenance of weight loss than those groups made up of children only. The parent–child weight-loss groups also reported more satisfaction with the program than the others.

Research indicates that children have an intrinsic natural need to be physically active. Young animals, including humans, are inherently active (French et al., 1994). Therefore, children will be active if given encouragement and opportunity. Childhood activity often is intermittent and sporadic in behavior (Bailey et al., 1995). Thus, children likely will not do prolonged exercise without rest periods. Physical activity patterns vary with children of different developmental and ability levels. Young children may not be attracted to high-intensity sports performance activities; older children may be (Borra et al., 1995). The amount of total daily activity (volume) is a good indicator of childhood activity. If given the opportunity, young children will perform relatively large volumes of intermittent physical activity (Bailey et al., 1995; French et al., 1994).

THE USE OF MUSIC AS A MOTIVATIONAL TOOL

Priest, Karageorghis, and Sharp (2004) investigated the presence of music as a motivational tool for exercise. It was found that motivational qualities of music are heightened when the music is delivered at a higher volume and that females reported the importance of music more highly than males. Additionally, the participants reported that the music facilitated their performance on cardiovascular equipment more so than on any other equipment. The researchers also found an effect of music compared with age. Although older adults (36–45 years) preferred noncurrent music, the youngest age group (16–26 years) preferred current music and dance music (Priest et al., 2004).

Key Points: Music Is a Motivational Tool for Physical Activity

- The motivational qualities of music are heightened when the music is delivered at a higher volume.
- Females reported the importance of music more highly than males.
- Music facilitates performance on cardiovascular equipment more so than on any other equipment.
- There is an effect of music compared to age:
  - Older adults (36–45 years) preferred noncurrent music.
  - Younger age-groups (16–26) preferred current music and dance music.

Source: (Priest, Karageorghis, & Sharp, 2004)

TEAM (GROUP) VERSUS INDIVIDUAL PHYSICAL ACTIVITY

Researchers suggest that a task-oriented approach to physical activity and sport will promote higher levels of moral reasoning in children (Kylo & Landers, 1995). With this approach, outcome goals such as winning or scoring are replaced with individual self-referenced criteria and mastery of specific skills. Individual goal-based sports may be better for overweight children than competitive team sports, especially during the initial stages of a weight management program (Sothern, 2006; Sothern et al., 2006). Research supports individual goal setting in sport and exercise as a reliable motivational technique, which improves exercise and sport performance (Kylo & Landers, 1995; Lerner & Locke, 1995). When engaging in individual goal-based activities, the child sets a personal goal for himself rather than one that depends on competing with another individual or team. For example, swimmers usually aim to exceed their personal best in any given event—meaning scoring better than their best score in previous attempts. Educators and health care professionals should focus the student's attention toward achieving personal goals as opposed to team competitive goals. Activities that offer children an opportunity to set individual goals include gymnastics, track and field, archery, golf, judo, karate, dance, tai bo, synchronized swimming (solo and duet), springboard diving, and ice skating. Ensure that the coach and teacher are aware of your child's special needs before signing him up (Sothern et al., 2001).

Talking Points: All Physical Activity Burns Calories (Verbal cues for patients or parents and family members)
Read through the following information with your patient or family members to help them to understand the exercise strategy used in the program.

Your child also burns calories in activities in which he doesn't break a sweat or become fatigued. Give him the opportunity to participate in less-challenging things he can do for hours at a time. Weekends are an especially good time for the entire family to play together. Try: golf, badminton, croquet, throwing passes, Frisbee, basketball free throw games (such as H-O-R-S-E), body toning classes, beach volleyball, line-dancing, modified yoga, games in the pool, playing tag, bowling, swinging on the swing set, pulling a wagon full of stuffed animals, gardening, yard work, housework, and more.

INDIVIDUALIZING PHYSICAL ACTIVITY PROGRAMS

King et al. (1989) suggested that exercise-promoting interventions be tailored specifically to the individual needs of each participant, especially as these needs relate to age, race, and gender. For example, overweight and obese children lack proficiency in mastering fundamental motor skills (Cliff, Okely, & Morgan, 2012; Maffeis, 2008). Therefore, successful intervention may depend on the use of specialized exercise programs designed to the obese child's specific needs (Sothern, 2001, 2004; Sothern et al., 1999, 2006; Neiman, 1990). If the student is cognitively ready to receive the information and physiologically capable of performing the physical task, then the instructor should experience success in the following: (1) motivating the obese child to participate in the physical activity, (2) encouraging the child to maintain increased physical activity patterns, and (3) promoting the student's acquisition of education concepts that support the physical activity (Sothern, 2006; Sothern et al., 1999, 2006).

Case in Point: Real Words from Real Patients and Their Families

I just wanted to write in to let you know how Matthew is doing. If you remember, he lost about 60 pounds on the program about 4 years ago. Well, he's 16 years old now and he just looks fantastic. His weight fluctuates up and down a little but he's managed to stay in the same size clothes this whole time. I just wanted to thank you for changing his life.

THE APPLICATION OF SOCIAL COGNITIVE THEORY TO PROMOTE PHYSICAL ACTIVITY IN MULTIDISCIPLINARY SETTINGS

Social cognitive theory (Bandura, 1986) provides training ideas that influence motivation to adopt any behavior (e.g., physical activity) based on individual self-efficacy beliefs. Self-efficacy beliefs are learned from four separate sources: (1) knowledge transfer; (2) emotional or physiological responses when associated with behavioral performance; (3) clear success or failure events, or mastery experiences; and (4) vicarious experiences through observational learning, or modeling and imitation (Hunter et al., 1990). Social cognitive theory recognizes a shared blend of these self-efficacy beliefs, which are interacting determinants of each other. An example of the use of these four separate sources of self-efficacy is found in an intervention by Sothern and colleagues (Sothern, 2006; Sothern et al., 1999, 2001, 2002, 2006).

Key Points: Parents and Teenagers

Social situations, emotions, and family events are often triggers to returning to underactive pursuits. These responses have become habitual. Younger children are more influenced by parents and family, but older ones seek autonomy and are more apt to listen to friends. Consequently, there may be times when parents must intervene to set appropriate limits for their teen and to help him deal with peer pressure to engage in sedentary pursuits. Sometimes when the parent becomes the "heavy," it takes the pressure off the teen.

When designing exercise programs for obese children, the instructor should consider activities that are mastered easily. Such activities will ensure that students experience initial success when participating in physical activity if adherence to the program is desired (Sothern, 2001, 2006; Sothern et al., 1999). Competitive programs with nonobese counterparts may not be appropriate because of the limited physiologic capacity of the obese child and the additional risk of injury due to excess weight on the premature musculoskeletal system (Brambilla et al., 2011; Cliff, Okely, & Morgan, 2011; Maffeis, 1998; Sothern, 2001; Van Vrancken-Tompkins, Sothern, & Bar-Or, 2006).

Talking Points: Keeping Parents Nurtured (Verbal cues for patients or parents and family members)
Read through the following information with your patient or family members to help them to understand the exercise strategy used in the program.

To prevent parental burnout, reach out to teachers, coaches, scout leaders, extended family, and friends to shore up support networks. Try a buddy system where you team up with a group of other parents of overweight kids to facilitate physical activities, educational sessions, and problem-solving dialogues. Consider creating a 24-hour telephone line with a recorded message to help inspire colleagues. Enlist the help of your community—local markets, skating rinks, shopping malls, or restaurants—and check out the programs offered by your local county or city recreation district facility. Almost all are geared toward families, run by volunteer parents, and are developmentally appropriate for children of different ages. Your local YMCA or religious organization may offer similar opportunities. The key is family support—and providing opportunities for fun and fitness for your child. We have often wondered whether these organizations even know they are helping prevent overweight problems in children—we thank them, and you as parents should become advocates for these programs. Show your gratitude and support for the healthy opportunities they provide. If you are one of the unlucky few whose community lacks such facilities and opportunities, consider organizing a parent rally to advocate them.

PUTTING RESEARCH INTO PRACTICE: LESSON PLANS TAILORED TO OVERWEIGHT AND OBESE YOUTH USING THE SOCIAL COGNITIVE THEORY

INCREASING DAILY ENERGY EXPENDITURES: THE MODERATE-INTENSITY PROGRESSIVE EXERCISE PROGRAM

The Moderate-Intensity Progressive Exercise Program (MPEP) is a fitness and behavior-modeling tool that provides immediate motivational instruction during the very first class. The initial class sets the stage for subsequent lessons in increasing daily energy expenditures. Students are instructed to stand erect, hold their shoulders back, and walk briskly around the room. Using Bandura's concepts described earlier, this session provides an example of his theory that may be applied to the exercise setting.

MASTERY EXPERIENCE

The participant becomes energized, feels taller, slimmer, and more in control through the action of lifting the chin, pulling the shoulders back, keeping the abdominal muscles tight, and taking quick, long steps. Additional motivation is given that more calories will be burned, weight will be lost, and they will feel and look fitter, taller, and healthier.

Talking Points: Breaking Old Habits (Verbal cues for patients or parents and family members)
Read through the following information with your patient or family members to help them to understand the exercise strategy used in the program.

As you work with your child to implement healthier behaviors, remind her that old habits can be difficult to change or modify. Like other learned behaviors that involve motor responses (such as learning to swim or ride a bike) it takes time, practice, and patience. Tell her that slip-ups will occur, just as falls are inevitable when learning to ride a bike. Remind her that you will be there to help her get back on track, and that eventually, she will master the new behaviors.

We have mentioned that positive reinforcement works more effectively than negative reinforcement to change behaviors. Positive reinforcement includes verbally acknowledging your child whenever she makes a healthy choice: "I noticed you came home after school and went straight to riding your bike."

KNOWLEDGE TRANSFER

Information on the value of increasing daily activity patterns is transferred through the illustration of the term: work. Work = Force × Distance; Force = Weight moved (simplified); Distance = Area covered in one step. When more space is covered in a step, more work is performed in the same amount of time, and thus more calories are burned. Sitting in a chair burns approximately 30–50 calories per hour; just walking casually burns 150–300 calories per hour.

PHYSIOLOGIC FEEDBACK

Participants are instructed to observe their muscles as they contract, relax, and stretch. They are instructed that diets will quickly take weight off. Unless the amount of activity each day is increased, however, the weight will be back in a very short time. Any time an individual moves a body part one or more muscles contract or become shorter. The human body needs energy or "calories" to make the muscles do this. The body gets these calories either from the food that is eaten or from the stored fat in the body (Table 5.1).

 Talking Points: Constructive Responses and Imposing Consequences (Verbal cues for patients or parents and family members)
Read through the following information with your patient or family members to help them to understand the exercise strategy used in the program.

The most constructive responses to unhealthy behavior are to ignore it, redirect the child's attention elsewhere, or problem solve. So, for example, if your child is watching television when she shouldn't be, instead of arguing with or shaming her, simply turn it off and tell her it is time for a bike ride. Or, if walking is part of her fitness routine—but she just doesn't like it—turn to problem solving. Offer a new iPod so she can listen to music or a story while she walks.

If, on the other hand, your child simply refuses to participate in the prescribed exercises, you may want to impose consequences—for example, remove phone privileges. A consequence like having to go to bed early, or reducing her allowance for a week, is more effective than nagging, arguing, or demeaning. Your child will be more likely to respond with increased energy and commitment to the program, rather than sullenly obeying your orders.

BODY MOVEMENT AWARENESS: MUSCULAR STRENGTH AND ENDURANCE—THE MPEP PUMP!

The second exercise program objective is based on the assumption that if an individual becomes competent at knowing which part of the body is responsible for a particular movement, he or she then will be able to identify safe and effective exercise. A balanced, symmetrical physique will promote long-term health in several ways. Injury will be deterred by the prevention of weak areas in the muscles. Balanced training will improve posture, resulting in a taller appearance. Through an improved perception of body size, the individual will experience increased self-esteem. He or she will be able to discriminate between movement that will enhance fitness and appearance and that which may injure. This body movement awareness will contribute to a feeling of control over the student's near environment enabling him or her to know precisely which muscles are responsible for certain movements. With this knowledge comes the power to gain self-control, self-discipline, and a healthy mind and body.

Muscular strength and endurance are discussed as the instructor passes around plastic models of lean tissue and fat tissue for the students to observe and feel. The function of the muscle as a shortening unit to lift and lower body parts is illustrated.

Table 5.1 Illustrations of the Six Basic Areas of the Exercise Component and Examples in Each of the Four Social Cognitive Theory Concepts

Physical activity patterns	Mastery	Knowledge	Role models	Physiological feedback
The MPEP STEP increasing daily energy	Participant becomes energized, feels taller and thinner	Movement burns calories; definition of work	Individuals who walk briskly	Body parts moving as muscles contract; brisk pace is energizing
Body locomotion: The engines of the body Metabolic systems: Aerobic and anaerobic	The concept of the body as an engine is easily understood	Anaerobic and aerobic metabolism	Olympic power lifters, marathon runners, track and field stars, basketball stars	Rate of perceived exertion (RPE); student can identify vigorous or mild activity
Cardiorespiratory endurance: Aerobic exercise	Low impact aerobics are easy to perform	Many activities are aerobic; how to take a heart rate	Sport celebrities, mother and father, teacher	Students feel different muscles working; they feel the heart rate pulse
The MPEP pump: Muscular strength and endurance	Student's muscles control movement; strength exercises are easy to execute	Trained muscles are stronger and burn calories	Television and movie celebrities; the muscles of the body Negative: Fat tissue model	Feeling muscles shorten to move limb; visualizing muscles as tight, strong
Stretch and flex: Muscular flexibility (the stretch test)	Posture is enhanced; feeling of well-being	Balanced posture and body symmetry	Negative: Poor posture; lordosis, kyphosis	Observe personal body imbalance
Body composition	Students will feel successful after losing fat weight	Healthy ranges of fat in the body	Athletes and people who exercise frequently	Clothes feel loose; muscles feel tight

MASTERY AND PHYSIOLOGICAL FEEDBACK

Mastery is achieved immediately as students realize the muscular control they possess, naturally, to move the individual body parts. Likewise, there is instantaneous physiological feedback as the students "feel" the muscles shorten and lengthen. The strength circuit exercises are easy to execute when performed with the recommended amount of weight or resistance. Students are amazed at how easily they can achieve the prescribed number of repetitions with the hand and leg weights.

KNOWLEDGE TRANSFER AND ROLE MODELING

Knowledge of how the muscles function is transferred through the class discussion. The importance of practice or repeating the movement to "teach the muscles" to become stronger, more dense, and tighter achieves both knowledge transfer and physiological feedback.

The plastic fat and lean tissue models serve as desired and undesired outcomes. Positive role models, such as television and movie celebrities, are used to motivate the students.

The muscles themselves become role models, taking on an animated character of their own, through the verbal cues described earlier (Table 5.1).

When conducting exercise sessions, educational content should be organized in a developmentally appropriate manner that is comprehended easily by students of all ages. In this way, instruction will be designed to better serve the emotional and cognitive, as well as physiologic, needs of obese individuals. By providing activities that illicit initial success, it is proposed that instruction will improve mastery concepts and thereby increase self-efficacy beliefs. Because knowledge of the positive outcome of the desired behavior change is central to the application of social learning theories ("learning" is even in the title), instruction includes activities that transfer knowledge during the exercise session. The complete lesson plans may be found in Chapter 6 of this textbook.

Case in Point: Real Words from Real Patients

For a long time, I didn't want to admit I was overweight. I kept calling myself extra muscular. I didn't want to exercise, and I didn't want to make changes. My parents tried a few things, but they didn't work. Then one day, I saw myself in a photograph with my friends and I realized that I wasn't just heavyset; I was overweight. It upset me, but my mom said it was okay, and that I should start this program. I lost weight in the first week. It made me so happy and gave me self-assurance. And I started thinking about the fact that if I stayed heavy, it could affect my health. So I kept with it and now I know I can do just about anything. Before, I didn't think I could, but now I know I can.
—Female patient, 15 years old

SUMMARY

Motivating overweight and obese children to increase physical activity is challenging. Altering poor health habits requires both motivation and self-regulatory skills. Overweight and obese children and adolescents should be taught how to monitor their health behaviors and use proximal goals to motivate them to increase physical activity. Realistic, attainable goals are desired and, therefore, information concerning the initial health, abilities, fitness levels, and interests of the child is essential (Sothern, 2006; Sothern et al., 2006). Social support from family and peers will help sustain their efforts as long as it provides the type of support that enhances their self-efficacy.

Overweight and obese youth often are teased by their peers because of their physical appearances; they often are subjected to peer rejection, ostracism, and physical and verbal victimization. These actions result in decreased physical activity in overweight or obese and normal weight youth (Losekam et al., 2010; Salvy et al., 2012). Weight criticism during physical activity and other verbal, physical, and relational manifestations of victimization are shown to be predictive of increased depressive symptoms, time spent alone, feelings of loneliness, and reduced sports enjoyment (Salvy et al., 2012). Thus, the actual experience of engaging in physical activity, if not carefully structured and monitored, may promote negative outcomes. It may be that overweight and obese children should first obtain the skills necessary to successfully participate in individual goal-based sports, and then after time, gradually be mainstreamed into team-based activities with healthy weight youth. Physical activities for overweight individuals should be appropriate to their specific physical and emotional needs. The health care professional must provide ongoing supervision and guidance. Education and behavioral counseling activities should be based on well-established curriculum design principles to ensure successful motivation and a positive learning environment (Sothern, 2006; Sothern et al., 2006).

REFERENCES

Ajzen, I. (1991). The theory of planned behavior. *Organizational Behavior and Human Decision Processes*, 50, 179–211.

Bailey, R. C., Olson, J., Pepper, S. L., Porszasz, J., Barstow, T. J., Cooper, D. M. (1995). The level and tempo of children's physical activities: An observational study. *Medicine and Science in Sports and Exercise*, 27(7), 1033–1041.

Bandura, A. (1986). *Social Foundations on Thought and Action: A Social Cognition Theory*. Englewood Cliffs, NJ: Prentice-Hall.

Bandura, A. (2004). Health promotion by social cognitive means. *Health Education and Behavior*, 31(2), 143–164.

Bandura, A., Cioffi, D., Taylor, C. B., Brouillard, M. E. (1988). Perceived self-efficacy in coping with cognitive stressors and opioid activation. *Journal of Personality and Social Psychology*, 55(3), 479–488.

Baranowski, T., Cullen, K. W., Nicklas, T., Thompson, D., Baranowski, J. (2003). Are current health behavioral change models helpful in guiding prevention of weight gain efforts? *Obesity Research*, 11(Suppl), 23S–43S.

Barriers to guideline adherence. Based on a presentation by Michael Cabana, MD. (1998). *American Journal of Managed Care*, 4(12 Suppl), S741–S744; discussion S745–748.

Belanger-Gravel, A., Godin, G., Vezina-Im, L., Amirealt, S., Poirier, P. (2010). The effect of theory-based interventions on physical activity participation among overweight/obese individuals: a systematic review. *Obesity Reviews*, 12, 430–439.

Borra, S. T., Schwartz, N. E., Spain, C. G., Natchipolsky, M. M. (1995). Food, physical activity, and fun: Inspiring America's kids to more healthful lifestyles. *Journal of the American Dietetic Association*, 95(7), 816–823.

Brambilla, P., Pozzobon, G., Pietrobelli, A. (2011). Physical activity as the main therapeutic tool for metabolic syndrome in childhood. *International Journal of Obesity*, 35(1), 16–28.

Chalip, L., Csikszentmihalyi, M., Kleiber, D., Larson, R. (1984). Variations of experience in formal and informal sport. *Research Quarterly for Exercise and Sport*, 35(2), 109–116.

Cliff, D. P., Okely, A. D., Morgan, P. J. (2011). Movement skills and physical activity in obese children: Randomized controlled trial. *Medicine and Science in Sports and Exercise*, 43(1), 90–100.

Conner, M., Norman, P. (2005). *Predicting Health Behavior: Research and Practice with Social Cognition Models* (2nd ed.). New York, NY: Open University Press: McGraw-Hill Education. Retrieved from http://www.scribd.com/doc/51975529/Predicting-Health-Behaviour

Crawley, F. E., Koballa, R. R. (1994). Attitude research in science education: Contemporary models and methods. *Science Education*, 78(1), 35–55.

Deforche, B., Haerens, L., Bourdeaudhuij, I. (2011). How to make overweight children exercise and follow the recommendations. *International Journal of Pediatric Obesity*, 6(Suppl 1), 35–41.

DiLillo, V., West, D. (2011). Motivational interviewing for weight loss. *Psychiatric Clinics of North America*, 34, 861–869.

Dishman, R. K. (1994). The measurement conundrum in exercise adherence research. *Medicine and Science in Sports and Exercise*, 26(11), 1382–1390.

Duncan, S. C., Duncan, T. E., Strycker, L. A. (2005). Sources and types of social support in youth physical activity. *Health Psychology*, 24(1), 3–10.

French, S. A., Perry, C. L., Leon, G. R., Fulkerson, J. A. (1994). Food preferences, eating patterns, and physical activity among adolescents: Correlates of eating disorders symptoms. *Journal of Adolescent Health*, 15(4), 286–294.

Glanz, K., Rimer, B., Viswanath, K. (2008). *Health Behavior and Health Education: Theory Research, and Practice* (4th ed., pp. 167–210). San Francisco, CA: Jossey-Bass.

Godin, G., Shephard, R. J. (1985). Gender differences in perceived physical self-efficacy among older individuals. *Perceptual and Motor Skills*, 60(2), 599–602.

Gordon, P. M., Heath, G. W., Holmes, A., Christy, D. (2000). The quantity and quality of physical activity among those trying to lose weight. *American Journal of Preventive Medicine*, 18(1), 83–86.

Haugen, T., Ommundsen, Y., Seiler, S. (2013). The relationship between physical activity and physical self-esteem in adolescents: the role of physical fitness indices. *Pediatric Exercise Science*, 25(1), 138–153.

Hassink, S., Kessel, S. (2010). Implications for pediatricians of the shaping America's youth findings. *Pediatrics*, 126(Suppl 2), 95–97.

Holm, K., Wyatt, H., Murphy, J., Hill, J., Odgen, L. (2012). Parental influence on child change in physical activity during a family-based intervention for child weight gain prevention. *Journal of Physical Activity and Health*, 9, 661–669.

Hunter, S., Johnson, C. C., Little-Christian, S. (1990). Heart smart: A multifactorial approach to cardiovascular risk reduction for grade school students. *American Journal of Health Promotion*, 4, 352–360.

Jakicic, J. M., Wing, R. R., Butler, B. A., Robertson, R. J. (1995). Prescribing exercise in multiple short bouts versus one continuous bout: Effects on adherence, cardiorespiratory fitness, and weight loss in overweight women. *International Journal of Obesity and Related Metabolic Disorders*, 19(12), 893–901.

Keller, C., Fleury, J., Gregor-Holl, N., Thompson, T. (1999). Predictive ability of social cognitive theory in exercise research: An integrated literature review. *Online Journal of Knowledge Synthesis for Nursing*, 6(2).

King, A. C., Taylor, C. B., Haskell, W. L., DeBusk, R. F. (1989). Influence of regular aerobic exercise on psychological health: A randomized, controlled trial of healthy middle-aged adults. *Health Psychology*, 8(3), 305–324.

Knowlden, A., Sharma, M. (2012). Systematic review of family and home-based interventions targeting paediatric overweight and obesity. *Obesity Reviews*, June(13), 499–508.

Kushner, R. F., Weinsier, R. L. (2000). Evaluation of the obese patient. practical considerations. *Medical Clinics of North America*, 84(2), 387–399, vi.

Kylo, B., Landers, D. (1995). Goal setting in sport and exercise: A research synthesis to resolve the controversy. *Journal of Sport and Exercise Psychology*, 17, 117–137.

Lerner, B., Locke, E. (1995). The effects of goal setting, self-efficacy, competition, and personal traits on the performance of an endurance task. *Journal of Sport and Exercise Psychology*, 17, 138–152.

Losekam, S., Goetzky, B., Kraeling, S., Rief, W., Hilbert, A. (2010). Physical activity in normal-weight and overweight youth: Associations with weight teasing and self-efficacy. *Obesity Facts*, 3, 239–244.

Maffeis, C. (2008). Physical activity in the prevention and treatment of childhood obesity: Physio-pathologic evidence and promising experiences. *International Journal of Pediatric Obesity*, 3 (Suppl 2), 29–32.

McInnis, K. J., Franklin, B. A., Rippe, J. M. (2003). Counseling for physical activity in overweight and obese patients. *American Family Physician*, 67(6), 1249–1256.

Metcalf, J. A., Roberts, S. O. (1993). Strength training and the immature athlete: An overview. *Journal of Pediatric Nursing*, 19(4), 325–332.

Milteer, R. M., Ginsburg, K. R., Council on Communications and Media, Committee on Psychosocial Aspects of Child and Family Health. (2012). The importance of play in promoting healthy child development and maintaining strong parent-child bond: Focus on children in poverty. *Pediatrics*, 129(1), e204–e213.

Moore, L. L., Nguyen, U. S., Rothman, K. J., Cupples, L. A., Ellison, R. C. (1995). Preschool physical activity level and change in body fatness in young children: The Framingham children's study. *American Journal of Epidemiology*, 142(9), 982–988.

Mummery, W. K., Spence, J. C., Hudec, J. C. (2000). Understanding physical activity intention in Canadian school children and youth. An application of the theory of planned behavior. *Research Quarterly for Exercise and Sport*, 71(2), 116–124.

Neiman, D. (1990). *Fitness and Sports Medicine: An Introduction*. Palo Alto, CA: Bull Publishing.

Nixon, C., Moore, J., Douthwaite, E., Gibson, E., Vogele, C., Kreichauff, S., Wildgruber, A., Manios, Y. (2012). Identifying effective behavioral models and behavior change strategies underpinning preschool and school-based obesity prevention interventions aimed at 4–6 year olds: A systematic review. *Obesity Reviews*, 13(Suppl), 106–117.

Nolen-Hoeksema, S., Girgus, J. S., Seligman, M. E. (1986). Learned helplessness in children: A longitudinal study of depression, achievement, and explanatory style. *Journal of Personality and Social Psychology*, 51(2), 435–442.

O'Brien, S. J. (1989). How can I help my preadolescent? *Childhood Education*, 66(1), 35–36.

Priest, D. L., Karageorghis, C. I., Sharp, N. C. (2004). The characteristics and effects of motivational music in exercise settings: The possible influence of gender, age, frequency of attendance, and time of attendance. *Journal of Sports Medicine and Physical Fitness*, 44(1), 77–86.

Prochaska, J. O., DiClemente, C. C. (1983). Stages and processes of self-change of smoking: Toward an integrative model of change. *Journal of Consulting and Clinical Psychology*, 51, 390–395.

Resnicow, K., Davis, R., Rollnick, S. (2006). Motivational Interviewing for Pediatric Obesity: Conceptual Issues and Evidence Review. *Journal of American Dietetic Association*, 106, 2024–2033.

Rosenkranz, R., Lubans, D., Peralta, L., Bennie, A., Sanders, T., Lonsdale, C. (2012). A cluster-randomized controlled trial of strategies to increase adolescents' physical activity and motivation during physical education lessons: the motivating active learning in physical education (malp) trial. *BMC Public Health*, 12, 834–853.

Salvy, S., Bowker, J., Germeroth, L., Barkley, J. (2012). Influence of peers and friends on over-weight/obese youths' physical activity. *American College of Sports Medicine*, 40(3), 127–132.

Seabra, A., Mendonca, D., Maia, J., Welk, G., Brustad, R., Fonseca, A., Seabra, A. (2012). Gender, weight status, and socioeconomic differences in psychosocial correlates of physical activity in schoolchildren. *Journal of Science and Medicine in Sport*, Oct.18.pii: S1440-2440(12)00193-4. Doi: 10.1016j.jsams.2012.07.008 [Epub ahead of print].

Silva, M., Vieira, P., Coutinho, S., Minderico, C., Matos, M., Sardinha, L., Teixeira, P. (2010). Using self-determination theory to promote physical activity and weight control: A randomized controlled trial in women. *Journal of Behavioral Medicine*, 33(2), 110–122.

Singh, G. K., Kogan, M. D., Siahpush, M., van Dyck, P. C. (2008). Independent and joint effects of socioeconomic, behavioral, and neighborhood characteristics on physical inactivity and activity levels among U.S. children and adolescents. *Journal of Community Health*, 33, 206–216.

Sonstroem, R. J. (1998). Physical self-concept: Assessment and external validity. *Exercise and Sport Sciences Reviews*, 26, 133–164.

Sothern, M. S. (2001). Exercise as a modality in the treatment of childhood obesity. *Pediatric Clinics of North America*, 48(4), 995–1015.

Sothern, M. (2004). Obesity prevention in children: Physical activity and nutrition. *Nutrition*, 20(7), 704–708.

Sothern, M. (2006). The business of pediatric weight management. In M. Sothern, T. K. von Almen, S. Gordon (Eds.), *Handbook of Pediatric Obesity: Clinical Management* (pp. 9–28). Boca Raton, FL: Taylor & Francis.

Sothern, M., Gordon, S. (2005). Family-based weight management in the pediatric health care setting. *Obesity Management*, 1(5), 197–202.

Sothern, M. S., Hunter, S., Suskind, R. M., Brown, R., Udall, J., Blecker, U. (1999). Motivating the obese child to move: The role of structured exercise in pediatric weight management. *Southern Medical Journal*, 92(6), 577–584.

Sothern, M., Schumacher, H., von Almen, T. K. (2001). *Trim Kids: The Proven Plan That Has Helped Thousands of Children Achieve a Healthier Weight*. New York, NY: HarperCollins.

Sothern, M., Schumacher, H., von Almen, T., Carlisle, L., Udall, J. (2002). Committed to kids: An integrated, four-level team approach to weight management in adolescents. *Journal of the American Dietetic Association*, 102(3), S81–S85.

Sothern, M., VanVrancken-Tompkins, C., Brooks, C., Thélin, C. (2006). Increasing physical activity in overweight youth in clinical settings. In M. Sothern, S. Gordon, T. K. von Almen (Eds.), *Handbook of Pediatric Obesity: Clinical Management* (pp. 173–188). Boca Raton, FL: Taylor & Francis.

Strong, W. B., Malina, R. M., Blimkie, C. J., Daniels, S. R., Dishman, R. K., Gutin, B., et al. (2005). Evidence-based physical activity for school-age youth. *Journal of Pediatrics*, 146(6), 732–737.

Sung-Chan, P., Sung, Y., Zhao, X., Brownson, R. (2012). Family-based models for childhood-obesity intervention: a systematic review of randomized controlled trials. *Obesity Reviews*, 14(4), 265–278.

Stralen, M., Yildirim, M., Velde, S., Brug, J., Mechelen, W., Chinapaw, M. (2011). What works in school-based energy balance behaviour interventions and what does not? A systematic review of mediating mechanisms. *International Journal of Obesity*, 35, 1251–1265.

Strong, W. B. (1990). Physical activity and children. *Circulation*, 81(5), 1697–1701.

Stucky-Ropp, R. C., DiLorenzo, T. M. (1993). Determinants of exercise in children. *Preventive Medicine*, 22(6), 880–889.

Taylor, W. C., Blair, S. N., Cummings, S. S., Wun, C. C., Malina, R. M. (1999). Childhood and adolescent physical activity patterns and adult physical activity. *Medicine and Science in Sports and Exercise*, 31(1), 118–123.

Tierney, S., Mama, M., Skelton, D., Woods, S., Rutter, M., Gibson, M. (2011). What can we learn from patients with heart failure about exercise adherence? A systematic review of qualitative papers. *Health Psychology*, 30(4), 401–410.

Trost, S. G., Saunders, R., Ward, D. S. (2002). Determinants of physical activity in middle school children. *American Journal of Health Behavior*, 26(2), 95–102.

U.S. Department of Health and Human Services. (2008). Physical activity guidelines for Americans. Retrieved June 25, 2009, from http://www.health.gov/paguidelines.

Van Itallie, T. (1992). Health implications of overweight and obesity in the United States. *Annals of Internal Medicine*, 103, 983–988.

Van Vrancken-Tompkins, C., Sothern, M., Bar-Or, O. (2006). Strengths and weaknesses in the response of the obese child to exercise. In M. Sothern, T. K. von Almen, S. Gordon (Eds.), *Handbook of Pediatric Obesity: Clinical Management*. Boca Raton, FL: Taylor & Francis.

Zimmerman, G. L., Olsen, C. G., Bosworth, M. F. (2000) A "stages of change" approach to helping patients change behavior. *American Family Physician*, 61, 1409–1416.

Chapter 6

PUTTING IT ALL TOGETHER

In the previous five chapters, you were provided with an overview of the existing scientific literature in support of individualized, tailored exercise prescriptions for overweight and obese children with comorbidities. In this chapter, we apply this information and provide specific guidelines for prescribing exercise to your patients along with verbal cues or "talking points," clinical reminders, and handouts to assist you with discussing the most appropriate exercise modality, intensity, frequency, and duration for each of your patient's individual needs. At the end of the chapter is a 40-week exercise curriculum, including lesson plans, which can be implemented in clinical, recreational or home-based settings.

TAILORING EXERCISE TO INDIVIDUAL NEEDS

Reducing overweight and related comorbidities, for example, hypertension, asthma, diabetes, and musculoskeletal disorders, with increased physical activity and healthier eating habits may help prevent or delay the development of cardiovascular disease (CVD) and type 2 diabetes in high-risk children and adolescents (McGavock, Sellers, & Dean, 2007). Therefore, it is imperative that children with a body mass index (BMI) greater than the 85th percentile for age and sex be counseled to increase physical activity and reduce weight gain while allowing for normal growth and development. Educators, researchers, and parents need to place a higher priority on increasing children's physical activity (McGavock et al., 2007).

Tailored exercise interventions utilizing strength training and progressive aerobic exercise consistently have been shown to reduce adiposity and improve metabolic profiles (Barbeau et al., 2007; Ben Ounis et al., 2010; Dao et al., 2004; LeMura & Maziekas, 2002; Loftin et al., 2001; Shaibi et al., 2006; Shaibi et al., 2009; Sothern, von Almen, & Gordon, 2006; Sothern, Loftin, Suskind, & Udall, 1999; Sothern, Loftin, Blecker, et al., 2000; Sothern, Loftin, Udall, et al., 1999, 2000; Yu et al., 2005). Children and adolescents at metabolic risk should partake in regular, moderate-intensity physical activity. This activity should be for at least 30 minutes, but preferably for 45–60 minutes, at least 5 days per week. It can be supplemented by an increase in physical exercise as part of daily lifestyle activities (Rosenzweig et al., 2008). For prevention and management of type 2 diabetes in children and adolescents, aerobic-based physical activity lasting 40–60 minutes daily for a minimum of 4 months is likely to enhance insulin sensitivity and may reduce the risk for type 2 diabetes.

Evidence-based recommendations for physical activity in school-age youth include participation in 60 minutes or more of moderate to vigorous activity. This activity should be enjoyable, developmentally appropriate, and involve a variety of activities (Milteer et al., 2012; Murray et al., 2013; Strong et al., 2005; U.S. Department of Health and Human Services [U.S. DHHS], 2008). The following evidence-based recommendations for physical activity in school-age youth are broken down by type and modality (Strong et al., 2005; U.S. DHHS, 2008).

Listed below are examples of developmentally appropriate physical activities.
- Preschool years: General movement activities (jumping, throwing, running, climbing)
- Prepubertal (6–9 years): More specialized and complex movements, anaerobic (tag, games, recreational sports)
- Puberty (10–14 years): Organized sports, skill development
- Adolescence (15–18 years): More structured health and fitness activities, refinement of skills.

Physical fitness, defined as an attribute that includes such fitness components as cardiorespiratory endurance, muscle strength and endurance, flexibility, and body composition

(Bovet, Auguste, & Burdette, 2007), is lower in obese versus healthy weight youth. In addition, several physiological and biomechanical differences may promote reduced physical activity in overweight and obese children (Brandou et al., 2005; Drinkard et al., 2007; Goran et al., 2000; Loftin et al., 2001, 2003, 2004, 2005; Nassis et al., 2005; Norman et al., 2005; Schultz, Sitler, Tierney, Hillstrom, & Song, 2009; Schultz et al., 2010, 2011; Sothern, 1998, 2001, 2002, 2004; Sothern & Gordon, 2003; Sothern, Gordon, & von Almen, 2006; Sothern, VanVrancken-Tompkins, et al., 2006; Sothern, Loftin, Blecker, et al., 1999a, 1999b; VanVrancken-Tompkins, Sothern, & Bar-Or, 2006). Musculoskeletal pain may occur in overweight children, especially in the lower extremities. Moreover, the extra energy cost of moving a greater body mass results in breathlessness or fatigue during exercise sooner than in their normal-weight counterparts. Gross motor competence and fundamental movement skills also are affected negatively by excess body fat in children and adolescents (Cliff et al., 2012; D'Hondt et al., 2013; Okely, Booth, & Chey, 2004). In addition to physiologic, metabolic, and biomechanical differences, children who suffer from overweight or obesity face greater psychological challenges when engaging in physical activities with leaner children (Losekam et al., 2010; Salvy et al., 2012; Schwimmer, Burwinkle, & Varni, 2003). Comorbidities associated with obesity place the child at greater risk during exercise. Childhood obesity health effects include, but are not limited to, type 2 diabetes, coronary artery disease, asthma, and mental health conditions (U.S. Centers for Disease Control and Prevention [CDC], 2012; Strong et al., 2005).

RECOMMENDATIONS FOR OBESE YOUTH WITH HYPERTENSION

Hypertension is independently related to cardiovascular disease risk, which is exacerbated in overweight and obese individuals (Kramer et al., 2009). This condition is routinely present in overweight and obese children (Jacobson, 2006). Children (5–17 years) with BMI greater than the 85th percentile who are considered to be at risk for developing obesity (this means that the BMI value is above the 85th percentile for age and gender according to CDC growth charts) are 2.4 times more likely to have elevated diastolic blood pressure and 4.5 times more likely to have high systolic blood pressure than healthy weight youth (Freedman et al., 2001).

Obese children and adolescents often demonstrate systemic hypertension at rest (Rowland & Loftin, 2006). Likewise, the level of resting blood pressure is related to the degree of adiposity. During exercise, hypertensive children and adolescents may display a heightened increase in blood pressure (Alpert, 2000). In several studies, however, hypertensive children and adolescents experienced no cardiovascular complications during either isometric or dynamic exercise (Alpert, 1999). In addition, systolic blood pressure at maximal exercise typically correlates with resting values. Thus, greater levels of systolic pressure can be expected during exercise testing of obese youth (Owens & Gutin, 1999). This makes it particularly challenging to those not trained in exercise science when selecting appropriate exercise modalities and intensities for obese children (Rowland & Loftin, 2006).

 Key Points: Hypertension

- Children with severe uncontrolled hypertension or target-organ involvement should not participate in competitive sports.
- Children with controlled hypertension and no target-organ disease may participate in moderate high-dynamic and low-static competitive sports.
- Children with controlled hypertension and evidence of left ventricular hypertrophy or renal impairment may participate in low-intensity activities, such as bowling or golf.

Source: From Goldberg, 1995.

The potential benefits of aerobic and muscular strength and endurance training (but not power-lifting) to youth with hypertension are well established (Janssen & LeBlanc, 2010; National High Blood Pressure Education Program [NHBPEP], 2004). Several studies document reduced blood pressure in obese youth following exercise training (Owens, 2006). In obese adolescents, 13–16 years of age, participation in an after-school exercise-plus-lifestyle program resulted in a significant reduction in diastolic blood pressure compared to those youth participating in lifestyle education (Kang et al., 2002). Furthermore, positive alterations in systolic blood pressure were significantly greater in the exercise plus lifestyle group. Recently, Mark and Janssen (2008) reported a positive dose response relationship between increased physical activity levels and blood pressure in children. Thus, exercise interventions should be considered a routine part of medical therapy for overweight children with hypertension provided that appropriate recommendations for intensity, duration frequency, and modality are followed. Guidelines for safe and effective exercise for youth with hypertension are outlined in Table 6.1 (McCambridge et al., 2010).

RECOMMENDATIONS FOR OBESE YOUTH WITH ASTHMA

Obesity is linked to several conditions, including asthma and cancer (Gonzalez, 2006; Koenig, 2001; Stunkard, 1996). The concomitant increase of asthma and obesity has led to the suggestion of a relationship between both entities. In fact, several studies have shown this association (Beuther & Sutherland, 2007; Gold et al., 1993; Luder, Melnik, & DiMaio, 1998; Shaheen et al., 1999).

Table 6.1   Recommendations: Children with Hypertension

- Lifestyle modifications, including daily physical activity and a well-balanced diet, should be discussed and encouraged at all well-child visits regardless of whether the patient has hypertension or normal blood pressure.
- The presence of prehypertension should not limit a person's eligibility for competitive athletics. Lifestyle modifications, including weight management, daily physical activity, and a well-balanced diet, should be discussed and encouraged. Patients with prehypertension should have their blood pressure measured every 6 months.
- Stage 1 hypertension in the absence of end organ damage, including left ventricular hypertrophy (LVH) or concomitant heart disease, should not limit a person's eligibility for competitive athletics. These athletes should have their blood pressure rechecked in 1–2 weeks to confirm the hypertension or sooner if they are symptomatic. Appropriate referrals to qualified pediatric medical subspecialists need to be made if patients are symptomatic, have LVH or concomitant heart disease, or have persistently elevated blood pressure on two additional occasions.
- Youth with stage 2 hypertension in the absence of end organ damage, including LVH or concomitant heart disease, should be restricted from high-static sports until their blood pressure is in the normal range after lifestyle modification or drug therapy. These athletes should be promptly referred and evaluated by a qualified pediatric medical subspecialist within 1 week if they are asymptomatic or immediately if they are symptomatic.
- When hypertension and other cardiovascular diseases coexist, eligibility for participation in competitive athletics usually should be based on the type and severity of the other cardiovascular disease.
- Medication, caffeine, drug, tobacco, and stimulant use should be reviewed with any athlete with hypertension because of the effects these substances may have on blood pressure.
- Although restricting sodium intake typically is recommended for those with hypertension, for some young athletes, rehydration often requires deliberate concomitant intake of additional salt-containing fluids and foods to ensure greater body-water retention and distribution to all fluid compartments.
- Care should be taken to appropriately diagnose and monitor athletes who are at higher risk for hypertension, such as obese athletes and athletes with spinal cord injuries.

Source: From McCambridge et al., *Pediatrics*, 125(6), 1287–1294, 2010. With permission.

Asthma is the most commonly diagnosed severe illness among pediatric patients in the United States (International Study of Asthma and Allergies in Childhood Steering Committee, 1998). It is estimated that 24.4 million people have been diagnosed with asthma in the United States and that more than a third of these people (at least 7.7 million) are children under 18 years of age. Asthma is the leading serious chronic illness and the number one cause of hospitalization and school absenteeism in the pediatric population. The overall prevalence of asthma in U.S children is estimated to be about 6.7% (Rodriguez et al., 2002). Children and adolescents considered at risk for developing overweight conditions are two times more likely to have asthma than healthy weight children.

In children older than 10 years of age who also have a family history of asthma, the prevalence of asthma is 31%. In children less than 10 years of age who also have a family history of asthma the prevalence of asthma is 15.6% (Third National Health and Nutrition Examination Surveys [NHANES III]; see Rodriguez et al., 2002).

Of great concern is the observation that obesity is shown to negatively affect asthma therapy in children with severe conditions (Carroll et al., 2006). In addition, pediatric obesity increases the duration of therapy during severe asthma exacerbations. Even more troubling is the finding that 77% of obese youth remained obese during adulthood (Freedman et al., 2001). Thus, obesity is likely to negatively affect asthma control throughout the life of these individuals.

Key Points: Asthma Considerations in Overweight and Obese Children

- Children with asthma typically have low fitness levels.
- Exercise triggers acute asthma, which may occur during but usually 5–10 minutes following the activity.
- Use standardized exercise tests to determine fitness and follow ACSM guidelines.
- Appropriate activities include:
  - Low-asthmogenic sports, such as tennis, handball, diving, karate, golf, baseball, sprinting, and gymnastics
  - Breathing and postural exercises to prevent "tight posture" associated with underused diaphragm

Source: From Goldberg, 1995.

Obesity has been suggested as a proinflammatory state in adults. There is increased evidence that obesity is accompanied by a chronic inflammatory response characterized by elevated blood levels of proinflammatory mediators, such as interleukin (IL-6), IL-1β, tumor necrosis factor alpha (TNFα), leptin, and C-reactive protein (CRP), and depressed blood levels of endogenous anti-inflammatory proteins, such as adiponectin (Baraldi & de Jongste, 2002; Bastard et al., 2000; Cook et al., 2000; Prochaska, Redding, & Evers, 2002; Visser, 2001; Visser et al., 1999, 2001; Yudkin et al., 2000). In children, especially before puberty, the relationship between obesity and inflammation is not as clear. Zabaleta and colleagues (2013) reported inverse correlations between body fat and TNFα, and between IL-8 and intramyocellular lipids in the soleus muscle of healthy prepubertal children 7 to 9 years of age. Leptin, a protein that is increased in the majority of obese adult individuals, also is shown to enhance the production of TNFα, IL-6, and IL-12 from stimulated macrophages in animal models (Considine et al., 1996). Similarly, weight loss is accompanied by a decrease in IL-6 in both adipose tissue and serum in adults and adolescents (Prochaska et al., 2002). Weight loss also improves asthma symptoms in conjunction with a decrease in inflammation.

Asthma is characterized by a state of airway hyper-responsiveness with infiltration of eosinophils, neutrophils, mast cells, and T lymphocytes (Busse & Lemanske, 2001; Jatakanon et al., 1999). The chronic inflammation leads to airway obstruction, airway hyper-responsiveness, and remodeling. Many inflammatory mediators have been found to play a role in asthma (and obesity), including IL-6, TNFα, leptin, and CRP (Bastard et al., 2000).

Table 6.2   Recommendations: Children with Asthma

- Children are able to participate in any physical activity if symptoms are well controlled. Swimming is less likely to trigger exercise-induced bronchoconstriction (EIB) than running.
- Children should keep an accurate history of symptoms, trigger exposures, treatments, and course of recovery from episodes of bronchospasm.
- Children should be diagnosed with EIB by a drop in forced expiratory volume in 1 second (10–15%) after a 6- to 8-minute exercise challenge and a positive response to beta-2 agonist medication. Eucapnic voluntary hyperventilation testing is recommended in athletes.
- Children should use leukotriene inhibitors, inhaled corticosteroids, or long-acting beta-2 agonists for optimal long-term disease control and avoid overuse of short-acting beta-2 agonists.
- Children should take inhaled beta-2 agonists 15–30 minutes before exercise.
- Children should not scuba dive if they have asthma symptoms or abnormal pulmonary function tests.
- Children who compete nationally or internationally require a therapeutic use exemption with confirmation of asthma or EIB to use certain medications. Consultation with a sport medicine physician is suggested.

Source: From Philpott, J. F., Houghton, K., Luke, A., *Clinical Journal of Sports Medicine*, 20(3), 167–172, 2010. With permission.

- Students with asthma can and should participate in physical education and sports.
- Students with asthma can fully participate in physical activity when they are symptom-free.
- Activity may need to be modified when a student's asthma is not well controlled (i.e., when the child has an upper respiratory infection).
- Asthma episodes can kill, so preventing asthma episodes and responding effectively to them are paramount.
- Premedication, if prescribed, and physical warm-ups are essential and can help prevent asthma episodes.
- Asthma action plans should include modified exercise recommendations from a personal physician.
- Appropriate school staff must have access to individual asthma action plans and individual asthma emergency protocol.

Source: From American Lung Association, Asthma-friendly schools initiative toolkit, New York, NY, 2007. With permission.

Because obesity is considered an inflammatory state, the condition is likely to negatively affect asthma control especially in those individuals with severe conditions. Thus, efforts to achieve and maintain a healthy body weight are essential to improving asthma severity in children and adolescents. These efforts should include the adoption of a healthy diet, behavioral therapy and appropriate exercise recommendations. The adoption of a regular exercise routine will initially result in an increase in inflammation, the result of increased energy expenditure, which is associated with higher oxidative stress (Niess & Simon, 2007). Long-term (more than 3 months) exercise training will lead to a reduction in inflammation, improved immune response, and lowered oxidative stress (Radak, Chung, & Goto, 2008). The guidelines in Table 6.2 should be followed when prescribing exercise to overweight and obese children with asthma (American Lung Association, 2007; Philpott, Houghton, & Luke, 2010).

RECOMMENDATIONS FOR OBESE YOUTH WITH TYPE 2 DIABETES

Metabolic disease may follow obesity during childhood (Daniels et al., 2005). Adiposity is a major determinant of type 2 diabetes in children and adolescents and is the most relevant modifiable diabetes risk factor in youth (McGavock et al., 2007; Ruzic, Sporis, & Matkovic, 2008; Schmitz et al., 2002). Obese children are developing type 2 diabetes at younger ages. In a study of 177 obese (more than 95th percentile BMI) youth, impaired glucose tolerance, or prediabetes, was detected in 25% of the 55 obese children (4–10 years of age) and in 21% of the 112 obese adolescents (11–18 years of age). In 4% of the obese adolescents, type 2 diabetes was diagnosed without any reported symptoms—for example, silent type 2 diabetes (Sinha et al., 2002).

Type 2 diabetes mellitus typically is preceded by insulin resistance (Ivy, Zderic, & Fogt, 1999). Studies performed in children and adolescents indicate that increased physical activity is significantly related to lower fasting insulin and greater insulin sensitivity (Nassis et al., 2005; Schmitz et al., 2002) even in the absence of reductions in body fat. Schmitz et al. (2002) observed the effect of physical activity on insulin resistance and other cardiovascular disease factors in 357 healthy weight children without diabetes (age range 10–16 years). They found a significant relationship between fasting insulin and insulin sensitivity and self-reported physical activity. Nassis et al. (2005) examined the effects of an aerobic exercise training program on insulin sensitivity in overweight and obese 9–15-year-olds. After 12 weeks of training, insulin sensitivity increased without changes in body weight or percent fat mass. Moreover, after the training, lower limb fat-free mass increased by 6.2%, a change that was significantly associated with enhanced insulin sensitivity (Nassis et al., 2005). Likewise, in a similar investigation, Kahle et al. (1996) observed a significant decrease in fasting insulin in obese adolescent males after 15 weeks of mild-intensity training. In a recent study, moderate aerobic exercise training was shown to improve overall glucose tolerance in adolescents (Thomas et al., 2009).

It has been proposed that physical activity may improve insulin sensitivity by enhancing glucose transport into muscle cells and increasing the production of muscle glycogen to replace the amount used during exercise (Corcoran, Lamon-Fava, & Fielding, 2007). Conversely, Kang et al. (2002) reported no significant changes in fasting insulin after 8 months of moderate to vigorous physical training in 80 obese youths. Additionally, no significant reductions in fasting insulin were observed by Treuth et al. (1998) over 5 months of resistance training in 12 obese prepubertal girls. Despite this earlier finding, recent investigations report significant metabolic benefits of aerobic and resistance training in children and adolescents. Zorba, Cengiz, and Karacabey (2011) reported reductions in insulin levels after a 12-week aerobic exercise training program, including walking and jogging exercise in obese children. Aerobic training improved insulin resistance and reduced visceral adiposity in sedentary overweight and obese children participating in an after-school program (Davis et al., 2012). In addition, a dose-response benefit was identified in those participating in 40 minutes versus 20 minutes of aerobic training daily. Shaibi et al. (2006) examined the effects of a 16-week resistance training program in 21 overweight Latino adolescent males randomly assigned to 2-week resistance training or a nonexercising control condition. Significant increases in strength as measured by one-repetition maximum (1RM) were observed in the resistance training group. More important, objectively measured insulin sensitivity measured by the frequently sampled intravenous glucose tolerance test was improved significantly (45.1 ± 7.3% in the resistance training group versus −.9 ± 12.9% in the control group). Remarkably, these results remained significant after adjusting for fat and lean mass by dual-energy x-ray absorptiometry (DEXA). Recently, Davis et al. (2011) reported similar benefits in Latina adolescent girls following circuit strength training. In another investigation, Benson, Torode, and Fiatarone Singh (2007) reported that poor upper body strength was an independent predictor of insulin resistance in a large cohort (N = 126) of children, 10–15 years of age even after adjusting for maturation, central adiposity, and body mass (Benson et al., 2007). Thus, resistance or strength training should be considered to be a safe and effective modality of exercise in children at risk for developing type 2 diabetes. This coincides with recent recommendations by the U.S. Government Physical Activity Guidelines for American Children and Adolescents, which include bone- and muscle-strengthening activities for inclusion into each day's minimum of 60 minutes of physical activity (U.S. DHHS, 2008).

Lifestyle modifications are necessary to manage established diabetes successfully and to lower the risk for type 2 diabetes in high-risk youth. In addition to diet, physical activity is a proven form of diabetes management and is considered a cornerstone in the prevention of diabetes (McGavock et al., 2007; Ruzic et al., 2008; Schmitz et al., 2002). In children with

Table 6.3   Recommendations: Children with Diabetes

Type 1 Diabetes
• Children and adolescents with type 1 diabetes should adhere to the Centers for Disease Control and Prevention and American Academy of Sports Medicine recommendations for a minimum of 30–60 minutes of moderate physical activity daily. • Blood glucose monitoring before exercise is recommended with a suggested intake of 15 grams (g) of carbohydrate (amount may need to be less in younger children; e.g., 10 g) for a blood glucose level below target range before exercise; for vigorous physical activity expected to be more than 30 minutes, an additional 15 g of carbohydrate may be necessary. • For prolonged vigorous exercise, hourly blood glucose monitoring during the exercise, as well as blood glucose monitoring after completion of exercise, is recommended to guide carbohydrate intake and prospective insulin dose adjustment for recurring exercise events. • At the onset of a new sports season, frequent blood glucose monitoring during the 12-hour postexercise period should be undertaken to guide insulin dose adjustments. • In the child or adolescent (particularly if overweight or obese), physical exercise should be encouraged and sedentary activity discouraged.

Source: From Silverstein J., et al., *Diabetes Care*, 28(1), 186–212, 2005.

diabetes, participation in physical activity provides numerous advantages (Riddell & Iscoe, 2006). By improving both insulin sensitivity and glucose uptake in skeletal muscle, physical activity may have the potential to reduce the incidence of type 2 diabetes in children and adolescents (McGavock et al., 2007; Schmitz et al., 2002). Specific exercise recommendations for children with diabetes are outlined in Table 6.3 (Silverstein et al., 2005). At the end of this chapter, detailed exercise prescriptions and lesson plans are provided for children with varied levels of obesity and family and medical histories.

RECOMMENDATIONS FOR CHILDREN WITH OBESITY-RELATED MUSCULOSKELETAL PROBLEMS

Musculoskeletal pain may occur in overweight children, especially in the lower extremities (Schultz et al., 2011; Taylor et al., 2006). In a recent investigation, bone and joint disorders were reported in 4.2% of obese children and only 1.5% of healthy weight children (Hadley, 2007). In obese children with private insurance the prevalence of bone and joint disorders was 13.2% versus only 2.6% in healthy weight children. The diagnosis rate is much lower in children who have Medicaid, however. In clinical evaluations, the most common musculoskeletal disorders identified are Blount disease (tibia vara), genu varum, and slipped capital femoral epiphysis (Krebs & Sothern, 2006). In particular, Blount disease and slipped capital femoral epiphysis are of greatest concern (Jacobson, 2006). Blount disease may occur with or without pain and is observed as a lateral outward bowing of the affected lower limbs. Symptoms of slipped capital femoral epiphysis include hip or knee pain, limp, and an externally rotated and abducted leg. Affecting primarily younger children with excessive weight, both of these conditions present a barrier to increasing physical activity as movement worsens the condition. As such, either of the two represents an orthopedic emergency and health care providers should recommend immediate surgical consultation for their patients (Jacobson, 2006).

Gross motor competence and fundamental movement skills also are affected negatively by excess body fat in children and adolescents (Cliff et al., 2012; Okely et al., 2004). In a recent study, a group of 43 eight-year-olds with an average weight of 40 kilograms (kg) took twice as long as healthy weight children to get out of a lounge chair. In some of the children, assistance was required for them to stand up from the seated position (Riddiford-Harland, Steele, & Baur, 2006). One of the authors, Professor Steele, reported that "[t]hey have flatter feet, collapsed arches.... We think they are just more uncomfortable all the time" (Riddiford-Harland et al., 2006).

Table 6.4 Recommendations: Children with Musculoskeletal Disorders

---

Children with Juvenile Idiopathic Arthritis (JIA)

- Can safely participate in sports without disease exacerbation.
- Should participate in moderate fitness, flexibility, and strengthening exercises.
- Can participate in impact activities and competitive contact sports if their disease is well controlled and they have adequate physical capacity.
- Should be encouraged to be physically active as tolerated. Those with moderate to severe impairment or actively inflamed joints should limit activities within pain limits.
- Should gradually return to full activity following a disease flare.
- Should take individualized training (especially for children with severe joint disease) within a group exercise format for physical–social benefit. Physiotherapists or pediatric rheumatology health care teams should coordinate individual exercise programs.
- Should have radiographic screening for C1–C2 instability before participation in collision or contact sports if they have neck arthritis. If present, further evaluation is required.
- Should wear appropriately fitted mouth guards during activities with jaw and dental injury risk (per general population), especially if they have jaw involvement.
- Should wear appropriate eye protection (per general population) during activities with ocular injury risk.

Source: From Philpott, J. F., Houghton, K., Luke, A., *Clinical Journal of Sports Medicine*, 20(3), 167–172, 2010.

In overweight and obese children who are at risk for developing musculoskeletal disorders, non-weight-bearing activities, such as cycling or resistance training, may provide the best option. In addition, the low levels of physical activity and reduced ability to participate in weight-bearing activities associated with musculoskeletal problems further place the overweight and obese child at risk for future osteoporosis and associated fractures later in life (Faigenbaum & Myer, 2010). Thus, it is important to consider alternative activities that do not require the weight to be supported during exercise, but likewise provide osteogenic stimulus during the pre- and postadolescent period of development. Resistance training provides the added benefit of producing mechanical strain, which may act concurrently with normal growth-related increases in bone development to maximize peak bone mass (Behm et al., 2008). Swimming also offers a good option, and rowing offers similar benefits. Provided that the special needs of overweight and obese children with musculoskeletal disorders are considered, safe and effective exercise recommendations may be implemented. One of the most common musculoskeletal disorders in children is juvenile arthritis. Guidelines for prescribing exercise to children with juvenile arthritis are outlined in Table 6.4 (Philpott et al., 2010).

TAILORING EXERCISE RECOMMENDATIONS TO AGE, OVERWEIGHT LEVEL, AND ASSOCIATED MEDICAL PROBLEMS

Identifying the most appropriate exercise modality, intensity, frequency, and duration for overweight and obese children, especially those with associated medical problems requires experience, knowledge and expertise in pediatric exercise medical science. Ideally, overweight and obese children should first be evaluated by a licensed physical therapist to determine musculoskeletal health and limitations and by a licensed clinical exercise physiologist to determine exercise tolerance, cardiorespiratory fitness, muscular strength, and endurance and flexibility capacity. Personal trainers, certified by the American College of Sports Medicine (ACSM), provide the next best option, but only provided they can demonstrate experience and knowledge of the individual needs of developing youth with regard to exercise. The majority of health care providers with basic medical knowledge in pediatrics, exercise, and behavioral science should be able to provide safe and effective exercise advice to their patients by following the information outlined in this book. Likewise, elementary and high school educators with a basic understanding of the physical and psychological needs of school-age youth will find that the recommendations and detailed instructions and lesson plans included in this book provide a safe and reasonable option for determining the most optimal plan of action for prescribing exercise for the overweight and obese child and adolescent.

According to the current scientific literature, physically inactive children and adolescents should take an incremental approach to reach the 60 minutes per day recommendation, increasing overall physical activity by 10% each week (Strong et al., 2005). Progressing too quickly likely will lead to excessive soreness, which will discourage children from continuing the exercise program. Also, excessive exercise may be counterproductive as overweight and obese children may experience overuse injuries if duration, frequency, and intensity are too challenging (U.S. DHHS, 2008).

Key Points: Evidence-Based Recommendations for Physical Activity in Sedentary Youth

Physically inactive youth:

- Incremental approach to reach the 60-minute-per-day recommendation
- Increase activity by 10% per week
- Progressing too quickly is counterproductive and leads to injury

Sources: Adapted from Strong et al., 2005; U.S. DHHS, 2008.

Key Points: American Heart Association Childhood Obesity Summit—Exercise and Overweight Youth

Overweight youth should be given realistic, easily obtainable physical activity goals and should not be compared with normal weight peers.

Source: From Daniels et al., 2009.

Key Points: Exercise Recommendations for Obese Children

Exercise prescriptions for obese children should involve family support activities that are doable and fun and that develop participatory skills.

Source: From Hassink et al., 2008.

Tables 6.5, 6.6, and 6.7 provide recommendations for frequency, duration, and activity for severely obese, obese, and overweight children and adolescents (Sothern, 2001; Sothern, Gordon, & von Almen, 2006; Sothern, Schumacher, et al., 2002; Sothern, VanVrancken-Tompkins, et al., 2006; Sothern, von Almen, & Schumacher, 2001; Sothern, von Almen, et al., 1993; Sothern, von Almen, et al., 1999; VanVrancken-Tompkins, Sothern, & Bar Or, 2006).

It is also important that overweight youth be provided with realistic, easily obtainable exercise goals (Daniels et al., 2009), which are fun and develop participatory skills (Hassink et al., 2008). This is especially relevant when engaging in activities with healthy weight children. Overweight and, especially, obese children should never be placed in situations in which their

Table 6.5 Moderate-Intensity Progressive Exercise Prescribed Duration of Exercise (minutes per session)

	Week 1	Week 5	Week 10
Overweight	30	45	60
Obese	25	40	55
Severely obese	20	35	50

Table 6.6   Moderate-Intensity Progressive Exercise Prescribed
Frequency of Exercise (days per week)

	Week 1	Week 5	Week 10
Overweight	3	4.5	6
Obese	2	4	5.5
Severely obese	1	3	5

exercise performance is compared with their healthy, leaner counterparts (Daniels et al., 2009). In a recent study, Lowry et al. (2007) reported that in overweight youth who need to increase physical activity, moderate-intensity activities provide opportunities with a low risk of injury.

The moderate-intensity, progressive exercise education intervention detailed in this chapter is based on the individual needs of children in different ranges of obesity (Sothern, 2001; Sothern et al., 2006; Sothern, Schumacher, et al., 2002; Sothern, VanVrancken-Tompkins, et al., 2006; Sothern, von Almen, & Schumacher, 2001; Sothern, von Almen, et al., 1993, 1999; VanVrancken-Tompkins, Sothern, Bar-Or, 2006). In each level, the activities described have been chosen because they are safe and effective for the child with a particular obese physical condition. The exercise guidelines contained in this chapter are conservative and progressive, increasing gradually over time. This is to ensure safety and to promote the attainment of mastery in the overweight students. The recommended intensity, duration, and frequency are specified for each obesity level and each comorbid condition (Sothern, 2001; Sothern, Gordon, & von Almen, 2006; Sothern, Schumacher, et al., 2002; Sothern, VanVrancken-Tompkins, et al., 2006; Sothern, von Almen, & Schumacher, 2001; Sothern, von Almen, et al., 1993, 1999; VanVrancken-Tompkins, Sothern, Bar-Or, 2006). These recommendations align perfectly with the most recent U.S. Guidelines for Physical Activity, the American Academy of Pediatrics, and the American Heart Association (Daniels et al., 2009; U.S. DHHS, 2008; U.S. Preventive Services Task Force, 2010). The program guidelines also are specific to the different levels of overweight—that is, initially the severely obese students have shorter beginning durations and frequencies than do the overweight or at-risk students.

 Key Points: Four-Level Progressive Exercise Program

The needs of the overweight child depend on his or her level of overweight. There are four distinct levels of the exercise program, each developed specifically for the individual needs of each level of obesity.

Level 1 (Red)

This is an inpatient or outpatient level that serves the needs of the child with severe obesity whose BMI exceeds 120% of the 95th percentile or an absolute BMI greater than 35 kg/m² for age and gender (AHA, 2013; CDC, 2012) or has other special medical indications.

Level 2 (Yellow)

This level is for children who are diagnosed as obese with a BMI greater than the 95th percentile but less than the 99th percentile, according to the CDC.

Level 3 (Green)

This level is for the child who is diagnosed with an overweight condition or a BMI greater than the 85th percentile but below the 95th percentile. This child is at increased risk for developing obesity.

Level 4 (Blue)

This level is for the healthy weight child with a BMI below the 85th percentile (CDC, 2012) or this level may serve as a maintenance program for formerly overweight children who achieve a healthy weight.

The exercise program also utilizes light to moderate intensity exercise initially and it is progressive, which means that the amount of exercise gradually increases over time. Light to moderate—not fast or hard—exercise is supported by several researchers as overweight and obese children can do moderate exercise for hours without getting too tired, which enables them to burn calories and fat (Brambilla, Pozzobon, & Pietrobelli, 2011; Daniels et al., 2009; Sothern, 2001; Sothern, Gordon, & von Almen, 2006; Sothern, VanVrancken-Tompkins, et al., 2006; VanVrancken-Tompkins, Sothern, & Bar-Or, 2006).

Talking Points: Duration, Frequency, and Intensity (Verbal cues for patients or parents and family members)
Read through the following information with your patient or family members to help them to understand the exercise strategy used in the program.

Duration means the amount of time you spend exercising at each session. Some basic rules about duration follow:

- You need to be physically active for at least 20 minutes most days per week to gain any health benefits from physical activity (it can be done in two 10-minute sessions).
- To lose weight and burn calories and fat, you should set a goal and start out slowly and work up to it.

Frequency refers to the number of exercise sessions you do in a given week. Basic rules about frequency include the following:

- You will need to exercise a minimum of 1–2 days per week to prevent losing your current level of fitness.
- If your goal is to improve your current level of fitness and shed some body fat, you should set a goal to work up to exercising 3–4 days per week.
- Those who are serious about losing body fat (that's you!) need to gradually work up to exercising 4–6 days per week. Our aerobic exercise goals each week automatically do this for you.

Intensity means how hard and fast you exercise. The intensity of your workout can change according to the speed, grade (steepness), muscles you use, and the force or resistance that you apply.

- Vigorous Intensity = more than 55–70% maximal oxygen uptake (VO_2max) or more than 65–80% maximal heart rate (MAXHR)
- Moderate Intensity = 45–55% VO_2max or 55–65% MAXHR
- Low Intensity = less than 45% VO_2max or less than 55% MAXHR

Glossary
Maximal Oxygen Uptake: the total amount of oxygen that individuals will consume when they are exercising at their maximum effort. Called VO_2max for short, it is well accepted as the best indicator of aerobic fitness.

Because excess fat weight places an increased burden on an individual's cardiorespiratory and musculoskeletal systems (Brandou et al., 2005; Drinkard et al., 2007; Goran et al., 2000; Loftin et al., 2001, 2003, 2004, 2005; Nassis et al., 2005; Norman et al., 2005; Schultz et al., 2009, 2010, 2011; Sothern, 1998, 2001, 2002, 2004; Sothern & Gordon, 2003; Sothern, Gordon, & von Almen, 2006; Sothern, Loftin, Blecker, et al., 1999a, 1999b; Sothern, VanVrancken-Tompkins, et al., 2006; VanVrancken-Tompkins, Sothern, & Bar-Or, 2006) the recommended exercise activities for the obese and severely obese children are arm-specific and less weight-bearing. Recommendations for healthy and overweight children include both weight-bearing and non-weight-bearing activities. Clinical, public health, fitness, and recreational professionals should use the information in the lists in Table 6.7 to guide patients and students toward the selection of the most appropriate type of aerobic activity for each of the three different overweight and obese levels.

Table 6.7 Activity Recommendations According to Body Mass Index (BMI) for Overweight, Obese, and Severely Obese Children and Adolescents

Overweight children (>85th–95th BMI), 7–18 Years	• Limited access to television, video games, computer • Recommended aerobic activities: Weight-bearing activities, such as brisk walking, treadmill, field sports, roller blading, hiking, racquetball, tennis, martial arts, skiing, jump rope, indoor or outdoor tag games • Parent training and fitness education • Pacing skills
Obese children (>95th–99th BMI), 7–18 Years	• Limited access to television, video games, computer • Recommended aerobic activities: Non-weight-bearing activities, such as swimming, cycling, strength or aerobic circuit training, arm ergometer (crank), recline bike, and interval walking (walking with frequent rests, as necessary) • Parent training and fitness education
Severely obese children (>120% of 95th BMI or absolute BMI >35 kg/m²), 7–18 Years	• Limited access to television, video games, computer • Recommended aerobic activities: Non-weight-bearing activities, such as swimming, recline bike, arm ergometer (crank), seated (chair) aerobics, and seated or lying circuit training • Parent training and fitness education • Other emotional and dietary concerns addressed during treatment

Throughout the implementation of the pediatric weight management program, the health care professional must provide ongoing supervision and guidance. Individuals with increasing levels of overweight conditions will respond differently to exercise of differing modalities and intensities (Brandou et al., 2005; Drinkard et al., 2007; Goran et al., 2000; Loftin et al., 2001, 2003, 2004, 2005; Nassis et al., 2005; Norman et al., 2005; Schultz et al., 2009, 2010, 2011; Sothern, 1998, 2001, 2002, 2004; Sothern & Gordon, 2003; Sothern, Gordon, & von Almen, 2006; Sothern, Loftin, Blecker, et al., 1999b; Sothern, VanVrancken-Tompkins, et al., 2006; VanVrancken-Tompkins, Sothern, & Bar-Or, 2006). By implementing the specialized developmentally appropriate recommendations detailed in this chapter and by closely following the guidelines in Chapter 2 as well as instructions for strength and flexibility exercises outlined in Chapters 3 and 4, safe and effective exercise for the prevention and management of pediatric obesity may be possible.

Although the learning activities are designed to be somewhat interchangeable, the instructor should not deviate from the recommended movement technique or intensity of an individual aerobic (Chapter 2), strength (Chapter 3), or flexibility (Chapter 4) exercise. Some activities may be interchanged, but only if their technical aspects and intensities are similar. Instructors also may introduce movement or activities of their own creation, but only if these are similar in technique and intensity to the recommended exercises, and if they are implemented cautiously. It is extremely important not to compromise safety for the sake of creativity. If the instructor is unsure whether a movement is safe or appropriate for the overweight or obese child, then another activity should be selected. The skills required for the activities at each level should be attained easily, to ensure that overweight and obese children will experience mastery, which will motivate them to continue the program. Throughout the program, if the instructor notices that any child is having difficulty, the activity should be adjusted accordingly.

It is important that health care professionals emphasize to the parents of their patients that they should assist their child with selecting the most appropriate exercise activities. They also should guide the child in deciding which days are best for planning the activities and how long they should participate.

Talking Points: Physical Activity Recommendations (Verbal cues for patients or parents and family members)
Read through the following information with your patient or family members to help them to understand the exercise strategy used in the program.

Each week, your child will participate in three types of activities:

1. Aerobic activity
2. Strength exercise routine
3. Stretching exercises

Each activity includes recommendations each week as to how often, and for how long, your child should perform it. These are meant to be realistic goals—they are also the minimal goals. If your child wants to do more, great! Usually if you give them less, they will do more. Then you can praise your child for going over and above. This really helps her achieve "mastery"—a feeling that she has accomplished something special. Just remember to have your child rest at least 1 day between strength work-outs so that her muscles can become stronger.

Let your child choose the activity she wants to do from the activities list on the goal-setting and exercise record (Tables 6.13–6.16). Then follow the recommendations for set-ting goals each week for how long and how often your child should perform the activity.

The exercise program also includes specific recommendations for children with obesity-related comorbidities, including hypertension, asthma, type 2 diabetes, and musculoskeletal disorders. These medical complications further limit the physical abilities of overweight and obese children. Therefore, considering these in the selection of the exercise modality, intensity, frequency, and duration is essential. Once the health care professional has identified associated comorbidities, he or she should use the information in the sidebar "Clinical Reminders for the Health Care Professional: Key Questions to Ask Your Patient about Exercise" to evaluate their patient's physical activity level, cardiorespiratory fitness, muscular strength, and endurance and flexibility level. Health care professionals also have the option of utilizing the measurement protocols outlined in Chapter 8 to more objectively evaluate these factors.

Clinical Reminders for the Health Care Professional: Key Questions to Ask Your Patient about Exercise

1. How much would you say you exercise each week?
   0–1 day (sedentary)
   2–3 days (moderately active)
   4–5 days (active)
   6–7 days (very active)
2. How easy is it for you to perform exercises like riding a bike, running, playing sports, or dancing?
   Very hard (very unfit)
   Hard (unfit)
   Easy (fit)
   Really easy (very fit)
3. How strong are you? Is it easy for you to pull yourself up on a bar or lift something heavy?
   Not strong at all—weak (poor)
   Sort of strong (average)
   Strong (good)
   Really strong (excellent)
4. How flexible are you? Is it easy for you to do stretches like touching your toes?
   Not flexible at all (poor)
   Kind of flexible (average)
   Flexible (good)
   Really flexible (excellent)

Table 6.8 Patient's Current Health Status (Select the level that best corresponds to the greatest number of selected categories.)

Color code	Weight level	Physical activity level	Cardiorespiratory fitness level	Muscular strength and endurance	Flexibility	Comorbidity (e.g., asthma, hypertension, diabetes)
Red	1, Severe Obesity	Sedentary	Unfit	Poor	Poor	Uncontrolled or severe
Yellow	2, Obesity	Moderately active	Moderately fit	Average	Average	Controlled or moderate
Green	3, Overweight	Active	Fit	Good	Good	Well controlled or mild
Blue	4, Healthy Weight	Very active	Very fit	Excellent	Excellent	No comorbidities

Health care professionals may review Table 6.8 to identify the factors, for example, overweight level, comorbidity, and so on, that are associated with their patient's current health status. They then may use this information to determine the category or level (1–4) that corresponds with the greatest number of factors identified. Then using this information, they will be able to advise their patients to begin the specific color-coded exercise program for that level. The health care professional also should refer to specific exercise recommendations for each obesity-related problem, for example, hypertension, asthma, and so on, outlined earlier in this chapter, and further adapt the program activities accordingly.

Clinical Reminders for the Health Care Professional: Tailoring Exercise to the Individual Needs of Your Patient

Determine the weight level or classification, then determine the physical activity, cardiorespiratory, muscular strength and endurance level, and flexibility level of your patient by asking the key questions in the handout or by using the objective measurements outlined in Chapter 8. Finally, determine the clinical level of control of the comorbidity, for example, uncontrolled or severe, controlled or well controlled. Once this assessment is complete, see Table 6.8. The exercise prescription color-coded level that you select should correspond to the highest number of selections that are identified.

For example, a severely obese (level 1, red) football player, with good strength and flexibility, excellent cardiorespiratory endurance, and well-controlled asthma should begin with the level 3 (green) exercise level program while also adhering to the specific guidelines for asthma patients (Table 6.1). On the other hand an overweight (level 3, green) sedentary, girl with high glucose levels, poor strength, and cardiorespiratory endurance but excellent flexibility should begin the level 1 (red) exercise program. When a patient's condition is identified as "in between" a color-coded level, health care provides always should select the lower of the levels to ensure initial success and reduce the risk of injury and overtraining.

Once the appropriate level and color program is identified for your patient, please see Tables 6.9–6.12 for specific recommendations for duration (how long), frequency (how many times per week), intensity (how hard or how fast), and modality (what type of activity) for each of the four levels. Use the information in these tables to prescribe specific guidelines and directions for exercise to your patient for each week over a 12-week period. When selecting the specific type of physical activity from the list provided for each exercise intensity level (e.g., light, moderate, moderate to vigorous), remember it is also important to consider the exercise limitations for each comorbidity—for example, hypertension (Table 6.1), asthma (Table 6.2), diabetes (Table 6.3), and juvenile arthritis (Table 6.4). For patients with comorbidities not covered in this chapter, physician review and approval of the exercise program is essential before engaging in the recommended activities.

Table 6.9 Initial 10-Week Recommendations for Sedentary Severely Obese Youth: Level 1, Red (>99th percentile BMI)

Week	Type		Frequency	Duration	Intensity			Suggested activities
	Non-weight-bearing activities	Weight-bearing activities	Days per week	Minutes per session	Light	Moderate	Moderate to vigorous	
1	X	X	2	20	X			Archery Bowling Watering garden
2	X	X	2	20	X			Setting the table Feeding animals
3	X	X	2	20–25	X			Stretching Modified yoga Tai Chi
4	X	X	2	20–25	X			Darts Billiards Miniature golf (Putt-Putt)
5	X	X	3	25–30	X			Playing fetch with your dog Visit a museum, aquarium, or zoo
6	X		3	25–30		X		Seashell hunting Boat riding
7	X		3	30–35		X		Playing pitch and catch with a friend Playing "dress up"—role play
8	X		3	30–35		X		Cycling (indoor and outdoor) Swimming Water exercise
9	X		4	35–40		X		Rowing (indoor and outdoor) Strength circuit training (seated)
10	X		4	35–40		X		Stomach crunches Horseback riding
11	X		5	40–45		X		Trip to the waterslide Jumping/diving into the pool
12	X		5	40–45		X		Wrestling Stretching while seated Seated aerobic dancing

Table 6.10 Initial 10-Week Recommendations for Sedentary Obese Youth: Level 2, Yellow (>95th–<99th percentile BMI)

Week	Type		Frequency	Duration	Intensity			Suggested Activities
	Non-Weight-Bearing Activities	Weight-Bearing Activities	Days per Week	Minutes per Session	Light	Moderate	Moderate to Vigorous	
1	Alternate between both non-weight-bearing and weight-bearing activities		2	20–25	X			Sailing Fishing
2			2	20–25	X			Playing in the waves Springboard diving Light housekeeping Playing outside
3			3	25–30	X			Nature walk Interactive computer game (WiiSports, bowling, or baseball)
4			3	25–30		X		Croquet Ping-Pong Kite flying
5			3	25–35		X		Making a snowman Making a sand castle Stretching on the floor
6			3	25–35		X		Laser tag Snorkeling Waterskiing
7			4	30–40		X		Water ballet Snow sledding Interval walking Line dancing
8			4	30–40		X		Ballroom dancing Low-impact aerobic dancing Gardening
9			4	35–45		X		Martial arts (karate, judo, etc.) Circuit strength training Tumbling
10			4	35–45		X		Sliding Baseball Volleyball
11			5	40–50		X		Family biking trip Interactive computer game (Wii Fit)
12			5	40–50		X		Family flag football Treadmill walking Aerobic circuit

Table 6.11 Initial 10-Week Recommendations for Sedentary Overweight Youth: Level 3, Green (>85th–<95th percentile BMI)

Week	Type		Frequency	Duration	Intensity			Suggested activities
	Non-weight-bearing activities	Weight-bearing activities	Days per Week	Minutes per session	Light	Moderate	Vigorous	
1	X	X	2	20–30	X			Golfing Shopping Swinging Badminton
2	X	X	2	20–35	X			Interactive computer game (Rock Star or Guitar Hero) Tubing down the river
3	X	X	3	25–40		X		Frisbee Walking the dog Pulling a wagon Stretching to music
4	X	X	3	25–40		X		Skipping rocks on a lake Scavenger hunt Playing tag outdoors
5	X	X	4	25–45		X		Climbing trees Yard work Skipping rope Mini-trampoline
6	X	X	5	25–45		X		Gymnastics Circuit strength training Aerobic dancing Brisk walking
7	X	X	5	35–50		X		Tennis Modified field sports* (football, hockey, soccer, etc.)
8	X	X	5	35–50			X	Interactive computer game (Dance, Dance, Revolution) Stair-climber
9	X	X	5	35–55			X	Elliptical machine Water polo Competitive swimming Synchronized swimming
10	X	X	5	35–50			X	Ice skating Swing dancing African dancing Jumping rope
11	X	X	6	40–60			X	Jogging Running Basketball Wall-climbing Spinning class
12	X	X	6	40–60			X	Fun runs Field sports (football, hockey, soccer, etc.)

*See the lesson plans at the end of this chapter for ideas to modify field sports for overweight children.

Table 6.12 Initial 10-Week Recommendations for Sedentary Healthy Weight Youth: Level 4, Blue (<85th percentile BMI)

Week	Type		Frequency	Duration	Intensity			Suggested Activities
	Non-Weight-Bearing Activities	Weight-Bearing Activities	Days per Week	Minutes per Session	Light	Moderate	Moderate To Vigorous	
1	X	X	7	60		X		Family hike Salsa dancing Yoga
2	X	X	7	60		X		Climbing on monkey bars Kick boxing
3	X	X	7	60		X		Jazz, tap, ballet, hip-hop dancing Cheerleading
4	X	X	7	60		X		Beach volleyball Cricket Swimming laps
5	X	X	7	60			X	Shooting hoops Softball Dancing freestyle to your favorite tune
6	X	X	7	60			X	Inline skating
7	X	X	7	60			X	Windsurfing Ice hockey Racquetball, handball, squash
8	X	X	7	60			X	Snow skiing (cross-country or downhill)
9	X	X	7	60			X	Field sports (football, soccer, hockey, etc.)
10	X	X	7	60			X	Surfing Wind-surfing Kiteboarding Swing dancing
11	X	X	7	60			X	Modern dance Sprinting Track and field events
12	X	X	7	60			X	Long-distance swimming Marathons Triathlons

Notice also that the recommended duration, frequency, and intensity for each level and color program automatically increase about 10% per week, which is the recommendation from the U.S. Government Physical Activity Guidelines (U.S. DHHS, 2008), the American Heart Association (Daniels et al., 2009), and others (Strong et al., 2005). In addition, suggested activities are provided for each week of the program.

Consider, for example, an obese (more than 95th percentile BMI to less than 99th percentile BMI) patient who is moderately active with an average aerobic fitness, strength, and flexibility and well-controlled hypertension. The patient's current health status places him or her in the level 2 (yellow) program (Tables 6.10 and 6.14). In weeks 1and 2, he or she will engage in both weight-bearing and non-weight-bearing light-intensity exercise, such as sailing, fishing, playing in the waves, springboard diving, light housekeeping, playing outside, or going on a nature walk, for 2 days at 20–25 minutes each session. Starting in week 3, he or she will increase the duration to 25–30 minutes and the frequency to 3 days per week, but will still select weight-bearing and non-weight-bearing light activities for 2 days that week. Beginning in week 4, the intensity of the exercise increases to a moderate level, and suggested activities such as laser tag, snorkeling, water skiing, water ballet, snow sledding, interval walking, line dancing, gardening, and martial arts (karate, judo, etc.) coordinate with this intensity. The duration of the exercise is maintained at 25–30 minutes per session and the frequency is maintained at 3 days per week. Care should be taken to monitor the patient's blood pressure routinely during this level of the program when the exercise intensity is increased. Once it is clear that the selected activities do not cause abnormal blood pressure increases, then the health care provider should follow the specific instructions for hypertensive youth engaged in physical activities outlined in Table 6.1. In weeks 5–12, the moderate intensity is maintained, but the duration and frequency of exercise increase a little (about 10%) each week, so that by the 12th week, your patient should be engaging in moderate-intensity activities that alternate between weight-bearing and non-weight-bearing exercise for 40–50 minutes per session and 5 days per week.

Health care providers should enlist the help of their patient's parent in explaining how best to follow the prescribed exercise activities. They should explain to the parent that his or her child will follow the recommendations for the designated color code (red, yellow, green, or blue) for 12 weeks. During this time, it will be best for the parent to set up monthly appointments so that the health care provider may evaluate the child's progress. At the completion of the 12-week program, the child's condition should be reevaluated to determine whether they have made enough progress to be prescribed the next level of the color-coded exercise program guidelines.

Talking Points: Four Color-Coded Levels (Verbal cues for patients or parents and family members)
Read through the following information with your patient and/or family members to help them to understand the exercise strategy used in the program.

Describe the four color-coded levels to your child; identify which one he or she is in, and explain that there is a different exercise program for each color. Let him or her know that when he or she reaches his or her first weight-loss goals, he or she will graduate to the next color code, and that the objective is to attain this long-term goal weight and be a lifelong member in the blue level. As you will see, our exercise plans are laid out according to your child's level.

Clinical Reminders for the Health Care Professional: Safety Tips

Be sure to emphasize these safety tips to your patient:

- Stop exercising if you feel any discomfort in a muscle or joint. It is normal to feel a gentle burning sensation, but if the pain is worse than that, stop immediately! You will need to report it to your teacher, coach, exercise physiologist, or me the next time I see you.

- Do the exercise exactly as instructed. The exercises have been designed especially for you and you should not change them.
- Be sure to record your daily activity on the Weekly Goal-Setting Form and Exercise Record (Tables 6.13–6.16).

Self-monitoring and goal setting are key components of successful exercise programs for overweight and obese children (von Almen, Sothern, & Schumacher, 2006). In this chapter, we provide easy-to-use forms for health care providers to give to their patient so that this process is user-friendly. There is a different form for each color-coded level and the recommendations from the previous tables are contained within each form to make it easy for patients to insert their weekly goals and record their successes (Tables 6.13–6.16). You will need 12 copies of this form on hand—one for every week. During each week of the program, fill out the form whenever you exercise.

Clinical Reminders for the Health Care Provider: Self-Monitoring and Goal Setting

After you weigh your patient ask to see the weekly report form (see Chapter 8). If the form is incomplete, assist your patient in filling out the form. Then be sure to review the past week's goals. Decide whether your patient has met or fallen short of the goal for the week. Provide praise or a small inexpensive reward for patients achieving their goals. If your patient did not achieve it, redirect him to set a new, more achievable goal.

Talking Points: Goal-Setting Tips (Verbal cues for patients or parents and family members)
Read through the following information with your patient or family members to help them to understand the exercise strategy used in the program.

Never ridicule or punish your child for not meeting his goal. Also, allow him to "plead the fifth," meaning that if he knows he did not meet his goal and feels too embarrassed to talk about it, just move on. Do not dwell on the mistakes of the past. Either way, set a new activity goal for the next week.

Talking Points: Self-Monitoring and Goal Setting (Verbal cues for patients or parents and family members)
Read through the following information with your patient or family members to help them to understand the exercise strategy used in the program.

At the beginning of each week, help your child write his or her goal in the weekly goal-setting and exercise record (Tables 6.13–6.16). You will need 12 copies of this form on hand—one for every week. During each week of the program, fill out the form whenever you exercise. This is the minimum amount of aerobic exercise that he or she should perform this week. Then help him or her to choose an activity from the list on the form. During the week, help your child to list the activities he or she accomplished this week and how long he or she did them in the spaces indicated. Check to ensure that your child is performing the activities for the length of time and the number of days per week from the goals. He or she should do them at a moderate or medium pace and be able to talk without strain while exercising. If his or her breathing becomes rapid or labored, instruct him or her to slow down. Remember: The exercise program establishes the minimum goals for each week to ensure that your child will be successful, which is crucial to her confidence and ongoing participation in the program. This week, make sure he or she can complete the activity without difficulty and that he or she is having fun.

Table 6.13 Patient Handout: Weekly Goal-Setting Form and Exercise Record: Level 1, Red

Weekly Goal-Setting Form and Exercise Record												
Patient Name:_____ Date:_____												

Level 1, Red (>99th percentile BMI)												
Recommended Goals and Suggested Activities												
Week	1	2	3	4	5	6	7	8	9	10	11	12
Times per Week	2	2	2	2	3	3	3	3	4	4	5	5
Minutes per session	20	20	20–25	20–25	25–30	25–30	30–35	30–35	35–40	35–40	40–45	40–45

Intensity	Light	Moderate
Suggested activities	Archery Bowling Watering the garden Setting the table Feeding animals Stretching Modified yoga Tai Chi Darts Billiards Miniature golf (Putt-Putt) Playing fetch with your dog Visiting a museum, aquarium, or zoo Seashell hunting Boat riding Playing pitch and catch with a friend Playing "dress up"—role play	Cycling (indoor and outdoor) Swimming Water exercise Rowing (indoor and outdoor) Strength circuit training (seated) Stomach crunches Horseback riding Trip to the waterslide Jumping/diving into the pool Wrestling Stretching while seated Seated aerobic dancing

Weekly Exercise Record Form		
Week No. ____ My goal this week is _____ times per week; _____ minutes per session.		
Day of the week	I've written below what kind of exercise I did each day:	This is how many minutes I did the exercise each day:
Sunday		
Monday		
Tuesday		
Wednesday		
Thursday		
Friday		
Saturday		

Table 6.14 Patient Handout: Weekly Goal-Setting Form and Exercise Record: Level 2, Yellow

<table>
<tr><td colspan="13">Weekly Goal-Setting Form and Exercise Record</td></tr>
<tr><td colspan="13">Patient Name:_____   Date:_____</td></tr>
<tr><td colspan="13">Level 2, Yellow (>95–<99th percentile BMI)</td></tr>
<tr><td colspan="13">Recommended Goals and Suggested Activities</td></tr>
<tr><td>Week</td><td>1</td><td>2</td><td>3</td><td>4</td><td>5</td><td>6</td><td>7</td><td>8</td><td>9</td><td>10</td><td>11</td><td>12</td></tr>
<tr><td>Times per week</td><td>2</td><td>2</td><td>3</td><td>3</td><td>3</td><td>3</td><td>4</td><td>4</td><td>4</td><td>4</td><td>5</td><td>5</td></tr>
<tr><td>Minutes per session</td><td>20–25</td><td>20–25</td><td>25–30</td><td>25–30</td><td>25–35</td><td>25–35</td><td>30–40</td><td>30–40</td><td>35–45</td><td>35–45</td><td>40–50</td><td>40–50</td></tr>
<tr><td>Intensity</td><td colspan="5">Light</td><td colspan="7">Moderate</td></tr>
<tr><td>Suggested activities</td><td colspan="5">Sailing
Fishing
Playing in the waves
Springboard diving
Light housekeeping
Playing outside
Nature walk
Interactive computer game (Wii Sports bowling, or baseball)
Croquet
Ping-Pong
Kite flying
Making a snowman
Making a sand castle
Stretching on the floor</td><td colspan="7">Laser tag
Snorkeling water skiing
Water ballet
Snow sledding
Interval walking
Line dancing
Ballroom dancing
Low-impact aerobic dancing
Gardening
Martial arts (karate, judo, etc.)
Circuit strength training
Tumbling
Sliding
Baseball
Volleyball
Family biking trip
Interactive computer game (Wii Fit)
Family flag football*
Treadmill walking
Aerobic circuit*</td></tr>
<tr><td colspan="13">Weekly Exercise Record Form</td></tr>
<tr><td colspan="13">Week No. _____ My goal this week is _____ times per week; _____ minutes per session.</td></tr>
<tr><td>Day of the week</td><td colspan="10">I've written below what kind of exercise I did each day.</td><td>This is how many minutes I did the exercise each day:</td></tr>
<tr><td>Sunday</td><td colspan="10"></td><td></td></tr>
<tr><td>Monday</td><td colspan="10"></td><td></td></tr>
<tr><td>Tuesday</td><td colspan="10"></td><td></td></tr>
<tr><td>Wednesday</td><td colspan="10"></td><td></td></tr>
<tr><td>Thursday</td><td colspan="10"></td><td></td></tr>
<tr><td>Friday</td><td colspan="10"></td><td></td></tr>
<tr><td>Saturday</td><td colspan="10"></td><td></td></tr>
</table>

Table 6.15 Patient Handout: Weekly Goal-Setting Form and Exercise Record: Level 3, Green

Weekly Goal-Setting Form and Exercise Record												

Patient Name:_____ Date:_____

Level 3, Green (>85th–<95th percentile BMI)

Recommended Goals and Suggested Activities

Week	1	2	3	4	5	6	7	8	9	10	11	12
Times per week	2	2	3	3	4	5	5	5	5	5	6	6
Minutes per session	20–30	20–35	25–40	25–40	25–45	25–45	35–50	35–50	35–55	35–50	40–60	40–60

Intensity	Light	Moderate	Moderate to Vigorous

Suggested activities	Golfing
	Shopping
	Swinging
	Badminton
	Interactive
	  computer game
	  (Rock Star or
	  Guitar Hero)
	Tubing down a
	  river
	Frisbee
	Walking the dog
	Pulling a wagon
	Stretching to
	  music
	Skipping rocks on
	  a lake
	Scavenger hunt
		Playing tag outdoors
		Climbing trees
		Yard work
		Skipping rope
		Mini-trampoline
		Gymnastics
		Circuit strength training
		Aerobic dancing
		Brisk walking
		Tennis
		Modified field sports*
		  (football, hockey, soccer, etc.)
		Interactive computer game
		  (Dance, Dance, Revolution)
		Stair-climber
		Elliptical machine
			Water polo
			Competitive swimming
			Synchronized swimming
			Ice skating
			Rock and roll dancing
			African dancing
			Jumping rope
			Jogging
			Running
			Basketball
			Wall-climbing
			Spinning class
			Fun runs
			Field sports (football,
			  hockey, soccer, etc.)

Weekly Exercise Record Form

Week No. _____ My goal this week is _____ times per week; _____ minutes per session.

Day of the week	I've written below what kind of exercise I did each day.	This is how many minutes I did the exercise each day:
Sunday		
Monday		
Tuesday		
Wednesday		
Thursday		
Friday		
Saturday		

Table 6.16 Patient Handout: Weekly Goal-Setting Form and Exercise Record: Level 4, Blue

Weekly Goal-Setting Form and Exercise Record												
Patient Name:_____ Date:_____												
Level 4, Blue (<85th percentile BMI)												
Recommended Goals and Suggested Activities												
Week	1	2	3	4	5	6	7	8	9	10	11	12
Times per week	7	7	7	7	7	7	7	7	7	7	7	7
Minutes per session	60	60	60	60	60	60	60	60	60	60	60	60

Intensity	Moderate	Moderate to Vigorous
Suggested activities	Family hike Salsa dancing Yoga Climbing on monkey bars Kick boxing Jazz, tap, ballet, hip-hop dancing Cheerleading Beach volleyball Cricket Swimming laps Shooting hoops Softball Dancing freestyle to your favorite tune	Inline skating Windsurfing Ice hockey Racquetball, handball, squash Snow skiing (cross-country or downhill) Field sports (football, soccer, hockey, etc.) Surfing Wind-surfing Kiteboarding Swing dancing Modern dance Sprinting Track and field events Long-distance swimming Marathons Triathlons

Weekly Exercise Record Form		
Week No. _____ My goal this week is _____ times per week; _____minutes per session		
Day of the week	I've written below what kind of exercise I did each day.	This is how many minutes I did the exercise each day:
Sunday		
Monday		
Tuesday		
Wednesday		
Thursday		
Friday		
Saturday		

The pediatric weight management exercise curriculum, which follows this section includes lesson plans and descriptions of activities in clinic and home settings based on developmentally appropriate recommendations, color-coded to level of obesity (Daniels et al., 2009; Milteer et al., 2012; Murray et al., 2013; Sothern, Gordon, & von Almen, 2006; Sothern, von Almen, & Schumacher, 2001; U.S. DHHS, 2008; U.S. Preventive Services Task Force, 2010).

CLINICAL OVERVIEW OF A TYPICAL MULTICOMPONENT WEIGHT MANAGEMENT PROGRAM FOR OVERWEIGHT CHILDREN

Multidisciplinary approaches, including exercise interventions, have long been employed in academic medical settings and as part of clinical research trials. And although the scientific findings of such approaches are positive (Kitzmann et al., 2010) and these approaches were recently recommended by the U.S. Preventive Services Task Force (2010), which was published in the scientific journal, pediatrics, the application of such interventions is sporadic, and inconsistent across the pediatric clinical community. There are many challenges to implementing pediatric weight management interventions (Sothern, Gordon, & von Almen, 2006). Several studies suggest that health care providers have significant difficulty in providing patients with plans to promote positive health-related behaviors or reduce negative behaviors (Barlow et al., 2002; Eisenmann, 2011). In addition, when proven methods for weight loss have been demonstrated, providers have difficulty in predicting those patients who most likely would adhere to these methods. In addition, they lack the time and support staff necessary for organizing the recommended multicomponent, moderate- to high-intensity behavioral interventions, which are most advantageous and cost-effective if delivered in group, family-based settings (Sothern, Gordon, & von Almen, 2006; Sothern, VanVrancken-Tompkins, et al., 2006). Last, insurance reimbursements for such programs are lacking (Gray et al., 2012; Simpson & Cooper, 2009) even though studies indicate that the public recognizes that pediatric obesity is a significant health problem and is supportive of interventions to manage obesity in children and adolescents (Evans et al., 2005). Many of these common barriers to implementing pediatric weight management programs can be addressed through education, careful planning, and the application of sound implementation strategies (Sothern, Gordon, & von Almen, 2006; Trick, 1990).

Case in Point: Real Words from Real Patients

Rene came to our clinic when she was 7 years old weighing 100 pounds more than what was ideal for her age and height. After losing about 25 pounds, she decided her problem was no longer severe enough to endure the rigors of our program, and she decided to drop out.

Ten years later, at age 17, she came back—carrying an extra 200 pounds. She had undergone surgery on her legs due to Blount disease (bowed legs from excess weight) and was hospitalized for weight-related breathing problems that doctors considered life-threatening. After becoming first involved in our hospital program, and then our outpatient program, Rene lost 135 pounds. Both she and her parents see the need for a lifetime commitment to healthy eating and activity. They have agreed to do just that.

Settling for temporary accomplishments will not help your child in the long run. Making healthy choices never ends. It is something all of us must do lifelong, whether or not we have a weight problem. It is even more crucial for a child at risk of overweight. When your child reaches his goal weight, celebrate by knowing that he will remain healthy for as long as the family remains committed to the new lifestyle. And celebrate by knowing your entire family will live a longer, healthier, and happier life together!

Key Points: U.S. Preventive Services Task Force Recommendation Statement, February 2010

Recommendations:

- Adequate evidence that multicomponent, moderate- to high-intensity behavioral interventions for obese children ages 6 years and older
- Multicomponent interventions included dietary, physical activity, and behavioral counseling
- Adequate evidence that the harms of behavioral interventions are no greater than small

Source: From U.S. Preventive Services Task Force, 2010.

PROGRAM OVERVIEW

Successful pediatric weight-management programs are comprehensive interventions, which are multidisciplinary and designed especially for the needs of the overweight and obese child age 7–17 years. The staff includes a team of medical, health, and nutrition professionals whose primary concern is the safety and success of the child in the program. Interactive sessions are delivered by these professionals during a once-weekly group, family-based setting (Sothern, Gordon, & von Almen, 2006; Sothern, von Almen, & Schumacher, 2001; Sothern, Schumacher, et al., 2002; von Almen, Sothern, & Schumacher, 2006).

 Key Points: American Heart Association Childhood Obesity Summit

The complex and multiple factors causing pediatric obesity warrant a multidisciplinary, collaborative approach:

- Engage professionals across multiple disciplines.
- National efforts include research, health, advocacy, education, media, and consumer advertising.

Source: From Daniels et al., 2009.

A pediatrician or family physician serves as the medical director for the program. He or she provides overall medical supervision and guidance. In severely overweight children, calorie restriction is recommended. A registered dietitian provides nutrition supervision and guidance for the program. He or she conducts weekly education sessions on nutrition topics and instructs patients in the proper administration of the clinic diet. Nutrition sessions are conducted in a group session with patients, parents, siblings, and extended family and friends in attendance.

A child development or behavior specialist provides instruction in behavior-modification skills and techniques for the program. He or she conducts weekly educational sessions on the psychosocial aspects of obesity in children. Behavior modification skills are introduced using discussion, modeling, role playing, and guided problem solving. Topics, such as self-monitoring, commitment, limit setting, habit formation, goal setting and action plans, decision-making skills, attitudes, and assertiveness training, are discussed.

An exercise physiologist or other pediatric exercise professional provides the exercise supervision and guidance for the program. He or she conducts weekly exercise sessions on various health and fitness topics and leads a weekly exercise class. Each session will be a mixture of sharing information on such topics as heart rate monitoring and injury prevention as well as the actual exercise. In addition, fitness counseling includes motivational techniques to increase daily activity levels and improve body movement awareness based on social cognitive theory (Bandura, 1986).

FAMILY INTERVENTION

Because successful behavior modification depends on what happens in the home, the pediatric weight-management program should include parents as an integral part of the weekly intervention. Research indicates that the child's successes are determined not only by the child's commitment but also by that of his or her parents (Sothern, Gordon, & von Almen, 2006). It is strongly recommended that at least one parent be required to attend the session, and siblings and extended family are encouraged to attend the weekly sessions with the overweight child. The parent's participation in the interactive nutrition, behavior, and exercise instruction is strongly promoted.

Talking Points: Enlisting Support (Verbal cues for patients or parents and family members)

Read through the following information with your patient or family members to help them to understand the exercise strategy used in the program.

Spread the news to friends, family, teachers, and others that your family has begun an exercise program to help him or her to achieve a healthier weight. Accept their praise and support. Most likely, everyone will want to see you succeed. Ask other overweight children if they would be interested in playing team sports once a week or join in other fun activities. Also, it is helpful for anyone who supervises your child to know that he or she is following the program.

FOUR-LEVEL PROGRESSION

The needs of the overweight child depend on his or her level of overweight. There are four distinct levels of the pediatric weight management program, each developed specifically for the individual needs of each level of obesity.

LEVEL 1 (RED)

This is an inpatient or outpatient level that serves the needs of the child with severe obesity or special medical indications.

LEVEL 2 (YELLOW)

This level is for children who are diagnosed as obese. Weekly outpatient sessions address issues of diet, behavior, and fitness.

LEVEL 3 (GREEN)

This level is for the child who is classified as overweight and is at risk for developing an obese condition. Weekly outpatient sessions are designed to arrest and reverse the onset of obesity through nutrition education, increased physical activity, exercise training, and behavior modification.

LEVEL 4 (BLUE)

This is the maintenance program. Weekly exercise sessions and monthly multitopic meetings reinforce the healthy habits learned in intervention levels 1, 2, and 3. The goal is for a lifetime of healthy eating and activity. This program also may serve as an obesity prevention program for healthy weight children with primary risk factors.

The results and intervention strategies of the pediatric weight management program within this chapter are widely published in a multitude of peer-reviewed scientific journals and proven to be successful in several studies (Carlisle, Gordon, & Sothern, 2005: Loftin et al., 2001, 2003, 2004, 2005; Sothern, 2006; Sothern & Gordon, 2005; Sothern, Hunter, et al., 1999; Sothern, Loftin, Suskind, et al., 1999; Sothern, Loftin, Blecker, et al., 2000; Sothern, Loftin, Udall, et al., 1999, 2000; Sothern, von Almen, & Schumacher, 2001; Sothern, Schumacher, et al., 2002; Sothern, Udall, et al., 2000; Sothern, VanVrancken-Tompkins, et al., 2006; Sothern, von Almen, et al., 1993, 1999; Suskind, Sothern, Farris, et al., 1993; Suskind, Sothern, von Almen, et al., 1996; Udall & Sothern, 2004; VanVrancken-Tomkins & Sothern, 2006; von Almen, Sothern, & Schumacher, 2006). After 10 weeks, a sample group of 55 children and adolescents showed a statistically significant decrease in weight from 81.7 ± 26.5 to 72 ± 23.9 kg, BMI from 32.9 ± 7.1 to 28.4 ± 6.4 kg/m^2, and percent of ideal body weight (% IBW) from 176.2 ± 33.9 to 150.6 ± 30.4% (p < .005) (Sothern, Udall, et al., 2000). These intervention methods have been published in the scientific textbook, *The Handbook of Pediatric Obesity: Clinical Management* (Sothern, Gordon, & von Almen, 2006) and in a popular press book for parents to use in conjunction with their pediatrician or family physician entitled *Trim Kids* (Sothern, von Almen, & Schumacher, 2001). The program is recognized by the National Cancer Institute as a Research Tested Intervention Program and recently was acknowledged by the U.S. surgeon general for its community dissemination in YMCA centers in Louisiana (http://www.surgeongeneral.gov/obesityprevention/communitychampions/index.html).

Pediatric weight management programs typically are held in a hospital, medical clinic, physician's office, or fitness or recreation club setting. Education materials are provided to the parents of the overweight or obese children (Sothern, von Almen, & Schumacher, 2001). Parents and children attend a weekly 2-hour comprehensive session for a recommended time period. Medical supervision and guidance are provided by a physician or nurse at each session to increase compliance and monitor side effects. During these sessions, the families receive dietary supervision, nutrition education, exercise instruction, fitness education, and behavioral counseling (Sothern, 2006; Sothern, Gordon, & von Almen, 2006; Sothern, Schumacher, et al., 2002; Sothern, von Almen, & Schumacher, 2001; von Almen, Sothern, & Schumacher, 2006).

SAMPLE WEEKLY CLINIC ACTIVITIES
Nutrition education and diet supervision
Nutrition education centers on identifying high-calorie and low-calorie foods in each food group for families and instructing them on appropriate serving sizes (Sothern, Gordon, & von Almen, 2006; Sothern, von Almen, & Schumacher, 2001). A series of learning activities are presented in each 12-week session that are specific to the needs of each group as they progress through the different stages of the treatment program. The children are provided with easy-to-use food frequency checklists to complete each week. Nutrition education sessions are conducted in a group session with family and friends in attendance. Patient participation is encouraged during the cooking demonstrations, calorie-counting, and food-measuring activities. During the early phases of the program, nutrition information is delivered in a simple, knowledge-based format. As the groups progress through the different levels, the activities require more advanced levels of comprehension and problem-solving skills. All activities are physically and cognitively appropriate for the children. By the end of the program, patients and their families are able to adequately identify, select, and prepare foods that are appropriate to continued weight maintenance and good health. Sessions for the children are limited to 30 minutes in duration. During this time, the dietitian conducts interactive sessions focused on the improvement of healthy food selection and discussions of the importance of portion control. Significantly overweight children receive individualized diet prescriptions and counseling on the specific number of servings and on appropriate serving sizes for each food group.

Exercise instruction and fitness education
Exercise instruction for the parents and children is conducted at each visit by an exercise physiologist or other certified pediatric exercise professional. Each session is a mixture of sharing information on such topics as heart rate monitoring and injury prevention as well as the actual exercise (Sothern, 2001; Sothern, Schumacher, et al., 2002; Sothern, VanVrancken-Tompkins, et al., 2006; Sothern, von Almen, & Schumacher, 2001). In

addition, fitness counseling includes motivational techniques to increase daily activity levels and improve body movement awareness (Sothern, Hunter, et al., 1999; Sothern, VanVrancken-Tompkins, et al., 2006). During each 12-week session of the program, the exercise activities correspond with the group's physical condition of obesity and ability to comprehend, synthesize, and apply health and fitness information to daily life situations. Children receive a Weekly Goal-Setting Form and Exercise Record (Tables 6.13–6.16) to record the type of activity and number of minutes of physical activity they perform each week. They are encouraged to select activities that they enjoy from a list of activities appropriate for their individual overweight level. Goals for how long and often they should exercise are provided. These goals become more challenging as they progress through the program. For example, in week 1, the recommendation is 2 days of exercise per week for 20 minutes. By week 5, the goal is 3 days per week for 35 minutes. By week 10, the goal is 4 days per week for 50 minutes. Compliance is monitored by observing these physical activity record cards and monitoring of heart and breathing rate. All activities are physically and cognitively appropriate for the children. Exercise education and motivational activity classes for the children are limited to 30 minutes in duration. During this time, the exercise physiologist conducts interactive sessions focused on the improvement of body composition, cardiorespiratory endurance, muscular strength, and endurance and muscular flexibility. The participants exercise in a playful, sporadic, and intermittent manner while the exercise physiologist discusses key concepts using symbols, music, and various props.

Behavioral counseling

Behavior change with reduced caloric intake and increased energy expenditure through exercise remains the mainstay of treatment for and prevention of obesity (Sothern, Gordon, & von Almen, 2006). Behavior modification and psychosocial education are integrated into educational sessions by a psychologist or other certified mental health or behavioral counseling professional. Behavior modification skills are taught, stressing how discussion, modeling, role playing, and guided problem solving are used. Topics such as self-monitoring, commitment, limit setting, habit formation, goal setting and action plans, decision-making skills, attitudes, and assertiveness training are discussed.

SAMPLE ACTIVITY DESCRIPTIONS

Group behavior—Goal setting

The behavior specialist will discuss with the participants how to set weekly, realistic behavior goals. They will be encouraged to record the goals on the Weekly Goal-Setting Form and Exercise Record (Tables 6.13–6.16) so that the specialist can revisit the goals during the next weekly class. Goals will be set in nutrition and physical activity. For example, a nutrition goal may be to replace two unhealthy snack foods with new vegetables. An exercise goal may be to perform 10 stomach crunches three times during the week or stretch while watching a favorite television program (Sothern, Gordon, & von Almen, 2006; Sothern, von Almen, & Schumacher, 2001).

Exercise—The Flex Test

The instructor will guide the parents through an evaluation of different areas of the body. Initially the parent will observe the child from a side view to determine whether the head and shoulders are aligned with the rest of the body. An appropriate area will be checked in the handout (see Chapter 4) if an imbalance is present. The child will then observe the parent. The instructor will discuss methods to correct the imbalances. He or she also will demonstrate corrective exercises. The parents will repeat this process with the other areas of the body (e.g., back, knees, etc.). The class will end with a stretching routine to music (Sothern, Gordon, & von Almen, 2006; Sothern, von Almen, & Schumacher, 2001).

Nutrition—Nutrition games: Fast-food follies

The instructor will review the fast-food list in the program book (Sothern et al., 2001). She will ask participants to volunteer to weigh food and help to calculate caloric and fat content of various fast-food meals. Compare best and worst choices: fried chicken dinner versus grilled chicken dinner, bacon-double cheeseburger with large fries and a regular drink versus grilled chicken sandwich with small fries and a diet drink. The instructor will measure and weigh items in class and have participants touch and feel the grease on the fried items.

 Key Points: Examples of Average Values

Fried chicken: 100 calories and 10 grams fat per ounce.
Fried hamburger: 100 calories and 10 grams fat per ounce.
Grilled chicken: 55 calories and 3 grams fat per ounce.
Cheese on sandwich: 100 calories and 10 grams fat per ounce (average).
French fries: 125 calories and 5 grams fat per ounce.
Average mayonnaise on sandwich (1 tablespoon): 135 calories and 15 grams fat per ounce.
Free toppings: mustard, ketchup, lettuce, tomato, pickles, onions.
Hamburger bun (2 starch/bread): 160 calories and 0–2 grams fat per whole bun.
Biscuit (average): 125 calories and 5 grams of fat per ounce.

Sources: Adapted from Sothern et al., 2001; Sothern et al., 2006.

Staffing

The pediatric weight management intervention should be supervised by a coordinator with experience in clinical intervention trials whose duties and responsibilities include the following:

1. Promotion and advertising
2. Ordering supplies
3. Recruitment
4. Phone screenings
5. Developing filing system for study participants, ensuring privacy, and securing approval and required documentation from referring or primary physician
6. Scheduling study participants and staff for testing and intervention
7. Recordkeeping and reporting
8. Data access, filing, and management
9. Set-up for weekly classes
10. Medical monitoring and weigh-in weekly (1 hour)
11. Compliance, attendance, and follow-up procedures
12. Regulatory (state and federal) procedures as necessary

Scheduling

The groups will meet on the same day at a location in two separate meeting areas; however, the groups will meet at different times so that staff members are able to coordinate schedules. Also, the schedule may be adjusted to account for the existing class schedule at the class location (see the sample schedule).

ORIENTATION

Individualized treatment accompanied by long-term educational follow-up is the most effective approach to the prevention and management of pediatric obesity. During the first orientation meeting, this concept should be discussed with the families of the overweight or obese patient.

It is important to stress that the intervention is closely supervised; thus, the child receives uncompromising care of the highest quality from the pediatric, behavior, exercise, and nutrition specialists. Also, by implementing a tailored approach in a supportive group setting, the child's physical and emotional well-being will be enhanced. Health care providers should emphasize to the families that weight loss and maintenance are the attractive side effects of the overall lifestyle focus of the program.

Talking Points: The "A" Factor (Verbal cues for patients or parents and family members)
Read through the following information with your patient or family members to help them to understand the exercise strategy used in the program.

We believe the success of the Pediatric Weight-Management Program is due to the "A" Factors:

- Availability of the highly committed program professionals. We are deeply concerned with the child's progress, health, and overall emotional well-being.
- Accountability of the child to the program staff. Each week, the parents and children report their progress to the staff and are responsible for compliance with the program guidelines. Written records of weight, exercise, and diet are examined by the staff every week, which we believe increases program compliance and success.
- Attention of only the positive kind. When the child does well, she or he receives strong positive reinforcement from the program staff. If the child does not do well, he or she receives encouragement to try harder the next week, but attention is quickly focused to another area of the program.

INITIAL EVALUATION

The objective of the medical component of the pediatric weight management program is to ensure that the intervention is safe and effective. This is determined by evaluating the program's impact on physiologic, metabolic, biochemical, and psychosocial parameters. Detailed protocols of these measures are found in Chapter 7 and Chapter 8.

Once the initial evaluation is performed, participants are assigned to groups 1 (red), 2 (yellow), or 3 (green) based on their initial BMI percentile. This level is also used to determine a recommended term of treatment. Children in level 1 are encouraged to attend the program for 1–2 years. Those in level 2 should participate in the program for at least 1 year and, children in level 3 are given a 6–12-month term of treatment.

WEEKLY INTERVENTION SESSIONS

During the first few months of the program, children and adolescents attend weekly 2-hour comprehensive sessions (Tables 6.17 and 6.18). During the medical monitoring period, students who are waiting can be directed to an outdoor park area that includes stationary park equipment and outdoor game supplies, such as jump ropes, balls, and Hula-Hoops. This will provide an additional opportunity for the families to engage in physical activity. An indoor nutrition and fitness activity center also may be set up with nutrition books, puzzles, games, and indoor physical activity supplies, such as jump ropes, softballs, mats, music, and videos, in case of inclement weather. This center also will serve as a demonstration area to encourage parents to create environments for play inside and outside of their own homes. Parents are instructed to supervise the children in the center during the free-play sessions.

Weekly sessions begin with group discussion highlighting the patients' accomplishments for the week (Sothern, von Almen, & Schumacher, 2001; Sothern, Schumacher, et al., 2002; Sothern, von Almen, et al., 1999; Sothern, von Almen, et al., 1993; von Almen, Sothern &

Table 6.17 Sample Weekly Clinic Intervention Schedule

Week	Topic	Activity
1	Getting ready for change	MPEP Step (Exercise Group) Veggie Tasting (Diet Group) Commitment Rating (All)
2	Warming up and cooling down, monitoring Dietary exchange system Hunger versus craving	Imitation Aerobics or Metabolic Engines of the Body: Pacing Skills—Varied Ethnic Music (Exercise Group) Stop-and-Go Foods (Diet Group) Goal Setting (All)
3	Mood and weight loss Goal setting The dairy group	Be a Goal Getter Family Relay (Exercise Group) Plan-a-Meal Circle (Diet Group) Behavior Bingo (All)
4	Reading labels Understanding limitations Role modeling	Fast-Food Lab (Diet Group) Cue Elimination (All) Family Aerobic Softball (Exercise Group)
5	Aerobic versus anaerobic metabolism Portion Control Planning meals	Aerobic Equipment Orientation (Exercise Group) Fun in the Kitchen: Low-Fat Chicken Tenders (Diet Group) Role Play: Positive Parenting (All)
6	Aerobic field sports Fruits and sugars Principles of behavior	Aerobic Soccer (Exercise Group) Food Lab: Fruit Group (Diet Group) Role Play: Problem Solving (All)
7	Healthy snacks Muscular flexibility	Snack Jeopardy (Diet Group) The Flex Test Stretch-and-Flex Series (Exercise Group) Social Sabotage (All)
8	Stepping out—Tips for dining outside the home Outdoor family fitness activities	Family Flag Football (Exercise Group) Role Play: Restaurant (Diet Group) Good/Bad; Healthy/Not (All)
9	Strength (MPEP-PUMP) Protein food group	Indoor Strength Circuit (Exercise Group) Food Lab: Meat Group (Diet Group) Role Play: After School (All)
10	Nutrition facts Aerobic exercise	Fast Food Follies or Nutrition Wheel of Fortune (Diet Group) African Dance (Exercise Group) Relapse Prevention (All)
11	Evaluation day	Evaluation Day
12	Awards Field day	Awards Field Day

Sources: Sothern, M., von Almen, T. K., Gordon, S. (Eds.), *Handbook of Pediatric Obesity: Clinical Management*, Taylor & Francis, Boca Raton, FL, 2006; Sothern, M. S., von Almen, T. K., Schumacher, H., *Trim Kids: The Proven Plan That Has Helped Thousands of Children Achieve a Healthier Weight*, Harper Collins, New York, NY, 2001.

Table 6.18 Typical Weekly Clinic Schedule

Time	Nutrition group activity	Exercise group activity
4:30–5:00 PM	Behavioral therapy	Medical monitoring and weigh-in
5:00–5:30 PM	Medical monitoring and weigh-in	Behavioral therapy
5:30–6:30 PM	Nutrition class	Exercise class

Schumacher, 2006). Positive reinforcement is given for trying new vegetables, turning down high-calorie snacks, or participating in physical activity. Goals are set for the next week and behavior modification skills are introduced using discussion, modeling, role playing, and guided problem solving.

Patients with psychological problems should be referred to a therapist for additional individual counseling while continuing in the program. Award certificates, inexpensive sports equipment, and other incentives items are given quarterly as positive reinforcement for achieving short-term goals. Special events, such as roller skating parties, park and field days, and holiday parties are organized during the one-year program to encourage continued participation.

At the beginning of the program, the participants receive education materials and Weekly Goal-Setting Forms and Exercise Records (Tables 6.13–6.16), which are color-coded to their level of overweight (Sothern, Gordon, & von Almen, 2006; Sothern, von Almen, & Schumacher, 2001). The color coding of the forms and records is used as positive reinforcement as participants move from one weight level into another.

PROCEDURES FOR ABSENTEES
Absentees are handled as follows: After one absence children should be telephoned and encouraged to come in the next week. After two absences, they should again be telephoned and reminded that they do not have to report their weight during the meeting. They will be encouraged to provide nutrition and physical activity accomplishments during the following meeting. It is very important at this point that the patient be handled in a positive manner he or she they returns. Instructors should refrain from giving negative attention to their re-gain or lack of compliancy. After three absences, the patient's physician should be notified and encouraged to telephone the patient. Also, the staff behavioral specialist or psychologist should be notified.

After four absences, the family should be scheduled for a group consult with all of the members of the staff. After this meeting, if attendance does not improve, the patient should be asked to leave the program. A follow-up questionnaire should be filled out before his or her departure that explains his or her reason for leaving. Every attempt should be made to avoid negative reinforcement of poor attendance or relapse. Words such as "cheating" or "fat" should not be used when interviewing patients. Exercise staff (instructors, interns, and assistants), nutrition staff (dietitians, interns, and assistants), and medical staff (nurses and physician) should confine questions and comments to exercise, nutrition, and medically related issues. Behavior issues should be addressed by the behavioral specialist or psychologist experienced in counseling families.

FOLLOW-UP EVALUATION
To determine whether the program intervention is safe and effective, an evaluation of the program's impact on physiologic, metabolic, biochemical, and psychosocial parameters should be implemented. Detailed protocols of these measures are found in Chapter 7 and Chapter 8. After attending 10 sessions, the children should again participate in the measurements outline in the initial evaluation. It is important to ensure that the same equipment is being used to measure height, weight, and waist circumference. Ideally the children should have the same clothes on as they did during the first session. Take a picture of the children and keep a copy in the student file and give one to the parents. If you did not take a picture during the first measurement session, ask the parents to bring in a "before" picture for you to keep in the file. After the follow-up evaluation is performed, fill out the Quarterly Evaluation Form in Chapter 7. This form compares the child's measures before and after completing the first 12-week session. Give one copy to the parents, send one to the pediatrician or family physician, and keep one in the student chart. Encourage the parents to bring the child in to see the family physician or pediatrician to discuss the results. Also, if the doctor recommends repeat blood tests, ask the parent to bring in the results so that you can discuss accomplishments.

Many of the children have prediabetes and it is likely that they will have positive changes in glucose and insulin. Most children will show improvements in cholesterol (see Chapter 9).

Although the students who just completed this first 10-week session (continuing students) are participating in measures, the newly enrolled children should be participating in the orientation class, which you should conduct as you did for the first 12-week session. Explain to the new students that next week they will have their measurements taken to determine the color level where they will begin.

QUARTERLY AWARDS FOR EXERCISE ACCOMPLISHMENTS

After the 10th class is completed, determine which of the children attended all the sessions. These children should receive an award for perfect attendance. Use the Weekly Goal-Setting Form and Exercise Record (Tables 6.13–6.16) to figure out which boy and girl participated in the most minutes of exercise during the past 10 weeks. During week 12, provide an inexpensive, physically active toy or sports equipment to the children with: (1) perfect attendance, (2) most minutes of exercise (one boy and one girl), and (3) most vegetables (one boy and one girl). Using the newly calculated BMI, determine which of the children grew enough or lost enough weight to graduate to the next color level. Usually, if the child has good attendance, reports a large number of exercise minutes and vegetables, and reports being able to run faster and exercise longer, then we graduate him or her to the next level. Most children will fall into this category. Explain to the children who did not graduate that sometimes it takes 6 months to graduate and to be patient and continue participating. Strongly encourage the children to continue in the program. Explain to them that those children who complete 1 year of the program are the ones who typically maintain their weight loss. Usually at 3 months, most children are about 25% of the way toward meeting their goals; at 6 months, they are at 50%, and after 1 year of consistent participation, most children easily achieve their goals.

While the continuing students are receiving their rewards, the new students are participating in measurements. Do not forget to take a "before" picture and make sure that you are taking an accurate height reading. This is very important as for every 1 inch the child grows he or she can weigh 3 to 5 more pounds. So, if a child does not lose any weight on the scale after 12 weeks, but he or she grows 2 inches, he or she has really lost 6 to 10 pounds.

MANAGING TWO GROUPS (NEW AND CONTINUING STUDENTS) SIMULTANEOUSLY

All students, new and continuing, weigh in as usual and show their food and physical activity records to the staff. During the group discussion, all of the students and their families, new and continuing, will sit together to report their accomplishments. After this, the new students along with their families will go to the behavior session and the continuing students along with their families will go to the nutrition session. After about 20–30 minutes, the sessions should swap, new students will go to the behavior session and continuing students will go to the nutrition session. Afterward, they will all participate in exercise together. During exercise, it is a good idea to have the children who are in the red and yellow program grouped together on one side of the room and those in the green and blue on the other side. This way, the instructor can better help the students pace their exercise intensity so that they do not get tired too fast.

Afterward, determine how best to stagger the sessions so that each of the groups is able to learn the material outlined in the educational materials (Sothern, Gordon, & von Almen, 2006; Sothern, von Almen, & Schumacher, 2001). For example, in week two the new students will require the entire time to learn about the meal plan, the continuing students could play one of the behavior games (Sothern, Gordon, & von Almen, 2006), or they could review the commitment rating, goal setting, and self-monitoring. It also may be beneficial during these classes, to keep the groups together, especially if a new cooking demonstration is planned. There are no strict rules, just arrange the schedule so that the continuing students always are engaged with some kind of learning. It also is appropriate, however, for the continuing students to participate in a review occasionally. The exercise sessions also can be staggered with the behavior and nutrition, especially when you are introducing newer advanced material that the new students may not be able to master.

Throughout each session, there should be 1–2 weeks when the behavioral counselor is available to speak with the parents on their own without the children and vice versa. This activity, however, should not take the place of having the parents exercise with the children. Instead, have the children attend a fun cooking demonstration while the behavioral counselor covers some of the parenting tips or have the parents discuss new recipes while the behavior counselor speaks to the students about how to deal with teasing from other children.

 Key Points: Tips for a Successful Multidisciplinary Pediatric Weight Management Program

1. Make sure the sessions are both fun and educational for the children. Remember the children are not mini-adults. They need to be entertained to keep their interest and they have short attention spans. Keep the sessions to 20 minutes most of the time and never keep them seated for more than 30 minutes (remember the 30-Minute Rule). If the parents report to you that their child does not want to come, then try to find out why. If more than one of the students in any one class expresses that they do not want to attend, then the classes probably are not entertaining enough.
2. Continue to stress to the students and their families that this is a program designed to help children achieve a healthier lifestyle. If they accomplish this, then they should also achieve a healthier weight. But because they are growing, they are not likely to see large weight losses over short periods of time. Stress that rapid weight loss is unhealthy and that some children may just "grow into" their weight.
3. Allow children who decided not to continue into another session to come in periodically to check in. If they gain weight encourage them to re-enroll; however, be very positive and understanding. This is not the time to scold them, rather tell them they just had a "lapse" and that to prevent a "relapse," they should recommit to the program for another session. Tell them your door is always open to their recommitting to a healthier life.
4. If you have one of more families that show signs of emotional problems, its best to refer them to their pediatrician or family physician for help. Their doctor can refer them to outside counseling, if necessary. It usually is recommended that they continue in the program while they are seeing the counselor with their doctor's approval.
5. Conduct staff debriefing sessions on a regular basis to discuss some of the challenges and propose solutions.
6. Once you become more experienced, you may want to implement new exercise activities that you develop, just ensure that they are safe and entertaining for children.

The maintenance level (blue) will begin after a participant achieves his or her goal weight, which is determined quarterly after each evaluation by the dietitian and the physician. Once the goal weight is achieved, subjects are encouraged to continue to attend weekly 2-hour sessions for the remainder of their recommended term of treatment.

SUMMARY
Pediatric weight management programs should integrate medical, nutrition, behavioral, and exercise recommendations into tailored, family-based interventions that are both educational and entertaining. The child–family group dynamics and peer modeling are primary components of successful management of obesity in youth. Several factors contribute to the success of such approaches (Sothern, 2006; Sothern & Gordon, 2005; Sothern, Gordon, & von Almen, 2006; Sothern, Schumacher, et al., 2002; Sothern, von Almen, & Schumacher, 2001; Sothern, von Almen, et al., 1993, 1999):

- Sessions are designed to entertain the children and promote initial success.
- Educational components feature parent-training methods in short, interactive sessions.
- Tailored dietary counseling results in noticeable weight loss, which motivates the patient to continue and improves exercise tolerance, thus, enabling increased physical activity.
- The program team provides consistent feedback. The patients and their families receive results and updates every 3 months. Most important, the program is conducted in groups of families.

Talking Points: Tips for Parents (Verbal cues for patients or parents and family members)

Read through the following information with your patient or family members to help them to understand the exercise strategy used in the program.

- Realize that young children have immature metabolic systems. Do not impose adult exercise regimens or goals on children.
- Encourage participation in aerobic activities appropriate for the child's age and size.
- Provide opportunities for young children to safely climb, run, and jump to encourage the development of muscular strength and endurance.
- Families that play together, stay healthy together. Reserve at least half a day of each weekend for family physical fitness.
- Gradually replace television, computer, and video games with indoor and outdoor play.

Clinical Reminders for the Health Care Professional: Childhood Obesity Recommendations

- Obesity is a chronic disease. Treatment should be lifelong. When the treatment is withdrawn, the patient usually regains the weight lost.
- All pediatric obesity management programs should be supervised by a pediatrician or family physician.
- Consult a registered dietitian for specific nutrition recommendations.
- Praise children when they engage in healthy behaviors.
- When unhealthy behaviors emerge, ignore, redirect, or problem solve.
- Set short-term, achievable goals and reward the child's successes.
- Reevaluate the child's condition every 3–6 months.

40-WEEK EXERCISE CURRICULUM FOR GROUP, FAMILY, CLINICAL, AND HOME-BASED EXERCISE INSTRUCTION

The moderate-intensity, progressive exercise educational curriculum is based on the individual needs of children in different ranges of obesity (Sothern, 1998, 2001, 2006; Sothern & Gordon, 2005; Sothern, Gordon, & von Almen, 2006; Sothern, Schumacher, et al., 2002; Sothern, von Almen, & Schumacher, 2001; Sothern, von Almen, et al., 1993, 1999). In each level, the activities described have been chosen because they are safe and effective for the child with a particular obese physical condition. The following section includes lesson plans and descriptions of activities, which may be performed during the clinic or at home and which are based on developmentally appropriate recommendations, color coded to level of obesity, medical condition, and training status (Daniels et al., 2009; Milteer et al., 2012; Murray et al., 2013; Sothern, 2001, 2006; Sothern, Gordon, & von Almen, 2006; Sothern, von Almen, & Schumacher, 2001; U.S. DHHS, 2008; U.S. Preventive Services Task Force, 2010). A list of lesson topics can be found in Table 6.19. Chapters 2, 3, and 4 provide specific

Table 6.19   Lesson Topics at a Glance

Level 1, Red (Severe Obesity)
1. Orientation, Exercise Benefits, Safety, Increasing Your Daily Activity (MPEP Step), and the Homework Rule
2. Warm-Up (MPEP Prep), Metabolic Systems (aerobic exercise to music—different intensities), Cool Down after Exercise
3. Cardiorespiratory Endurance, Monitoring Heart Rate, Proper Use of Aerobic Equipment, Low-Impact or Chair Aerobics
4. Muscular Strength and Endurance, Weightlifting Technique (MPEP Pump)
5. Planning for Holidays, Family Field Sports (flag football)
6. Flexibility: Flex Test, Flex-and-Stretch Series
7. Individual Differences (body types and composition), Spinning (cycle) Class or Aerobic Circuit Class, Abdominal Crunch Challenge
8. Metabolic Rates, Maximize Your Workout, Water Aerobics
9. Exercise Myths, Specialty Theme Aerobics, or Line Dancing (guest instructor)
10. Park Day: Outdoor Play (bring your bikes, scooters, skateboards)

Level 2, Yellow (Obese)
1. Increasing Your Daily Activity: Creating Outdoor Play Areas, Obstacle Course
2. Cardiorespiratory Endurance, Family Field Sports (aerobic volleyball)
3. Metabolic Engine Review, Rockin' to the Oldies
4. Strength Facts: Muscle Fibers, Strength Circuit Class
5. Cross-Training: Body Sculpting or "Toning" Class
6. Flex Test, Modified Yoga, Relax Your Back
7. Fat Metabolism, Steady-State Activities, Aerobic Circuit with Exercise Equipment, Abdominal Crunch Challenge
8. Raising Activity Levels: Family Team Sports (aerobic soccer)
9. Guest Instructor: Ballroom or Theme Dancing
10. Park Day: Walking Aerobics

Level 3, Green (Overweight)
1. Increasing Daily Activities: Inside When the Weather Is Bad, Imagination Station, Balloon Games, Classy Moves, 30-minute Rule
2. Specialty Aerobics: Salsa/Latin Dance, Review Metabolic Systems
3. Cardiorespiratory Endurance: The Fit Kit Walking Program, Neighborhood or Nature Walk
4. Muscular Strength and Endurance, Advanced Resistance Training, Pull Your Own Weight Series
5. Planning for Family and Holiday Events: Aerobic Musical Chairs, Easter Egg Charades
6. Flex Test 1: Pilates (guest instructor)
7. Interval Training and Periodization: Relays (indoor or outdoor), Be a Goal Getter
8. Getting the Most Out of Your Workout, 20 Ways to Burn 20 Calories, Combined Strength and Aerobic Circuit
9. Family Field Sports (aerobic softball)
10. MPEP Step Contest: Fun Walk or Run in the Park

Level 4, Blue (Healthy Weight)
1. Increasing Daily Activities: Exercising on the Road, Roller or Inline Skating, Field Trip
2. MPEP Ultimate Workout, Beach Party Aerobics with Beach Balls
3. Cardiorespiratory Endurance, Aerobic Equipment Triathlon
4. Muscular Strength and Endurance: Band-Aid for Out-of-Shape Muscles
5. Family Field Sports: The Family Hike (if it rains, play laser tag or go roller skating)
6. Flex Test: Martial Arts (guest instructor)
7. Family Field Sports (basketball)
8. Exercise Techniques: Tennis Lesson and Drills
9. Power Sports: Discussion, Guest Speaker (professional athlete)
10. Family Field Sports: Field Day (annual)

instructions, illustrations, and recommendations for aerobic, strength, and flexibility activities included in the following lessons plans:

PUTTING RESEARCH INTO PRACTICE: WEEKLY EXERCISE LESSON PLANS TAILORED TO OVERWEIGHT AND OBESE YOUTH

LESSON 1, LEVEL 1 (RED)

Table 6.20   Overview: Lesson 1, Level 1 (Red)

Suggested time: 20–40 minutes (Total time)	Activities	Materials and staff needed
5–10 minutes	Introduction: Orientation, Exercise Benefits, Safety	Parents and patients' educational materials and books (Sothern, von Almen, & Schumacher, 2001)
10–20 minutes	Activity I: Increasing Your Daily Activity: PEP Step	
5–10 minutes	Activity II: The Home Work Rule	Exercise attire Staff: Exercise trainer

Objectives
After participation in this lesson the student will be able to:
1. Gain knowledge concerning the benefits of exercise and increasing daily physical activity to health.
2. Recognize safe methods to engage in exercise.
3. Identify the benefits to walking briskly with good posture.
4. Gain time management skills necessary to include daily physical activity into the home and family routine after school.

INTRODUCTION
The instructor will briefly describe the benefits of exercise to overall health and provide tips for ensuring a safe workout. Methods to encourage overweight and obese children to increase their overall daily energy expenditure are an integral component of pediatric weight management programs. One method that will help patients achieve this goal is to encourage them to walk more briskly, with better posture.

BENEFITS OF EXERCISE
Regular physical activity is shown to lessen the burden of obesity-related comorbidities, including reductions in blood pressure, increased insulin sensitivity, and decrease in hepatomegaly (Hassink et al., 2008). Vigorous, intermittent physical activity is shown to reduce components of the metabolic syndrome in prepubertal children (Barbeau et al., 2007; Kahle et al., 1996; Nassis et al., 2005; Shaibi et al., 2006; Yu et al., 2005). Moreover, physical activity improves metabolic health in obese youth independent of adiposity change (Shaibi et al., 2009). Significant improvements in body composition are associated with exercise programs, including low- to moderate-intensity aerobic and high-repetition strength training (LeMura & Maziekas, 2002). Regular physical activity reduces depression, and childhood obesity is associated with depression (Erickson et al., 2000). Regular participation in exercise reduces inflammatory cytokines (Radak et al., 2008), and childhood obesity is associated with inflammation and asthma (Arshi et al., 2010). Furthermore, physical activity lifestyle changes positively alter satiety factors in youth (Balagopal et al., 2010). In contrast to these outcomes of regular physical activity, chronic sustained periods of muscular unloading

(sitting) reduce contractile stimulation, suppress muscle lipoprotein lipase, triglyceride and glucose uptake, and high-density lipoprotein production (Bey & Hamilton, 2003; Thomas et al., 2005).

The benefits of chronic exercise training to the ability of the body to use fat as a fuel (e.g., fat oxidation) are numerous. Endurance-trained muscle stores more glycogen and fat than untrained muscle (Byrne & Wilmore, 2001). In addition, as exercise training is continued, oxidative enzyme activity and free fatty acid levels increase (Hurley & Hagberg, 1998; Kelley et al., 1999). Over time, there is an increased use of fat as an energy source and a sparing of muscle and liver glycogen (Talanian et al., 2007). Eventually after 6–8 weeks of consistent exercise training, the lactate threshold increases, reflecting an improved ability to perform exercise aerobically at higher intensities (Tonkonogi et al., 2000). Once an individual reaches this status, fitness levels will be maintained as long as the training is consistent.

Key Points: Consistent Training

In formerly sedentary individuals, following consistent training the following improvements in fitness may be expected:

Training Duration (weeks)	Percent Improvement in Fitness
6–12	~25%
12–24	~50%
24–36	~75%
36–52	~100%

After 1 year of consistent training, untrained individuals may reach their individual genetic potential.

Clinical Reminders for the Health Care Professional: Safety Tips

Be sure to emphasize these safety tips to your patient:

- Stop exercising if you feel any discomfort in a muscle or joint. It is normal to feel a gentle burning sensation, but if the pain is worse than that, stop immediately! Your will need to report it to your teacher, coach, exercise physiologist, or me the next time I see you.
- Do the exercise exactly as instructed. The exercises have been designed especially for you and you should not change them.
- Always warm up before exercise and cool down and stretch after exercise. In the next lesson we will show you how.

ACTIVITY I. INCREASING YOUR DAILY ENERGY EXPENDITURES AND THE PEP STEP

The instructor should begin by asking the children to walk around the room so parents can watch. Most children will shuffle slowly with their heads down and shoulders rolled forward. The instructor then should ask the parents to watch their son or daughter during this activity.

Once the children have walked around the room, the instructor should ask them to stand side by side at the front of the room. Then, the instructor should drop his or her head, roll shoulders forward, and walk slowly in front of the children several times. The instructor should use the following verbal cues:

Talking Points: The PEP Step (Verbal cues for patients or parents and family members)
Read through the following information with your patient or family members to help them to understand the exercise strategy used in the program.

"OK, now watch this"
Instructor walks slowly in front of the students with head and shoulders down.
"Does this look familiar? Who do I look like? Do I look very tall? How tall do I look?"
One or more of the children will typically respond, "Four feet tall!" Use this moment to engage the families by laughing along.
"Do I look important and like I know where I'm going? Can you even see my face? When your head is down and your shoulders are hunched forward, no one can see your pretty face! You appear shorter and more overweight."

Demonstrate how to do the PEP step. Lift your head and hold your shoulders back. Walk forward briskly, while smiling widely in front of children and their parents. Use the following verbal cues:

Talking Points: The PEP Step (Verbal cues for patients or parents and family members)

"Now who do I look like?" "A supermodel (or super athlete or movie star), right?"
The children and families will typically laugh at this point.
"Maybe not, but I do look taller and more important, don't I? Actually, I look about five to six inches taller just because I lifted my head. And because of that, I also look about 25 to 30 pounds lighter. "When you walk with your chin up, shoulders back in a brisk manner, you appear taller, fitter, more in control. You look like you know where you are going. You look important!" And, you also look 25–30 pounds lighter, too. This is why this program works so well; because everyone loses about 25–30 pounds in the first week!"
Everyone laughs.
"O.K. now it's your turn to do the PEP step. Follow me."
Students now walk briskly around the room with head and shoulders back.
"Now grab mom (or dad, grandmother, other family member) by the hand and get her to follow you and do the PEP step, too."
Family members follow their son or daughter.

Participants will become energized, feel taller and fitter, and gain more control through the action of lifting the chin, pulling back the shoulders, tightening the tummy, and taking quick, long steps. Also, the participants will gain instantaneous mastery over the environment, a newfound feeling of self-control, and hope for future success. The class ends with instructions for the kids to walk in this manner on their way home as well as for the rest of the week. Additional motivation for the kids is that brisk walking burns more calories and results in more weight loss, and the kids will feel and look fitter, taller, and healthier.

Key Points: Increasing Daily Physical Activity

Information on the value of increasing daily activity can be transferred through illustration of the term "work." Work is equal to the force times the distance; force is equal to the weight moved (this is a simplification) and distance is equal to the area covered in one step. When more space is covered in one step, more work is performed in the same amount of time, and therefore more calories are burned.

Talking Points: Walking Briskly Increases Physical Activity (Verbal cues for patients or parents and family members)
Read through the following information with your patient and/or family members to help them to understand the exercise strategy used in the program.

Think about large people. Do they move fast? Usually not, and that may be one reason why they are large. When you move slowly, you do not burn many calories. You also do not use many muscles, and those you do use are not used effectively. Now, think of people who walk briskly. They are usually fitter, taller, and appear more energetic. They automatically burn up more calories simply because they move faster and cover more ground in less time. It is amazing how simply walking faster, taking bigger strides, and holding your chin up a little higher can make you look and feel lighter and more effective. And that feels good!

We want you to burn as many calories as you can as often as you can. To do that, you will have to work your body more effectively on a regular basis. Now, when you hear the term "work," it will refer to how much energy you expend to burn calories. One way to work more effectively is to walk more briskly, covering as much ground as possible. By walking faster, you automatically increase your daily activity, which will help you lose—and keep off—the weight.

Case in Point: Real Words from Real Patients

Melissa [10 years old] was a participant in our program and lost 2 pounds in the first week just by walking with the PEP Step. She also reported that others reacted differently toward her, she accomplished more, and she felt much more energetic.

The instructor should review the four-level program with the patients and parents and then provide the Weekly Goal-Setting Form and Exercise Record (Tables 6.13–6.16). He or she then should discuss the goals and appropriate activities for the level that has been assigned to the patient.

ACTIVITY II. THE HOMEWORK RULE
The instructor should reemphasize to the patient that he or she should be moving around as much as possible. This also includes when he or she gets home from school. The following verbal cues should be used:

Talking Points: The Homework Rule (Verbal cues for patients or parents and family members)
Read through the following information with your patient or family members to help them to understand the exercise strategy used in the program.

Put off homework until after you exercise. When you get home from school, you may feel tired, but it is your brain that's pooped, not your body!

As soon as you get home from school, drink a big glass of ice water. Maybe you are tired because you are thirsty or dehydrated (not having enough water in your body can cause fatigue).

If the weather's nice, go outside and play. Ride your bike, skate, or walk the dog, or play ball, tag, or jump rope. If the weather is bad, come inside to your new play area, turn on some music, and dance. Whatever you do, it has to be active!

You need be active for at least 30 minutes before you start your homework. An hour would be even better! This will give your brain a chance to rest from the long school day. After you exercise, do homework. There may be time before dinner for television. You can do your Strength-and-Flex Exercises while you watch your favorite show.

Talking Points: Indoor and Outdoor Active Play (Verbal cues for patients or parents and family members)
Read through the following information with your patient or family members to help them to understand the exercise strategy used in the program.

Encourage your child to do as much playing as possible. Let him or her know that playing burns even more calories than structured exercise. Weave his or her favorite playful activities into daily life. Work with him or her to create indoor and outdoor play areas where he or she will want to spend time. Be imaginative! Resist the urge to push, thinking more will be better. If he or she can do it, great. But if you assign him or her less to do, he or she may do more.

LESSON 2, LEVEL 1

Table 6.21   Overview: Lesson 2, Level 1 (Red)

Suggested time: 45–60 minutes (Total time)	Activities	Materials and staff needed
5 minutes	Introduction	Parents and patients' educational materials and books (Sothern, von Almen, & Schumacher, 2001) Exercise attire Music player Staff: Exercise trainer or guest aerobic dance instructor
5 minutes	Activity I: Warming Up	
25–35 minutes	Activity II: Metabolic Engines of the Body	
5–10 minutes	Aerobics and Anaerobic Exercises	
5 minutes	Activity III: Cooling Down	

Objectives
After participation in this lesson the student will be able to:
1. Identify safe methods to warm up the body prior to engaging in an exercise session.
2. Identify differences between aerobic versus anaerobic exercise.
3. Gain knowledge concerning the benefits of aerobic exercise to health.
4. Develop pacing skills to monitor exercise performance to increase duration.
5. Identify movement and exercises that will improve cardiorespiratory (aerobic) endurance.
6. Identify safe methods to cool down the body after engaging in an exercise session.

INTRODUCTION

The instructor will discuss the importance of warming up before participating in physical activity. He or she will lead the patients in a 3–5 minute warm-up routine to music. The instructor then will lead the students in a 30–45 minute low-impact aerobic class while instructing them about the different metabolic engines of the body (e.g., aerobic and anaerobic). The class will end with a discussion of the importance and demonstration of cooling down after exercise.

ACTIVITY I. TECHNIQUES FOR WARMING UP

The instructor should discuss the importance of warming up before beginning any exercise using the following verbal cues:

Talking Points: Warming Up (Verbal cues for patients or parents and family members)
Read through the following information with your patient or family members to help them to understand the exercise strategy used in the program.

You have just tied your sneakers and are about to go for an easy walk or bike ride around the park. Before you do any type of exercise, you will need to warm up for at least 5 minutes before each session. Warming up is simple: Move each part of your body in a slow, controlled manner. When you slowly move an arm, a leg, or a shoulder, your heart sends blood to that body part, delivering fuel to the muscles and tissues that are in motion. Moving your arms and legs helps the heart pump blood throughout your entire body, preparing your body for more movement. Try the suggestions below, or make up your own!

Some Warm-Up Suggestions:

- March in place for 3–5 minutes while moving your arms up and down.
- Do arm circles forward, then back, 20 times.
- Do 10 modified jumping jacks or "side jacks" (instead of jumping, alternate placing each heel out to the side on the floor while the arms go above the head).
- Tap each foot 20 times; then rise on your toes 10 times.

If you fail to "warm up" before you begin to exercise, you may deprive the arms and legs of essential fuel. Without enough fuel, the muscles cannot perform very well and they may even become injured. Now let's do some warm-up movements to music.

The instructor should play music that has a slow to moderate tempo and lead the students through several warm-up movements for about 3–5 minutes.

Case in Point: Real Words from Real Patients

My mom and dad are divorced. I live with my mom but I see my dad almost every day. My dad is really fit, and he kept bugging me about my weight. He'd make me go jogging with him and he'd get mad if I couldn't keep up. I started my exercise program last week. I was really happy when my teacher said that I didn't have to keep up with my dad anymore. Now my dad and I do fun things like basketball and bike riding. Sometimes I even beat him in bike races—I think he lets me win, but that's ok. I've already lost 12 pounds! Dad is so proud of me.

—Female patient, age 10

ACTIVITY II. METABOLIC ENGINES OF THE BODY—AEROBIC AND ANAEROBIC ACTIVITIES

During this activity, the instructor will discuss the metabolic system with the children and their families.

Young children are perfectly suited for short bursts of high-energy movement. Any mother of a preschool child knows this first-hand. Outdoor tag is a good example (burning about 350–400 calories per hour). Unfortunately, the spontaneous activity of young children decreases as they get older. Scientists do not know whether this is a natural occurrence or whether it is a result of their changing environment. For overweight and obese children and adolescents, activity may be less frequent because they are unable to keep up with the demands of certain sports, dance, or group games. In addition, their metabolic systems—the engines of their bodies—are different. Using a car as a metaphor, overweight and obese children run out of gas sooner because the excess weight makes their engine run harder when they move forward; just as a small car can go farther on the same amount of gas as a large truck.

Regardless of weight, a child's body has three types of engines (or metabolisms), much like a car has three different gears: one for fast takeoffs, one for start-and-stop driving, and one for highway driving:

Medium-slow

This engine enables movement for long stretches of time. This is the engine that is fired up for aerobic exercises. It uses a combination of oxygen, fat stored in the body, and sugar (or carbohydrates) for fuel. After about 20 minutes of activity at the same speed, the child's body begins to use more of the stored fat for fuel. If children have not eaten for several hours, their metabolic engines will utilize even more of that stored fat. The longer a child maintains the medium-slow speed, the more calories and fat will be burned.

Because overweight and obese children have more stored fat than others, they can exercise in the medium-slow engine for hours without running out of gas as long as their pace stays low and consistent. But they must keep it slow and steady for a long period of time. It is all right to move into the fast engine for a moment as long as it is brief and they return to the easier pace.

Fast

This engine taps into the body's anaerobic capabilities. "Anaerobic" means "without air"—this engine depends not on oxygen, but primarily on sugar stored in the muscles (glycogen) for its fuel source. Children use this engine whenever the speed of their activity increases to a higher level.

An overweight and obese child can use the fast engine until the workload becomes too difficult. At this point, a substance called lactic acid will build in his or her muscles. This substance will make his or her muscles burn and feel tired. The breathing rate will increase because he or she is trying to take in more oxygen in order to shift gears and begin using the medium-slow engine again. Unfortunately, because the fast engine is anaerobic, trying to take in more oxygen by breathing faster will not help. The child's body will not allow him to shift to the medium-slow aerobic engine unless he or she slows down.

 Key Points: The Engines of the Body

The fast engine has a very small fuel tank. It only takes between 3 and 5 minutes for a child to run out of gas. Unless activity is reduced to a speed or level to allow the child to shift to the medium-slow engine again, he or she will be physically unable to continue.
The fast engine is great for short periods of exercise that promote strength and power. Sprinting is one example. So are stomach crunches.

Super fast

Skilled and powerful athletes such as Olympic weightlifters, jumpers, or sprinters use the super-fast engine. It relies on chemicals made from fuel stored directly in muscle fibers and immediately ready for use. The tank of the super-fast engine is even smaller than the fast engine. When children turn on that engine, they will run out of gas in only 10 seconds.

Children can increase the size of the tanks in each of these engines by engaging in regular exercise training, increasing how often ("frequency") and how long ("duration") he or she spends being physically active during any given week. By doing this, eventually, the child will be able to exercise for longer periods in all of the metabolic engines.

 Clinical Reminders for the Health Care Professional: Excess Weight Is Physically Disabling

It is very important to listen to your overweight or obese patient. When they are exercising and say that they are tired, it means that they really are tired. If they say they are hurting, that means they really are hurting. Allow them to slow down or stop to catch their breath. Then, gently encourage them to begin moving again at a pace that is more comfortable. Do not make the mistake of thinking that your patient is faking his or her discomfort, because he or she probably is not. Most important, don't get irritated with your patient's limitations. Remember: His or her excess weight is physically disabling; he or she needs encouragement, not criticism.

It is important not to rush the process. The heavier the overweight or obese child is, the longer it will take for him or her to comfortably use and improve his engines. Obese children take at least 3 months to experience a noticeable change, and at least 6 months to reach their full potential for improvement. Severely obese children will take longer. Be patient, and always refer to the color-coded guidelines in the exercise plan detailed in this book as you gradually add more exercise into his or her routine. Help your patient practice taking his heart rate to help him better pace his effort. Please refer to the instructions in Lesson 3.

Case in Point: Real Words from Real Patients

My wife and I never realized that just by walking a couple days a week, stretching and flexing with our son, that we would see such dramatic effects. We're all happier, healthier and thinner because of it. Even Sophie, our dog, has started to run in the backyard again!

—Father of 7-year-old male patient

Key Points: Exercise Intensity

The body uses different fuel systems for different levels or "intensities" of work:

Initiation of Movement

Very Vigorous: When movement is first initiated from a resting position or when activity increases to an extremely vigorous pace for 0–10 seconds, the body uses a fuel called adenosine triphosphate (ATP), which is stored in the muscles.

Vigorous: From 10 seconds to 5 minutes, the body uses a fuel called glycogen, which also is stored in the muscles. After exercising vigorously for about 5 minutes, the muscles produce lactic acid, which causes muscles to feel tired and burn.

Low to Moderate: After 5 minutes, and for hours and hours after as long as the pace is kept to this level, the body uses glycogen plus oxygen in the air plus fat to make fuel and breathe out carbon dioxide.

During this exercise activity, the instructor will demonstrate how the metabolic system works with the children and their families using engines as the metaphor and music as the motivator. He or she will select three different pieces of music with varying tempos: one slow, one medium-fast, and one very fast. After several minutes of playing music with a slower beat, he or she will change it to a song with a faster beat and then one with a very fast tempo. The instructor will vary the pace of movement to match the beat of the music and encourage the children and families to do the same. The instructor will use the following verbal cues:

Talking Points: The Metabolic Engines of the Body (Verbal cues for patients or parents and family members)
Read through the following information with your patient or family members to help them to understand the exercise strategy used in the program.

"When you exercise, your body depends on three different engines to move. Your body has three engines. Engine 3 is the slowest engine, but it is the best one for getting rid of fat because you can do it for longer periods of time. Engine 2 is faster than Engine 3, and it works well for becoming stronger and more powerful. Engine 1 is the super-fast engine and is used by very powerful athletes such as Olympic weightlifters and jumpers. I am going to put on some music and you dance around to it."

After several minutes of dancing to one kind of music, the instructor should change it to another, and so on. After moving to each tempo, the instructor should ask the following:

"What type of engine are you using now?
How long do you think you can use this engine?

If you are using Engine 2, the fast engine, you will only be able to keep moving for up to about 5 minutes. If you are using Engine 1, the super-fast engine, you can only keep this up for about 10 seconds. But if you are using Engine 3, the slow engine, you can go on for hours because all this engine needs for fuel is your breathing (oxygen, stored fat, and some of what you have eaten) to make it run. This is the engine you use when exercising at a moderate intensity."

Talking Points: Aerobic Exercise (Verbal cues for patients or parents and family members)
Read through the following information with your patient or family members to help them to understand the exercise strategy used in the program.

Explain to your child that when doing aerobic exercises, he should use Engine 3 to burn the most calories. If he kicks into Engine 1 or 2, he is engaging in anaerobic exercise, which will not burn as many calories simply because he will not be able to sustain the pace for long enough time periods.

The instructor should review the following information so patients and families will grasp the difference between the two types of exercise using the following cues:

Talking Points: Aerobic Versus Anaerobic Exercise (Verbal cues for patients or parents and family members)
Read through the following information with your patient or family members to help them to understand the exercise strategy used in the program.

The word "aerobic" means with oxygen. "Anaerobic means" without oxygen. When you do aerobic activities, you send oxygen to the muscles. There, the oxygen mixes with glucose, a sugar that your body produces from carbohydrates and fats. Together, they produce fuel so your body can continue to participate in the aerobic activity. The stronger and better trained your cardiorespiratory system becomes from doing aerobic exercise, the more oxygen is delivered to your exercising muscles, and the more exercise you can do with more ease. The more trained your muscles are, the more they can accept and use that oxygen to make you go.

When you move into Engine 2 or an anaerobic pace, your body only uses the glucose—not oxygen—for fuel. You can do this for only between 3 and 5 minutes because when you burn glucose, a substance called lactic acid builds in your muscles. That is what creates a burning sensation in your muscles and, after a short time, depletes your muscles of energy. The more intensely you exercise, the faster the muscle fatigue occurs. At that point, you have to either slow down so that the oxygen demand is lower and the lactic acid is absorbed, or your body will be physically unable to continue.

The point at which your body shifts from aerobic to anaerobic exercise is called the anaerobic threshold. When you exercise hard enough to activate the anaerobic metabolism, your muscles will burn, you will be out of breath, and you will feel tired all over.

This does not mean anaerobic exercise is bad for you. In fact, to become stronger and more fit, you will have to use your anaerobic system to do quite a few activities.

Aerobic versus Anaerobic Activities

Aerobic	Anaerobic
Walking	Running, high speed
Jogging	Body toning (e.g., Pilates)
Cycling	Strength or resistance training
Treadmill or stair-climber	Gymnastic stunts
Lap swimming	Interval training
Aerobic dance	Wrestling
Long-distance field events	Sprints

ACTIVITY III. COOLING-DOWN TECHNIQUE

The instructor will provide direction to the children on the techniques for cooling down after exercise. About 5–10 minutes before your patient completes an exercise session—whether it is riding a bike, jogging, swimming, walking, or dancing—he or she will need to start cooling down. The child should do this gradually until he or she is maintaining a slow, easy pace. It is important that children continue at this pace for the last 10 minutes or so of their workout. Cooling down is important because your patient's body needs time to return to its normal heart rate and breathing pattern. Otherwise, the blood traveling to his or her exercising muscles will pool, or remain in the muscles. This can make your patient feel dizzy or nauseous, and he or she may experience painful muscle cramps. The instructor should use the following verbal cues:

Talking Points: Cooling Down (Verbal cues for patients or parents and family members)
Read through the following information with your patient or family members to help them to understand the exercise strategy used in the program.

The sign says 2 miles to the end of the park walking track. You are walking at a very brisk pace while swinging your arms vigorously. You are in your target heart rate zone. You know you only have 5–10 minutes left in your training session. What do you do now?

Slow down gradually to a very slow, easy pace for the remaining time. Why do you need to slow down your pace?

Your body needs time to return to its normal heart rate and breathing pattern. If you suddenly just stop in the middle of your training zone, the heart and lungs do not have time to adjust.

Cooling down is just like warming up. You simply move your arms and legs slowly after exercising, and your blood leaves the muscles and returns to the heart and lungs. Your legs even have a built-in pump to help with that process, but you have to keep them moving for the pump to work.

Slowing down before stopping your exercise also helps bring your temperature back to its normal range. That is why it is called cooling down!

No matter what exercise you are doing, always slow the pace for the last 5–10 minutes.

LESSON 3, LEVEL 1

Table 6.22   Overview: Lesson 3, Level 1 (Red)

Suggested time: 45 minutes (Total time)	Activities	Materials and staff needed
5–10 minutes	Introduction	Parents and patients' educational materials and books (Sothern, von Almen, & Schumacher, 2001)
10–15 minutes	Activity I: Cardiorespiratory Aerobic Exercise	
30–35 minutes	Activity II: Proper Use of Aerobic Equipment or Low-Impact or Chair Aerobics	Exercise attire Chairs Music player Staff: Exercise trainer or aerobic guest dance instructor

Objectives
After participation in this lesson the student will be able to:
1. Identify safe methods to participate in exercises to improve aerobic endurance.
2. Gain knowledge concerning the benefits of aerobic endurance training to health.
3. Gain knowledge and experience in techniques to identify intensity of exercise through heart rate monitoring.
4. Safely participate in an exercise session using aerobic equipment or chair aerobics.

INTRODUCTION

The instructor will introduce the term, cardiorespiratory endurance, and explain how to identify whether an activity will increase this fitness component. He or she will discuss the importance of properly using exercise equipment, provide instruction for each specific exercise machine and guide the patients as they exercise on the different machines. This can be done in a circuit format with patient's moving to the next exercise apparatus after 5–10 minutes of practice. If exercise equipment is not available, then the instructor may lead the class in a low-impact exercise routine to music. Provide chairs to severely obese children so that they may continue to perform arm motions if they become too fatigued to continue leg movements.

ACTIVITY I. CARDIORESPIRATORY AEROBIC EXERCISE

The instructor will use the following verbal cues to discuss cardiorespiratory or aerobic exercise:

Talking Points Exercise Activity Ideas (Verbal cues for patients or parents and family members)
Read through the following information with your patient or family members to help them to understand the exercise strategy used in the program.

Cardiorespiratory endurance exercise is a type of workout, which demands that your large muscles move at moderate or high intensity for long stretches of time. It is also called aerobic exercise and examples include walking, jogging, dancing, and swimming. Cardiorespiratory training can strengthen your heart and lungs, improve your stamina, keep your body in good, toned shape, and improve your outlook on life.

ACTIVITY II. PROPER USE OF AEROBIC EQUIPMENT

The instructor will educate the children in a group on methods to properly use treadmills, cycle ergometers, stair-climbers, rowing machines, or other similar equipment. He or she will emphasize moderate intensity and safety and will discuss the mechanisms on each apparatus that control intensity. The children will be allowed to try each of the machines for a 5- to 10-minute period.

Talking Points: Exercise Equipment (Verbal cues for patients or parents and family members)
Read through the following information with your patient or family members to help them to understand the exercise strategy used in the program.

If left up to children, most would prefer to burn calories while outside playing tag, swinging, chasing balls, or throwing themselves in a pile of fallen leaves. Older kids go outside for different reasons: to participate in sports, go for a bike ride, walk to the mall, or engage in a game of football. Sometimes, however, it is nice to have an option to exercise inside. Exercise machines can provide a good workout while your child watches television or reads. Younger kids are not as inclined to take these machines seriously, but it is not out of the question. A 10-year-old participant in our program loves the stationary bike. He rides it every day because it is the only time his mother lets him watch television!

Handout for Patients: Rate the Exercise Equipment

You increase the number of calories you burn by using more muscle groups at once. We have rated these exercise machines according to their calorie-burning potential.

***** Treadmill, cross-country ski machine, exercise cycle with handles, rowing machine

**** Stair-climber with handles and support

*** Outdoor cycle, exercise cycle (incline or upright), stair-climber with support rails

** Arm ergometer (arm crank)

* Abdominal crunch machine

No way! Avoid gadgets, typically advertised by celebrities on television and in magazines, that promise quick fixes, and other unrealistic claims.

The instructor should use the time while the children are using the exercise equipment to demonstrate the proper way to monitor intensity by taking their heart rate.

Handout for Patients: Testing Your Child's Heart Rate

When your child is moving, observe her breathing. Is she having difficulty? Is she red in the face? Is she complaining of being hot and tired? These are cues that she may be going too fast. It is a good reason to teach your child how to take her heart rate so that she will know the safest speed for her circumstances.

Resting Heart Rate: Get a watch or clock with a second hand. Ask your child to sit quietly for 5 minutes. Find her pulse by placing the middle three fingers of one hand on the underside of the opposite wrist. If you have difficulty locating her pulse this way, place the same three fingers on either side of her throat just below the point of the jaw, in between the Adam's apple and the neck muscle. There you will find the pulsing carotid artery. Be careful not to press it too hard. Once you feel her pulse, refer to the second hand of your watch and count the number of pulse beats during a 10-second interval.

Record the number of beat over 10 seconds: _____.
× 6 = _____ (Multiply the number by 6.)
Record the resting pulse rate: _____ .

(This figure represents your child's resting pulse rate in beats per minute.)

Active Heart Rate: After your child has been moving around for 10 minutes or more, repeat the process, but ask your daughter to remain standing and to keep her feet moving from side to side.

Record her active heart rate over 10 seconds: _____.
× 6 = _____ (Multiply this number by 6.)

Use this table to see whether she is in the correct range:

Your child is:	Level 3 (Green) Overweight	Level 2 (Yellow) Obese	Level 1 (Red) Severely Obese
Heart rate in beats per 10 seconds	26–28	23–26	19–23
Heart rate beats per minute	156–168	138–156	114–138

Clinical Reminders for the Health Care Professional: Guidelines for Exercise

The exercise program detailed in this book has adopted the guidelines developed by the American College of Sports Medicine (ACSM) for cardiorespiratory fitness, body composition, muscular strength, endurance, and flexibility. We suggest that only children who graduate to the maintenance phase or level of the program should follow these guidelines; other children should work toward them gradually. The program outlined in this book does this automatically.

LESSON 4, LEVEL 1

Table 6.23   Overview: Lesson 4, Level 1 (Red)

Suggested time: 40–60 minutes (Total time)	Activities	Materials and staff needed
5–10 minutes	Introduction: Muscular Strength and Endurance	Parents and patients' educational materials and books (Sothern, von Almen, & Schumacher, 2001) Exercise attire Hand weights and ankle weights Exercise mats Resistance bands Fat and lean weight models Staff: Exercise trainer
10–15 minutes	Activity I: Muscle and Fat Weightlifting (resistance training) Demonstration and Instruction (MPEP Pump)	
25–35 minutes	Activity II: Muscular Strength and Endurance Strength Training Circuit	

Objectives
After participation in this lesson the student will be able to:
1. Identify safe methods to participate in exercises to improve muscular strength and endurance.
2. Gain knowledge concerning the benefits of resistance training to health.
3. Safely participate in a resistance training circuit under the supervision of a parent or other adult
4. Gain knowledge concerning the specific muscle or muscle group that is responsible for varied types of body movement.

INTRODUCTION

The instructor will discuss the benefits of strength training and factors that affect the results. Proper technique and methods will be emphasized. Strength or resistance training may be used safely to enhance the efforts to prevent and reverse childhood obesity and other chronic pediatric diseases in clinic-based interventions (Bar-Or & Rowland, 2004; Faigenbaum & Myer, 2010; Faigenbaum et al., 2009; LeMura & Maziekas, 2002; Metcalf & Roberts, 1993; Stratton et al., 2004).

Key Points: Benefits of Resistance Training

Resistance training is defined as weight training, strength training, circuit weight training, isometrics, and isokinetics. This type of training involves exercising the muscles against moderate to heavy loads, generally with few repetitions, and results in varying degrees of muscle size increase (hypertrophy), increased lean body mass, and increased strength and power. For many years, resistance weight training evoked a negative image and was avoided by athletic and medical professionals. However, recently major research studies determined that this type of training using moderate loads (50–70% of one-repetition maximum) and following prescribed regimens produced the following benefits:

- Improvement in both strength and cardiovascular endurance
- Safe and effective exercise conditioning in cardiac and hypertensive patients when set guidelines are followed
- Significant decreases in resting blood pressure; possibly successful antihypertensive therapy
- Improvement in body composition by increase of lean muscle mass and decrease of fat stores
- Prevention of musculoskeletal disorders, especially in the back area
- Improvement of self-image and self-efficacy (feeling of control over one's situation)
- Acceleration of heart rate and blood pressure responses within clinically acceptable levels during exercise

- Favorable modification of risk factors for coronary artery disease
- Possible provision of up to 15% increase in aerobic endurance (maximum oxygen uptake—VO_2max)
- Possible promotion of the use of glucose and fat by muscles, improving insulin sensitivity, lipoprotein lipid profiles, and blood pressure, and increase of high-density lipoprotein cholesterol

ACTIVITY I. MUSCLE AND FAT

The instructor should pass around models of muscle tissue and fat tissue for the kids to feel and observe using verbal cues:

Talking Points: Muscle and Fat (Verbal cues for patients or parents and family members) *Read through the following information with your patient or family members to help them to understand the exercise strategy used in the program.*

This is only one pound of fat. Notice how big it is, but it is very light. This is 2 pounds of muscle. Notice how small it is but that it is much heavier than fat. When you have too much fat it makes you look very large. But, if you have a lot of muscle you will look lean.

Muscles have very little brains—they remember only after being shown many times. They will stay tight without you telling them to, if you exercise them with weight at least twice a week.

The most important thing is that a muscle that you have exercised becomes a trained muscle. Trained muscles burn calories even when you are not exercising them. Fat tissue just hangs around.

Strength training can improve blood pressure, body composition, and promotes strong bones.

ACTIVITY II. DEMONSTRATION AND INSTRUCTION

The instructor reviews the technique for each of the strength exercises using the illustrations, descriptions, and instructions previously detailed in this chapter. Children should begin performing the exercises as instructed in the illustrations in this chapter without weight or resistance for a 4-week period. During the fourth week, the exercise physiologist will instruct the children on the proper technique during the scheduled weekly session. During the session, parents are enlisted as spotters to ensure safety. The children then are instructed to perform the exercise routine according to the illustrations in this chapter and as indicated on the Weekly Goal-Setting Form and Exercise Record, twice per week with at least 1 day of rest between sessions.

ACTIVITY III. MUSCULAR STRENGTH AND ENDURANCE— STRENGTH-TRAINING CIRCUIT

The children will participate in a circuit strength-training session. The strength-training stations will follow the exercises illustrated previously detailed in this chapter and on the Strength and Flexibility Workout Chart (Table 3.9; see also Chapter 4). During the circuit, the instructor will discuss facts concerning strength training.

As the children move from one station of the circuit to another, strength exercises, specifically designed for overweight children, are performed in *one set* of 8–12 repetitions. The movement time is 2–4 seconds concentric and 2–4 seconds eccentric through a full range of motion. Children under 14 years of age begin at the lowest intensity. Proper technique is emphasized. Participants increase load (weight or resistance) only when the 12th repetition is performed with ease and in perfect form.

The children initially use 1-pound weights in each hand and 1- to 3-pound weights on each ankle to perform the exercises. They initially perform eight repetitions per exercise, with an emphasis on proper technique. When eight repetitions are performed in perfect form with ease, the exercises are increased to nine repetitions. This pattern continues until 12 repetitions can be done in perfect form. The amount of weight to be lifted then is increased to 3 pounds for each hand and 5 pounds for each ankle and the repetitions are reduced to eight per exercise. The same progression is then repeated. Exercises for the upper and middle back muscles use an exercise band. Children use the band with lowest resistance initially and then progress through the same pattern of increased repetitions and intensity. The complete resistance training circuit, consisting of 8–12 different exercises, can be performed easily in 20–30 minutes.

Clinical Reminders for the Health Care Professional: Exercise Safety

Parents can be recruited as spotters for the kids, or the kids can be paired as buddies. As one child is executing the exercise the buddy or parent spots, and then they change places.

Talking Points: Safe and Effective Resistance Training for Youth (Verbal cues for patients or parents and family members)
Read through the following information with your patient or family members to help them to understand the exercise strategy used in the program.

Resistance weight training comes with a lot of different names and forms (weight training, strength training, circuit weight training, isometrics, and isokinetics). Generally it means that you exercise your muscles against moderate to heavy loads, with few repetitions. Depending on what you do, this is the method for building muscle size, increasing lean body mass, and increasing your strength and power. Ask your pediatrician about which kinds of strengthening activities are safe for your overweight child. His growing bones and developing joints may be at risk for injury if he asks too much of his body by strenuous lifting, pushing, jarring, or pulling. Even jumping could cause harm. Severely obese children should only participate in strength exercises that offer good support for their joints. The exercises outlined in this chapter were designed especially for overweight children. In Week 4, your child should start the process of exercising with weights. Children under 14 years old should begin at the lowest intensity. No matter what the child's age, you should focus on the child's technique. Upon getting your pediatrician's approval and making sure the equipment you are using is in good repair, encourage your child to strengthen his or her muscles by following the guidelines in this chapter.

Key Points: Guidelines for Resistance Training

Force and Weight Aspects

Individuals should begin the program at 60% of maximum strength threshold. This weight should be maintained until 8–12 repetitions can be performed at specified velocities and in perfect form (technique). At this time an increase in weight of 5–10% is recommended.

Speed of Movement (Velocity)

A 2- to 4-second count for both the lifting and lowering phases with constant movement throughout is recommended. The movement should be performed with no rest and with a slight hold at the highest-force resistance. The velocity can be increased slightly when using free weights, and a hold is not necessary.

Frequency

Untrained individuals should begin the program at a frequency of once per week with twice per week the maximum. Trained individuals can begin the program at a frequency of twice per week, with a minimum of once per week to prevent a loss in strength and muscle size. A minimum of 1 day between workouts is necessary to guarantee enough rest to promote strength gains. For individuals working at peak workloads, 2–3 days of rest between workouts is advisable. This will help to prevent overwork and injury. It is inadvisable to work out with weights more frequently than three times per week.

Duration

A period of 1–2 minutes per station is suggested. Each station should consist of one set of between 8 and 12 repetitions performed as specified. This will induce a balanced workout of muscular strength, muscular endurance, and slight VO₂ improvement provided there is a minimum rest period with no more than 1 minute between stations (a 15 to 30-second rest is recommended).

Technique

Body alignment should follow ACSM guidelines with positioning for maximum isolation of designated muscles or muscle groups. The general technique for all exercises is as follows:

Movement should occur only in the joint adjacent to the muscle(s) being contracted. All other body parts should be stationary and relaxed.

As the movement begins, the individual should focus on the muscle(s) being worked, and fully contract (squeeze and shorten) the muscle into the holding point. When extending the weights, a maximum range of motion should be achieved.

There should be a light grip on the handles unless specifically working the forearm. This prevents an unnecessary elevation in blood pressure.

Technique specific to each exercise should be illustrated by a weightlifting instructor or trainer.

Breathing should be continuous and at a normal rate throughout the exercise with no specific inhalation or exhalation phase. To aid in concentration a quiet, nondistracting atmosphere is recommended. Warm-up should consist of approximately 5 minutes of low-impact jogging moves, range of motion without weight, and gentle stretching. Cooling down should be a similar process with more intense stretching.

Safety

At least one spotter is required on all free-weight stations. A spotter is encouraged on all stations to aid the subject, especially through the latter repetitions of maximum force.

Injury Prevention

It is suggested that exercises be performed only as specified. It is advisable that a spotter be utilized to correct faulty technique as muscle reaches fatigue.

Muscle Soreness

Slight muscle soreness and tightness are normal 1–2 days following weight training. Research suggests that this may be due to the muscle-rebuilding process. Proper cooling down and adequate stretching are encouraged to prevent soreness. If the soreness is light, gentle stretching and range-of-motion exercise are beneficial, along with elevation and ice for swelling. If there is no swelling, then a warm bath and massage are beneficial. For severe soreness, the RICE method—rest, ice, compression, and elevation—is recommended.

Clinical Reminders for the Health Care Professional: Strength Training for Overweight and Obese Youth

Appropriate strength training for overweight and obese children should include the following:

Moderate-high intensity (60–80% of one-repetition maximum)

- A balanced routine of 8–12 exercises specifically designed for obese children

- One set of 8–12 repetitions
- Movement time: 2–4 seconds concentric; 2–4 seconds eccentric

Children under 14 years begin at the lowest intensity. Proper technique is emphasized. Participant increases load (weight or resistance) only when the 12th repetition is performed with ease and in perfect form.

Glossary

Muscular Strength and Endurance: the maximum force that a muscle or group of muscles can generate (strength), or the ability of that muscle or group of muscles to repeat contractions over time (endurance). Strength training, sometimes called weightlifting, increases both muscular strength and endurance.

LESSON 5, LEVEL 1

Table 6.24   Overview: Lesson 5, Level 1 (Red)

Suggested time: 35-45 minutes (Total time)	Activities	Materials and staff needed
5 minutes	Introduction: Planning for Holidays	Parents and patients' educational materials and books (Sothern, von Almen, & Schumacher 2001) Exercise attire Flags and belts or napkins (one different color for each team) Staff: Exercise trainer
30–40 minutes	Activity I: Flag Football	
Objectives After participation in this lesson the student will be able to: 1. Identify ways to organize family events to include exercise activities. 2. Identify safe methods to participate in family field sports. 3. Gain knowledge concerning the proper technique and rules for the game of flag football. 4. Safely participate in a flag football game with family members. 5. Gain knowledge concerning how to pace exercise activities to reduce fatigue by alternating positions on the field.		

INTRODUCTION

The instructor will discuss methods to encourage physical activity during holiday time with families. One way to do this is to organize a game of flag football with patients and their family members (no tackling or use napkins or flag belts if available). During holidays, such as Thanksgiving, Christmas, and New Years, this is an effective way to get your patients, their parents, siblings, and cousins outside and away from the football games on television during the first and third quarters. Then they can all gather around the television to watch the second and last quarter.

Ask parents to plan weekends around family fun and fitness. Have them commit to spending at least one weekend day doing something active. A trip to the water park or a venture to the mountains provides opportunities where the family can fish, row a boat, ride a horse, or rent a bicycle. City life offers plenty of choices, too. Families can spend the day at the zoo, tour a children's interactive museum, or visit a laser tag center. When planning next year's family vacation, ask parents to consider a beach with kid-friendly pools, swimming with dolphins, cross-country skiing, or a hiking trip.

A televised sports event can spark family-oriented physical activity. For example, on the day that a football game is scheduled, ask parents to take the family outside and spend the first quarter tossing a football. Then, allow the family to go inside and watch the second quarter. During half-time and the third quarter, encourage them to resume the family game outside. After that, they may watch the fourth quarter so they know who wins.

Remind parents that participating in sports is far healthier than watching them. Studies show that if parents engage in physical activities, their children will grow up to be active, too. Likewise, if parents spend their leisure time being observers, that is, watching sports on television, then chances are, their kids will grow up to be observers, too.

Social situations, emotions, and family events are often responsible for why children remain underactive. These responses have become habitual. Parents and their children will need to work together to develop healthier solutions so the child does not avoid physical activities and develop a poor self-image. For example, one of our patients provided an example for how to alter habitual responses. He had always wanted to play football, but, because of his weight, he was never picked at recess games and lacked the confidence to try out for the playground teams—so he eventually quit trying. After 1 month on the program, however, he lost 8 pounds and became more confident about his physical skills. He and his father began passing the football each evening, and the whole family participated in weekend football games. He knew his skills were improving, and soon enough, he developed the confidence to try out for his neighborhood park team. Next thing he knew, he was playing tackle for the team and was being chosen regularly for pick-up games during school recess.

Clinical Reminders for the Health Care Professional: Parent Participation

The parents may serve as goal posts by holding their arms in a "letter L" position facing inward to each other. The instructor will need to have a parent serve as quarterback to help explain the rules of the game to the inexperienced younger children.

ACTIVITY I. FLAG FOOTBALL

Purchase inexpensive table napkins in two different colors. Divide your patients and their family members into two teams and ask everyone to tuck one of the colored napkins into their waistband.

Key Points: Organizing Teams

When organizing teams try this method: Tell the kids and parents to make a "train" behind you. Then assign every other participant to a different color. For example: Red team, Blue team, Red team, and so on. Assign the Red team to the outfield and the Blue team to home plate.

Play a game of football with these aerobic rules: Allow 20 seconds only to prepare for the kick-off. Allow only 10 seconds for the huddle. The ball must be snapped for the next play no more than 10 seconds after it is down. Switch player position every 15 minutes: quarterback and running back, defense and offense. These rules keep the game moving and the calories burning.

LESSON 6, LEVEL 1

Table 6.25   Overview: Lesson 6, Level 1 (Red)

Suggested time: 35–45 minutes (Total time)	Activities	Materials and staff needed
10–15 minutes	Introduction: Flexibility	Parents and patients' educational materials and books (Sothern, von Almen, & Schumacher, 2001) Exercise attire Floor mats Staff: Exercise trainer
25–30 minutes	Activity I: Flex Test, a Balancing Act	
Objectives After participation in this lesson the student will be able to: 1. Identify movements that will increase muscular flexibility. 2. Gain knowledge concerning the benefits of muscular flexibility to health. 3. Identify imbalances in the posture that lead to bone and joint problems. 4. Identify movement and exercises that will improve posture, muscular flexibility and reduce the risk of injury.		

INTRODUCTION

The instructor will discuss the importance of flexibility. Flexibility refers to the maximum ability to move a joint through its full range of motion. Flexibility keeps your body in balance. Stretching will help you improve and maintain flexibility. If you neglect flexibility in your training, you may acquire muscle or joint injuries or chronic disorders. One of these disorders, pronation distortion syndrome is characterized by knee flexion, internal rotation, and adduction (knock-kneed) and excessive foot pronation (flat feet). Individuals with this condition develop patterns of injury including plantar fasciitis, posterior tibialis tendinitis (shin splints), patellar tendinitis, and low back pain. Obese individuals are at higher risk (Irving et al., 2007; Kaufmann et al., 1999; Moen et al., 2009). Stretching will help you improve and maintain flexibility.

Talking Points: Flexibility and Balance (Verbal cues for patients or parents and family members)
Read through the following information with your patient or family members to help them to understand the exercise strategy used in the program.

Aerobic exercise is great for healthy hearts and lungs. But if your child only engages in aerobic exercise, she will be missing two critical components: strength and flexibility. What good is a car with a great engine but that has no tires, hood, top, or doors? Muscles provide the framework for your child's engine and must be strong to protect her from injury. A car runs more efficiently when it is in alignment. The same holds true for the human body. The function of flexibility is to maintain balance. When your child was born, she was in perfect proportion. She was symmetrical—the left side was identical to the right. The front of the body was in balance with the rear. After years of using one part of the body more than another, imbalances occur. This can result in poor posture, unfit appearance, or injury and pain in a bone or joint.

ACTIVITY I. FLEX TEST

Students will be guided through the Flex Test sequence in partners. The instructor will emphasize the importance of balance as it relates to flexibility and strength. Students should be shown how to keep the knees slightly bent or "soft" and not overextended during activities. Corrective exercises, designed to improve the imbalanced areas of the body, will be introduced. The program flexibility exercises in this chapter will then be reviewed to music.

Stretching and flexibility are important to your patient's exercise routine to maintain good posture and overall balance. Using the car as a metaphor helps children understand the value of good posture and a balanced body. Individuals cannot drive a car that has a flat tire—it is unbalanced. In the same regard, children cannot achieve a healthy lifestyle if they do not have a balanced body. When children are born, their body was a perfectly designed machine—just like a brand new car. It was symmetrical, meaning that the left side was identical to the right, and the front was in balance with the rear. But after years of using one part of the body more than the other parts, it can get out of balance. Although, children do not have flat tires to show them that they are out of balance, they do have poor posture, or worse, an injury or pain in their bones and joints.

Talking Points: Importance of Balance (Verbal cues for patients or parents and family members)
Read through the following information with your patient or family members to help them to understand the exercise strategy used in the program.

If you overtrain or neglect to stretch your chest muscles or undertrain your back area, you could walk around looking like a gorilla (instructor demonstrates)! Additionally, your back could begin to hunch over and you will start to look like a very old outerspace alien (instructor demonstrates)! But if your chest is flexible and your back is strong, you will appear taller, thinner, and stronger. This is why you have been doing Stretch-and-Flex exercises since the first week. Do these exercises whenever and wherever you can, It is easy to do them while you are watching television, playing outside, or relaxing in your room after you warm up for 3–5 minutes.

The Flex Test is a way to determine whether your patient has any of these imbalances. Flex exercises can help correct those imbalances and prevent others from occurring.

Guide the patient and their parent through the following Flex Test. Then continue with the information that follows.

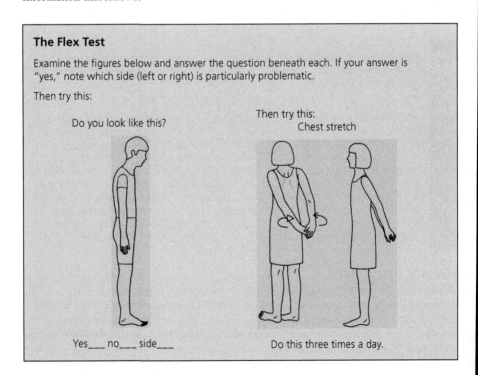

The Flex Test

Examine the figures below and answer the question beneath each. If your answer is "yes," note which side (left or right) is particularly problematic.

Then try this:

Do you look like this?

Then try this:
Chest stretch

Yes___ no___ side___

Do this three times a day.

Rowing, low

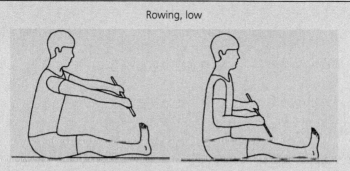

Do 8–12 repetitions two to three times per week.

Do you look like this?

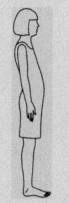

Yes___ no___ side___

Then try this:

Stomach crunch and pelvic tilt

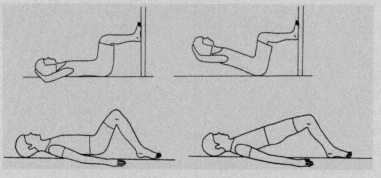

Do 8–20 repetitions two to three times per week.

Do you look like this?

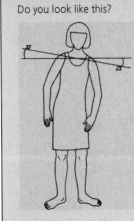

Yes___ no___ side___

Then try this:
Shoulder stretch

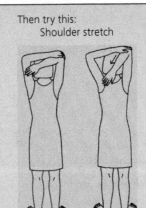

Do this three times a day.

And try this:
Upper back stretch

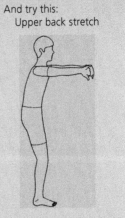

Do this three times a day.

Do you look like this?

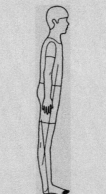

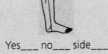

Yes___ no___ side___

Then try this:

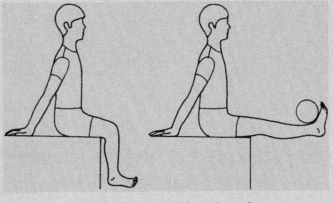

Leg extension, sitting and leg curl, standing

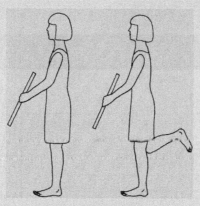

Do these three times per week.

And try this:

Lying Quad Stretch

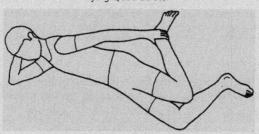

Do this three times a day.
Important: Keep knees "soft" or slightly bent when standing
(do not lock or hyperextend the knees). This automatically takes
stress off the knee joints and the lower back.

Do you look like this?   Do you look like this?

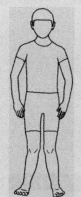

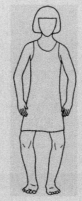

Do you look like this?

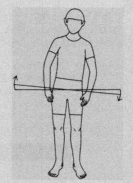

Yes___ no___ side___   Yes___ no___ side___
         or   or   Yes___ no___ side___

Then see your pediatrician or family physician. He or she will likely refer you to an orthopedic specialist.

LESSON 7, LEVEL 1

Table 6.26   Overview: Lesson 7, Level 1 (Red)

Suggested time: 45–60 minutes (Total time)	Activities	Materials and staff needed
10 minutes	Introduction	Parents and patients' educational materials and books (Sothern, von Almen, & Schumacher, 2001) Exercise attire Music player Indoor cycle ergometer for each student Stopwatch Staff: Exercise trainer or guest spinning instructor
25–35 minutes	Activity I: Body Composition Discussion Activity II: Body Types Activity III: Spinning (cycle) Class to Music	
10–15 minutes	Activity IV: Abdominal (stomach) Crunch Challenge	
Objectives After participation in this lesson the student will be able to: 1. Gain knowledge concerning individual body types and how these affect exercise performance. 2. Safely participate in a cycle spinning class to improve aerobic endurance. 3. Identify methods to set individual goals to improve abdominal strength through participation in a timed stomach crunch exercise bout.		

INTRODUCTION
The instructor will introduce one of the four components of fitness: body composition. He or she will then lead the class in a spinning (indoor cycle) activity to music. The class will end with the patients participating in the abdominal crunch challenge.

ACTIVITY I. BODY COMPOSITION DISCUSSION
Our bodies are made up of many different tissues. Body composition refers to the percentage of your body weight composed of fat, and the percentage of body weight composed of lean tissue and bone. Fat is a soft tissue primarily found underneath your skin. The rest of our tissues—muscles and bones—are classified as lean body mass. Exercise burns fat tissue and helps to maintain or improve lean muscle tissue. Body composition changes after you begin exercising regularly and by engaging in different types of exercise.

Talking Points : Body Fat (Verbal cues for patients or parents and family members)
Read through the following information with your patient or family members to help them to understand the exercise strategy used in the program.

Your doctor can help you to measure your body fat percentage. You then can compare your body fat percent with the accompanying chart to find out whether you were lean optimal, healthy, overweight or obese. You will check again with the doctor in another 3 months to see how your percentage of body fat and classification has changed.
　　Percent Body Fat Classification: Use the following chart, which works for all ages, to help you determine your body percent fat classification:

Classification	Male (% fat)	Female (% fat)
Lean	<8	<16
Optimal	8–15	16–22
Healthy	16–20	23–28
Overweight	21–25	29–35
Obese	>25	>35

Athletes (because they are avid exercisers, they have optimal percentage of fat levels):

Long-distance runners	4–9	6–15
Wrestlers	4–10	10–17
Gymnasts	4–10	10–17
Body Builders (elite)	6–10	10–17
Swimmers	5–11	18–24
Basketball Athletes	7–11	18–24
Canoers/Kayakers	11–15	18–24
Tennis Players	14–17	19–22

ACTIVITY II. BODY TYPES

The instructor will describe the different types of body types—mesomorph, ectomorph, and endomorph—and discuss the benefits of tailoring exercise routines to these different types. The following information also includes recommendations that will help you select sports and recreational activities that best align with your patient's individual body type.

Mesomorph

These people have a high muscle-to-fat ratio and tend to have an hourglass-shaped body. The best exercises for mesomorphs include activities that require strength, power, and endurance, such as football, baseball, martial arts, boxing, wrestling, weightlifting, shot put, discus, long jump, ice skating, ice hockey, water polo, sprinting events in track and field, swimming, springboard diving, gymnastics, and tumbling.

Endomorph

This group has a higher fat-to-muscle ratio. They tend to be pear shaped, round and soft. Endomorphs do well in all types of middle-distance or moderate intensity activities, such as swimming, synchronized swimming, dance, or brisk walking. They are also well suited for the individual sports of martial arts, tennis, archery, bowling, sailing, golf, softball, hiking, snorkeling, scuba diving, water skiing, and middle-distance field events.

Ectomorph

These bodies are long and rectangular-shaped, typically low in weight and fat. They excel at long-distance events, such as field sports, basketball, soccer, football (running back), ice hockey (offense), field hockey, track and field long-distance runs, pole vaulting, marathons, triathlons, swimming long distance, cross-country running, and skiing.

Talking Points: Body Types (Verbal cues for patients or parents and family members) *Read through the following information with your patient or family members to help them to understand the exercise strategy used in the program.*

Just as no two snowflakes are alike, so too no two human bodies share exactly the same genetic makeup or body proportions. You may have one overweight child among five lean siblings. But just because your overweight child may have a genetic predisposition to heaviness, it does not mean she has to live a lifetime of overweight, poor nutrition and exercise habits, and medical problems.

Identifying body types can help determine which physical activities are best suited for your child. Remember: no matter what the size or shape of your child, she needs to experience a variety of physical activities in a supportive environment. To begin, figure out which somatotype—or genetically determined body type—your child inherited. Your doctor or health care professionals can assist you.

Exercise that is right for your patient's age, size, and genetic makeup is determined by many factors. One of these factors is muscle fiber types. Muscle fibers generally are classified as slow twitch or fast twitch. The percentage we have of each is genetically determined. Those with more slow-twitch muscle fibers are better equipped to partake in moderate- to vigorous-intensity, long-duration exercises, such as those defined for ectomorphs (like basketball). Those with more fast-twitch muscle fibers are well suited to high-intensity, short-duration exercises, such as those suggested for mesomorphs. People with an equal number of both slow-twitch and fast-twitch muscle fibers typically excel at middle-distance or moderate-intensity events, although they are typically competent in all types of sports or activities.

Talking Points: Selecting the Best Physical Activity (Verbal cues for patients or parents and family members)
Read through the following information with your patient or family members to help them to understand the exercise strategy used in the program.

After determining which body type your child has, notice the activities she gravitates to—those that she likes and is able to master with ease. She probably will independently select those best suited to her innate ability, personal preferences, and positive feedback she receives from coaches, parents, and peers. You may be tempted to limit activities to those she likes most and that are compatible with her body type, but it is important to expose her to many different exercises—all in a nonintimidating and nurturing environment. Respect your child's passion for the activities she chooses. Try not to impose your personal preferences. Even short, stocky athletes can excel in basketball if they love the game.

Every body type benefits from a variety of exercises, although those benefits may manifest differently. Genetics determines skin thickness and where fat tissue is stored. So, even if your patient has a consistent strength-training component to his or her routine, genetics may prevent him or her from ever appearing as lean as kids with different genetic profiles, skin, and muscle tissue. Help your patient accept the body he or she was born with while encouraging activities of all kinds.

Key Points: Developing a Tailored Exercise Program

Aerobic exercise burns large amounts of fat. The longer you do an aerobic activity, the more your body draws from its fat stores for fuel. It is much better for kids to do an activity that is easy to sustain for long periods of time than to do something more intense for short periods. When you maintain an even level of intensity in an activity, you reach what is called steady state.
      Steady-state activity is best for older children and adults who want to lose fat, so encourage your older child not to change the intensity of her exercise during the workout. Younger children will naturally start and stop during physical activity, since their body engines are immature and are better suited for intermittent activities. When a young child plays tag (a start-and-stop activity) for a few hours, her total caloric expenditure will be the same as that of an older child performing a steady-state (nonstop) biking session for a slightly shorter or sometimes an equal amount of time.

It is healthy to accept your body type. Genetics determine not only fat distribution and muscle fiber types, but also bone density and heaviness. Some ethnic groups have larger bones and, therefore, carry more weight. Help your patient accept the size of her body frame whether it is small, medium, or large.

Consider the size of your patient's frame when selecting physical activities. Large-framed girls with dense, heavy bones excel in sports requiring strength and endurance such as volleyball, baseball, and basketball. Small-framed boys do well in martial arts, gymnastics, and soccer and other sports requiring speed, agility, and strength. Always provide the opportunity to try as many different activities as possible, even those that do not appear well suited to your patient's physical make up.

Most important, remember that all activity burns calories and improves overall health.

Even though individualizing your patient's exercise program according to somatotype may help him or her, remember that he or she feels mastery when he or she successfully partakes in a behavior in which he or she engages and will almost certainly carry out that behavior again.

Clinical Reminders for the Health Care Professional: Positive Reinforcement

Provide positive reinforcement. Kids will do anything for attention, and the type you give (positive or negative) is thought to drive and maintain the child's behavior. So, for example, if you give attention for positive actions, chances are your patient will repeat that behavior in the future. Likewise, if you respond to unhealthy action, chances are your patient will repeat that behavior in the future. It is essential to focus on positive behaviors that reinforce weight-loss goals while ignoring, redirecting, or consciously problem solving negative behaviors.

ACTIVITY III. SPINNING (INDOOR CYCLE) OR AEROBIC CIRCUIT CLASS

Patients and family members will participate in a spinning (indoor cycle) class to music. If exercise cycle equipment is not available, then the instructor may choose to have the patients and family members participate in an aerobic station routine to music. A different aerobic move will be described on a card, which will be placed at each of 10–12 stations. Each student will begin at one of the stations. After 2 minutes of movement to music, the instructor will call "rotate" and the students will move in a clockwise fashion to the next station. This continues until all stations have been visited.

ACTIVITY IV. ABDOMINAL CRUNCH CHALLENGE

Using the instructions for performing abdominal crunches located in Chapter 4, the instructor will demonstrate the technique. The patients then will participate in the abdominal crunch challenge. Each patient will have a family member serve as coach during this activity. The coach will monitor the exercise technique and provide verbal encouragement during the challenge. He or she will also count the number of crunch movements that the patient is able to complete in 5 minutes. This score will become the patient's personal best score, which he or she will refer to during the next 10-week session to determine whether abdominal strength is improving.

LESSON 8, LEVEL 1

Table 6.27 Overview: Lesson 8, Level 1 (Red)

Suggested time: 45–50 minutes (Total time)	Activities	Materials and staff needed
5–10 minutes	Introduction: Metabolic Rates, Maximize your Workouts	Parents and patients' educational materials and books (Sothern, von Almen, & Schumacher, 2001) Swimming attire Music player Towel Change of clothes Kickboards and arm floats for each participant Staff: Exercise trainer or guest water aerobics instructor
35–45 minutes	Activity I: Water Aerobics	

Objectives
After participation in this lesson the student will be able to:
1. Gain knowledge concerning individual metabolic rates and the factors that affect this rate.
2. Recognize safe methods to maximize aerobic activities to ensure positive impacts on metabolism.
3. Identify the benefits to participating in aquatic physical activities.
4. Safely participate in a water aerobics exercise class to music.

INTRODUCTION

The instructor will discuss metabolic rates and how to maximize exercise to receive the most benefit to improving metabolic health. He or she then will discuss the benefits of water sports and recreational activities to achieving and maintaining a healthy weight. Available activities include water aerobics, water polo, synchronized swimming (water ballet), competitive swimming (races), water skiing, surfing, rafting, snorkeling, scuba, windsurfing, sailing, and jet skis. Exercising in water is great for obese children, especially those with severe conditions because the water supports the child's weight while he or she is moving freely.

ACTIVITY I. WATER AEROBICS

Students will participate in a water aerobics class. Arm and leg movements to music will be performed in chest-deep water. The instructor will use the exercise to introduce the concept of metabolic rate—that is, the individual speed at which each student will burn calories.

 Talking Points: Metabolic Rate (Verbal cues for patients or parents and family members)
Read through the following information with your patient or family members to help them to understand the exercise strategy used in the program.

Your engines each burn the calories you eat and the fat stored in your body at different speeds. It depends on a lot of different factors. How fast your parents' engines burn calories affects your metabolic rate. How tall you are and how much you weigh will also affect the rate. If you are on a diet, this can slow down your engine. If you exercise, however, you can stop your engine from slowing down. The more muscles you have will also speed up your rate. Remember: Muscles, if they are trained, burn calories even when you are not exercising. Fat is just that lazy stuff that hangs around.

LESSON 9, LEVEL 1

Table 6.28   Overview: Lesson 9, Level 1 (Red)

Suggested time: 45–50 minutes (Total time)	Activities	Materials and staff needed
5–10 minutes	Introduction: Exercise Myths	Parents and patients' educational materials and books (Sothern, von Almen, & Schumacher, 2001) Exercise attire Music player Overhead or slide projector Staff: Exercise trainer or guest dance instructor
35–45 minutes	Activity I: Specialty Theme Aerobic or Line Dancing, Guest Lecture	

Objectives
After participation in this lesson the student will be able to:
1. Gain knowledge concerning common myths to participation in physical activity.
2. Recognize safe methods to engage in specialty theme aerobic exercise to music.
3. Identify the benefits of dancing to overall health and well-being.
4. Safely participate in a group dance class to improve aerobic fitness.

INTRODUCTION
The instructor will discuss some common myths about exercise.

ACTIVITY I. SPECIALTY THEME AEROBIC DANCE CLASS
A guest instructor will teach a specialty theme aerobics or line-dancing class. Some suggestions are country line dancing, Latin-beat music and moves, rockin' to the oldies, hip-hop aerobics, African dance, belly dancing.

Talking Points: Exercise Myths (Verbal cues for patients or parents and family members)
Read through the following information with your patient or family members to help them to understand the exercise strategy used in the program or in the patient handout.

Don't Be Fooled by These Exer-Myths!

Myth: No Pain, No Gain
Truth: During exercise, you should feel a gentle burning in your muscles, which indicates fatigue. If you feel pain or discomfort in a bone, joint, or muscle, stop the exercise immediately and consult a doctor.
Myth: Movie Star Exercise Equipment and Videos
Truth: These types of items are designed primarily for profit. They have not been researched and could cause severe injury. Stay away from them!
Myth: Fat-Burning Exercises
Truth: All exercises—except for high-intensity anaerobic activities—burn fat. The longer you exercise, the more fat you will burn. Fat loss is promoted by creating a caloric deficit, not by the type of exercise you do.
Myth: Spot Reducing
Truth: There are no exercises that can burn fat in one particular area of the body. You can, however, train a specific muscle or group of muscles for strength and endurance, resulting in a toned appearance. Being toned is a condition in which muscles remain contracted even when you do not consciously tighten them. So, doing abdominal crunches alone (without other

> calorie-burning activities or reducing how much you eat) will not melt away those inches around your waist, although they will help strengthen your abdominals.
>
> Myth: Strength Training Makes Big Muscles
> Truth: Strength training does not always result in larger muscles. Rather, genetic make-up, the type of strength training being performed, and the frequency of the training will determine the results. Women especially probably will not develop "big" muscles through strength training. They will create more dense and, therefore, more toned muscles that will make them look leaner and will increase the rate at which they burn calories. Parents, if you train once or twice per week with your son or daughter, you will be doing yourselves and your child a favor.

LESSON 10, LEVEL 1

Table 6.29   Overview: Lesson 10, Level 1 (Red)

Suggested time: 40–50 minutes (Total time)	Activities	Materials and staff needed
5–10 minutes	Introduction:	Parents and patients' educational materials and books (Sothern, von Almen, & Schumacher, 2001) Exercise attire Cabbage baseballs, bats, bases, home plate Staff: Exercise trainer
40–45 minutes	Activity I: Park Day	

Objectives
After participation in this lesson the student will be able to:
1. Gain knowledge concerning the benefits of group sports activities to overall health and well-being.
2. Recognize opportunities to engage in safe methods to participate in physical activities in an outdoor setting.
3. Safely participate in a softball game with friends and family members designed to maximize opportunities for movement to promote increased physical activity.

INTRODUCTION

The instructor will congratulate his or her patients and family members for completing the 10-week session. He or she should discuss how to prepare for the follow-up medical tests, which will determine their overall progress. Patients will be informed that rewards will be given out in 2 weeks for attendance and exercise compliance.

ACTIVITY I. PARK DAY

Family and friends then will be encouraged to join the patients in a Park Day of outdoor play. One week before the event, the instructor will inform the students to bring a bike, roller skates, roller blades, or skateboard to class on this day. The students, family, and friends will be allowed to circle the park in groups using whatever equipment they bring along. Water stations will be set up at 0.5- to 1-mile intervals. The instructor may choose to set up volleyball nets, soccer goals, and so on and bring extra balls along for those children who do not want to walk and do not have bikes or skates. This event requires a parent or additional staff member to supervise.

Talking Points: Exercise Activity Ideas—Family Fun and Fitness (Verbal cues for patients or parents and family members)
Read through the following information with your patient or family members to help them to understand the exercise strategy used in the program.

This week, come up with a list of half-day, weekend activities that the entire family can do together. Gather input from each family member, bring out the calendar, mark what you will do and on which weekend, and stick to it. Here are some of our favorite ways to spend time together burning calories and having fun:

Water sports: swimming, tubing down a river, fishing, body surfing and playing on the beach, water slide, and water polo

Ball sports: football, volleyball, tennis, basketball, soccer, croquet, golf, bowling, softball, and playing fetch with your dog

Mountain sports: cross-country or downhill skiing, snow-shoeing, hiking, caving, horseback riding, and biking

Around the neighborhood: Frisbee, tag, biking, walking, kick the can, walking the dog, pulling the wagon, and inline skating.

Talking Points: Monitoring Progress (Verbal cues for patients or parents and family members)
Read through the following information with your patient or family members to help them to understand the exercise strategy used in the program.

Congratulations! You have nearly completed the first 12 weeks of your exercise program! Chances are good that you have met with many successes and that your family is healthier and happier.

It is now time to evaluate your child's progress by visiting your pediatrician. The doctor can determine whether your child has either lost adequate weight or has grown enough to graduate to the next color-coded level. If she graduates, then reward, reward, reward! Also, set a new 3-month goal. Refer to your child's 12-week goals. Did she attain some of them? If so, reward her with special (nonfood) gifts, such as sports equipment, trips to the water slide, new and smaller size clothing, a camping trip, or other family adventure. If she is graduating to the next color-coded level of the program, consider printing up a graduation notice or certificate of achievement. These little steps go a long way to help rally enthusiasm for the next 12 weeks.

If your child was successful at not gaining weight, but needs to remain in the same color-coded level, give as much positive reinforcement as you can. Rave about the efforts she has made, and express your faith in her. As you begin a new 12-week program, brainstorm together an idea for a reward she will receive upon graduating after this new session.

If you discover, however, that the percentage of your child's overweight condition or body fat has increased from the time of her last visit, then you must recommit to new and more attainable weight-loss goals. Also, try practicing the strategies and behaviors that helped her when things went smoothly in the past.

Work with your child so she does not get angry, hopeless, or nervous. Taking a deep breath, reassessing long- and short-term goals, defining rewards, and recommitting to being healthy and happy is all it takes. And remember: Everyone who tries to lose weight has setbacks.

Do not be discouraged if you have to revolve through the program several more times before your child meets her goal weight. By now, you have a good handle on the program, know what incentives work for your child, what tempts her to make unhealthy choices, and how to deal with problems. The next 3 months will most likely be easier than the first 3 months. You are all beginning to master the program. It will simply take as long as it takes, but it is helpful to think in terms of 3-month intervals. It is natural that both your overweight child and the family may have a higher commitment to the program at the very beginning, and a lower one later on. This only becomes problematic if everyone falls back into sedentary behavior. The goal of each session is to integrate the lifestyle changes into your lives more fully and comfortably so that they become an expected and easy part of life.

Each time you begin a new session, practice every component of the program. Establish new goals for each level, for example, because old goals are no longer relevant. And do not trick yourself into believing that you do not need to make goals, continue praising your child, or working the program fully. It is the combination of these elements that make the program work—not isolated pieces. Eventually, if you continue participating fully, your child will reach her goal weight. Do not forget that she is always growing. That growth is her best friend. For every 1 inch she grows, her goal weight increases by 3–5 pounds.

Be sure to acknowledge accomplishments of other family members as you end this first session. Take time to celebrate by throwing yourselves a party with your new activities or taking an evening out together for some outdoor family fun.

Before embarking on another session or moving into maintenance, ask yourself these questions:

- As you review the previous 12 weeks, do you feel happy? Confident in your success? Some self-satisfaction?
- Is your child's behavior different? Is she more confident? Are her spirits higher?
- Are you all ready to go for the next 12 weeks?
- Are you committed to helping your child maintain her goal weight?

LESSON 1, LEVEL 2 (YELLOW)

Table 6.30   Overview: Lesson 1, Level 2 (Yellow)

Suggested time: 45–55 minutes (Total time)	Activities	Materials and staff needed
10–15 minutes	Introduction: Increasing Your Daily Activity	Parents and patients' educational materials and books (Sothern, von Almen, & Schumacher, 2001) Exercise attire Obstacle course equipment of your choice Staff: Exercise trainer
10 minutes	Activity I: Creating Outdoor Play Areas	
25–30 minutes	Activity II: Obstacle Course	

Objectives
After participation in this lesson the student will be able to:
1. Gain knowledge concerning the benefits of exercise and increasing daily physical activity to health.
2. Recognize opportunities to engage in safe methods to participate in physical activities in an outdoor setting.
3. Safely participate in an obstacle course activity in an outdoor setting.

INTRODUCTION

The instructor will introduce or review the PEP step activity from lesson 1, level 1 (red). He or she will discuss methods to create outdoor play areas. The patients and their family members will participate in an outdoor obstacle course. If reviewing the MPEP step activity, use the following additional information:

Talking Points: Observe Your Child's Behavior (Verbal cues for patients or parents and family members)
Read through the following information with your patient or family members to help them to understand the exercise strategy used in the program.

Take a moment to observe your child's demeanor. Notice her posture, how quickly or slowly she walks, her overall physique, and how it makes her look. Lots of overweight kids move slowly, with hunched shoulders, appearing as though they lack confidence. Improving the way your child walks can burn considerably more calories, and make her look and feel healthier. Teach your child that burning calories does not only happen when she is doing hard exercise or playing. She burns them all the time.

Talking Points: Brisk Walking (Verbal cues for patients or parents and family members)
Read through the following information with your patient or family members to help them to understand the exercise strategy used in the program.

Remember, slow movement does not burn very many calories. It does not use very many muscles. Notice people who walk briskly. They are usually fitter and appear more energetic. It is easier for them—their muscles are trained. They automatically burn more calories because they cover more area in less time. Therefore, they carry around less fat weight, making it easier to move. Become one of them—you will not believe how much weight you will lose by moving!

Participants are instructed to observe their muscles as they contract, relax, and stretch, with the following verbal cues:

Talking Points: Increasing Daily Activity (Verbal cues for patients or parents and family members)
Read through the following information with your patient or family members to help them to understand the exercise strategy used in the program.

Unless you learn to increase the amount of activity you do each day, you will gain the weight back in a very short time. Any time you move a body part it requires one or more muscles to contract or become shorter. Your body needs energy or calories to make the muscles do this. Your body gets these calories either from the food you eat or the fat stored on your body. If you move you will lose weight and keep the weight off!

Patient and Parent Handout: Activity Worksheet

You can calculate how many calories (kcal) you use in a day.	
Take the number of hours in a day:	24
Subtract sleeping hours:	−10
The hours that remain:	14
Let's calculate how many calories you would use . . .	
Walking casually:	
150 kcal/hour × 14 hours/day × 7 days/week	=
Sitting in a chair:	
50 kcal/hour × 14 hours/day × 7 days/week	=
The difference between sitting in a chair and walking casually . . .	
(walking calories) − (sitting calories)	=
−	
Remember: 3500 kcal = 1 pound of fat!	
If you walk briskly, just think how many calories you will burn this week!	

ACTIVITY I. CREATING OUTDOOR FUN

Ask parents to take an inventory of their yard. Is there a swing set? Sandbox? A wading pool? A sprinkler with an attachment for playing with water? If not, encourage them to get busy. Let them know that their child can engage in the great outdoors in so many ways. Her age will determine her interests. Older children love to climb rope swings or ladders leading to a tree fort in which they can play endlessly. They also enjoy competition, sporting games (basketball, baseball, badminton, croquet, miniature golf), and tag, tag, and more tag. Younger kids enjoy playing knights-in-shining armor with an open field for battle. They like balls of all sizes. Building makeshift houses out of cardboard boxes provides endless adventure. Or they will pull their wagon full of their favorite things.

Tell parents that they should enter into this process understanding that it may be a process of trial and error. Maybe for their child's first 6–8 years, watching television was her idea of fun. She may have to explore different corners of this new world of activity before she finds the right fit. Bear with her. Your patience will pay off enormously.

Tell parents that if they do not have a yard, find the nearest park. Even older kids enjoy monkey bars, swings, teeter-totters, tunnels, and the wonderful playground equipment so many parks offer. Encourage parents to take their children to the grassy area and throw a Frisbee, pitch some baseballs, or ride bikes around the periphery of the park. The only hard-and-fast rule to all this is that they need to find activities their child likes and do them.

ACTIVITY II. OBSTACLE COURSE

The instructor will set up an obstacle course indoors or outdoors for the kids to run through. Times are recorded for each attempt and prizes awarded to the participants with the best times. Local gymnastics training centers are good locations for obstacle courses, as well as outdoor parks

LESSON 2, LEVEL 2

Table 6.31   Overview: Lesson 2, Level 2 (Yellow)

Suggested time: 45–50 minutes (Total time)	Activities	Materials and staff needed
5–10 minutes	Introduction: Cardiorespiratory Endurance, Family Field Sports	Parents and patients' educational materials and books (Sothern, von Almen, & Schumacher, 2001) Exercise attire Volleyballs Volleyball net Whistle
35–40 minutes	Activity I: Aerobic Volleyball	
		Staff: Exercise trainer

Objectives
After participation in this lesson the student will be able to:
1. Identify safe methods to warm up the body before engaging in an exercise session.
2. Gain knowledge concerning the benefits of aerobic exercise to health.
3. Identify movement and exercises that will improve cardiorespiratory (aerobic) endurance.
4. Safely participate in a softball game with friends and family members designed to maximize opportunities for movement to promote increased physical activity.
5. Identify safe methods to cool down the body after engaging in an exercise session.

INTRODUCTION

The instructor will review the different types of cardiorespiratory (aerobic) exercises and discuss ways to make recreational and sports activities more physically active. The patients and their family members then will participate in an Aerobic Volleyball Game.

ACTIVITY I. AEROBIC VOLLEYBALL

Gather your patients and their family members and set up a volleyball game. You will need some music to make it complete—along with these few additional guidelines:

When the opposing team scores a point, the receiving team has to do 10 aerobic moves to the music, such as aerobic dance moves (like modified [side] jacks, the twist, the grapevine, and the cha-cha), while the ball is retrieved.

When the serving team gets a "side out" (they lose the point and the serve to the opposing team), they have to do 10 dance movements to the music.

It also is fun to ask those who fumble the ball to walk, jog, or dance around the court.

 Patient Handout: Rate the Aerobic Activity*

Best Calorie Burners

Swimming	Cross-country Skiing
30 yards/minute = 375 calories/hour	850–1200 calories/hour

45 yards/minute = 615 calories/hour

Low-impact Aerobics	Jump Rope
360–480 calories/hour	50–60 skips/minute = 455 calories/hour

Karate or Martial Arts
750 calories/hour

Second-Best Calorie Burners

Brisk Walking or Jogging	Handball, Squash, Racquetball
5.5 miles/hour = 585–660 calories/hour	600–660 calories/hour
Cycling	Soccer and Long-Distance Field Sports
12 miles/hour = 480–600 calories/hour	525–575 calories/hour

Roller or Ice Skating
360–420 calories/hour

Third-Best Calorie Burners

Football, Basketball, Hockey	Tennis Singles
5.5 miles/hour = 585 calories/hour	380–420 calories/hour
Volleyball	Windsurfing
300–330 calories/hour	280–400 calories/hour

Fourth-Best Calorie Burners

Golf without a Cart	Softball
240–300 calories/hour	300–360 calories/hour
Water Skiing	Sailing
240–300 calories/hour	180–240 calories/hour
Bowling	
240–300 calories/hour	

*This chart is based on a person weighing 150 pounds. Your child will burn fewer calories if he is smaller, and more if he is larger.

LESSON 3, LEVEL 2

Table 6.32   Overview: Lesson 3, Level 2 (Yellow)

Suggested time: 40–45 minutes (Total time)	Activities	Materials and staff needed
10–15 minutes	Introduction: Metabolic Engine Review	Parents and patients' educational materials and books (Sothern, von Almen, & Schumacher, 2001) Exercise attire Music player Staff: Exercise trainer or guest aerobic dance instructor
30–35 minutes	Activity I: Rockin' to the Oldies, Aerobic Class	
Objectives After participation in this lesson the student will be able to: 1. Identify differences between aerobic versus anaerobic exercise. 2. Gain knowledge concerning the benefits of aerobic exercise to health. 3. Develop pacing skills to monitor exercise performance in order to increase duration. 4. Safely participate in an aerobic exercise routine to music.		

INTRODUCTION

The instructor will introduce or review all of the metabolic systems. See lesson 1, level 1 (red), for information.

ACTIVITY I. ROCKIN' TO THE OLDIES AEROBIC DANCE CLASS

The instructor will then lead a low-impact aerobics class to 1950s and 1960s music. Fun old-ies moves include the twist, mashed potato, the hustle, the monkey, the skate, the pony, and partner jitterbug.

The instructor may choose to hire a guest instructor to teach this class. Suggested music includes Beach Boys Surfin' Music, Wipeout, Do You Love Me (Dirty Dancing), KC and the Sunshine Band, Ray Charles (Hit the Road Jack), and Aretha Franklin (Respect).

LESSON 4, LEVEL 2

Table 6.33   Overview: Lesson 4, Level 2 (Yellow)

Suggested time: 45–50 minutes (Total time)	Activities	Materials and staff needed
5–10 minutes	Introduction: Strength Facts—Muscle Fibers	Parents and patients' educational materials and books (Sothern, von Almen, & Schumacher, 2001) Exercise attire Hand weights Ankle weights Exercise stretch resistance bands Chairs Station markers Staff: Exercise trainer
35–40 minutes	Activity I: Strength Circuit Class	
Objectives After participation in this lesson the student will be able to: 1. Identify safe methods to participate in exercises to improve muscular strength and endurance. 2. Gain knowledge concerning the benefits of resistance training to health. 3. Safely participate in a resistance training circuit under the supervision of a parent or other adult. 4. Gain knowledge concerning the specific muscle fiber composition related to low and high intensity physical activity.		

INTRODUCTION

The instructor will review the benefits of strength training and review the proper technique for each of the exercises. He or she will discuss how different types of muscle fibers affect strength-training results. The patients and their family members will then participate in a strength-training circuit class.

MUSCLE FIBER COMPOSITION

Muscle fibers generally are classified as slow twitch or fast twitch. The percentage of each is genetically determined. Slow twitch equals low intensity, long duration. Fast twitch equals high intensity, short duration. Those with more slow-twitch muscles are better equipped to partake in moderate- to vigorous-intensity, long-duration exercises (like basketball). Those with more fast twitch muscles are well suited to high intensity, short-duration exercises. Individuals with an equal number of both slow-twitch and fast-twitch fibers typically excel at middle-distance or moderate-intensity events, although they typically are competent in all types of sports or activities.

Key Points: Classification of Muscle Fiber Types

Characteristic	Slow-Twitch Type I	Fast-Twitch(a) Type IIa
Aerobic capacity	High	Moderate
Anaerobic capacity	Low	High
Oxidation	High	Moderate
Glycolysis	Low	High
Force/size	Low	High
Fatigue time	Low	High

Sources: Adapted from Sothern, 2001; Wilmore & Costill, 1994.

MUSCLE FIBER SIZE AND NUMBER

The size of muscle fibers can be enlarged through strength training. This will result in both larger muscle cross-sectional areas and longer muscle fibers. Because muscles are more metabolically active, they are denser and more toned.

Patient Handout: How to Plan Your Own Resistance Weight-Training Program

Allow sufficient time in your routine for an adequate warm-up and cooldown, as recommended by your instructor.
Use this sequence of exercises:

- Start with your large muscle groups, preferably leg muscles, and do abdominal exercises at the end of the routine.
- Follow with exercises that work the upper body muscles in unison.
- Follow these with exercises that isolate specific arm muscles.
- Then do another exercise that works upper body muscles in unison and that is different from the earlier exercise.
- Do another large muscle group, such as abdominal muscles or oblique (waistline) muscles.
- Finally do exercises for the calf muscles.

If you feel pain during the performance of an exercise, stop immediately. This might indicate an existing injury, a structural problem, or improper technique. Ask your exercise instructor for assistance.

Remember to monitor your results. This is the only way you can determine whether a particular exercise and its duration and intensity are right for you.

Remember that genetic factors determine the results of your exercise program. Respect your own limitations and avoid comparing your progress with that of others.

When you are doing your exercise routine, be courteous to others who are performing an exercise circuit. Try to organize your workout so that it does not upset the rhythm of the majority.

ACTIVITY I. STRENGTH CIRCUIT CLASS

The students will participate in strength circuit class. The stations will follow the exercises illustrated in Chapter 4 of this book. During this circuit, the instructor will discuss facts concerning strength training. See lesson 4, level 1, for more information.

LESSON 5, LEVEL 2

Table 6.34 Overview: Lesson 5, Level 2 (Yellow)

Suggested time: 45–50 minutes (Total time)	Activities	Materials and staff needed
10–15 minutes	Introduction: Cross-Training	Parents and patients' educational materials and books (Sothern, von Almen, & Schumacher, 2001) Exercise attire Hand weights Ankle weights Music player Music Station markers Stopwatch Whistle Staff: Exercise trainer
30–35 minutes	Activity I: Toning or Body Sculpting	
Objectives	After participation in this lesson the student will be able to: 1. Gain knowledge concerning the benefits of participation in cross-training programs. 2. Identify safe methods to participate in cross-training activities. 4. Safely participate in a circuit class with varied aerobic exercise movements.	

INTRODUCTION

The instructor will discuss how to prevent activity burnout by engaging in cross-training. He or she will then lead the class in a body sculpting or "toning" class.

Talking Points: Cross-Training (Verbal cues for patients or parents and family members)
Read through the following information with your patient or family members to help them to understand the exercise strategy used in the program.

By now, your child is accustomed to regular activity and exercise. To keep him interested and to add variety to the routine, this is a good time to introduce cross-training. He will continue with a structured exercise program, but now he will integrate two or more different types of aerobic and endurance activities into his workout. Cross-training also burns more calories by targeting and using all different muscle groups (including slow- and fast-twitch muscle fibers), which results in an all-over toned appearance (or "buff," as your kids might call it).

There are four types of cross-training, including the following:

1. Continuous Cross-Training—a regimen without rest, such as jogging, swimming, walking, or cycling. Alternate types of activity by days or by weeks. Maintain intensity consistently throughout the session.

2. Interval Cross-Training—this workout draws from a variety of activities interspersed with rest periods, followed by repeating the activities. For example, run very hard for one lap, walk easily for two laps, jog moderately for one lap, run very hard for one lap, and so on. Intensity varies from very high to very low during the workout.

3. Fartlek Cross-Training—a more casual version of interval training, this free-form training typically occurs outdoors on trails or roads. The exercise–rest cycle is not predetermined or precisely timed or measured. Instead, it is based on how the individual feels. He could run uphill for 10 minutes, walk on a flat area for 5 minutes, slowly jog downhill and on flat land for 15 minutes, walk rapidly uphill for 20 minutes, and so on.

4. Circuit Cross-Training—this approach involves 10–20 stations of varying calisthenics and weight lifting exercise, coupled with running or walking.

Talking Points: Monitoring Activity and Providing Feedback (Verbal cues for patients or parents and family members)
Read through the following information with your patient or family members to help them to understand the exercise strategy used in the program.

As your child explores new types of exercises, observe his reactions so that you can monitor whether the routine is right for him or whether it is too challenging. Look for the following clues: Is he discouraged or sad? Is he breathing very fast, turning red in the face, and sweating profusely? Is he complaining that his ankles, knees, or other joints hurt? If so, the activity is too challenging. Refine the workout by reducing the time he spends performing the activity as well as the work level, speed, and or intensity. Allow him more time to rest, give him extra water, and make sure he is getting enough sleep. To grow properly, children need between 9 and 11 hours of sleep per night.

As your child enters this level of the program, negotiate specific rewards for her long-term exercise goals. Find out what she wants—new weights, new clothing for her fit body, a weekend trip to an activity park—in exchange for following her cross-training routine for a specified amount of time. Make the agreement formal by signing a contract that specifies her responsibilities and her reward. Then, see how powerful an incentive can be!

ACTIVITY I. TONING OR BODY SCULPTING

The instructor will lead a "toning" or "body-sculpting" class to music. The exercises will be done with or without weight, in a standing or a sitting position. Some of the exercises will be executed while lying on the floor. The exercises should be different from those illustrated in Chapter 4 or in lesson 4, level 1 (red). The instructor, however, should use caution when choosing exercises. Those that place the back, hip, leg, or arm joints at risk should be avoided. Kneeling or standing "donkey kicks" are not appropriate. Also avoid ballistic or fast movements. Some examples of appropriate exercises include side leg lifts, standing; all types of stomach crunches; standing modified squats; lying leg lifts; modified plié with hand weights performing overhead press; and biceps curl. All movements should be performed slowly to a four-beat count of the music. The instructor will discuss safety and injury prevention during the workout. He or she also will discuss how genetic influences determine how an individual responds to different types of muscle training. See lesson 7, level 1 (red), for more information.

Clinical Reminders for the Health Care Professional: Gender Differences

The body-sculpting exercises are especially preferred by adolescent females. If most of your class are boys, you may wish to choose another activity, such as basketball, biking, or field sports.

LESSON 6, LEVEL 2

Table 6.35 Overview: Lesson 6, Level 2 (Yellow)

Suggested time: 45–55 minutes (Total time)	Activities	Materials and staff needed
5–10 minutes	Introduction:	Parents and patients' educational materials and books (Sothern, von Almen, & Schumacher, 2001) Exercise attire Music player Staff: Exercise trainer or guest yoga instructor
10–15 minutes	Flex Test	
25–30 minutes	Activity I: Modified Yoga	
5 minutes	Activity II: Relax Your Back	

Objectives
After participation in this lesson the student will be able to:
1. Identify movements that will increase muscular flexibility.
2. Gain knowledge concerning the benefits of muscular flexibility to health.
3. Identify imbalances in the posture that lead to bone and joint problems.
4. Identify movement and exercises that will improve posture and muscular flexibility and reduce the risk of injury.
5. Safely participate in activities to improve muscular flexibility and reduce back pain and discomfort.

INTRODUCTION

The patients will again participate in the Flex Test illustrated in lesson 6, level 1 (red). The instructor will discuss the importance of flexibility exercise and relaxation techniques to reduce stress. Many relaxation techniques have stood the test of centuries, developed and practiced as inspirational healing traditions around the world. They often are based on breathing slowly and deeply until a sense of calm and well-being takes over. Some experts recommend visualization, soothing music, or positive self-talk to assist with the process and to keep from being distracted. The theory is that by visualizing a calm and serene scene, you cannot worry about daily stress and conflict. This can be difficult, however, if you do not yet know how to breathe slowly and deeply. Your patient should experiment with these tools only after he or she feels comfortable and confident with the breathing response. Review the relaxation technique in the patient handout with your patients and their families.

Patient Handout: Relaxation Rotation: How, When, and Why to Relax

By now, your child should be engaging in more activity, and learning to change his own behavior. That adds up to the heartening fact that he is gradually but steadily reversing the vicious cycle of his overweight condition. That is all good news, but even so, along the way, he (and you!) may experience some unexpected stress.

Learning to relax can be of great benefit to those seeking behavioral changes. Once you and your child learn the techniques in this section, the key then becomes to recognize precursors to stress and apply the relaxation technique before the stress plays out through underactivity.

Relaxing in a deep, influential way requires some initial dedication. Practicing for a couple of weeks will get you off to a good start. Follow these guidelines, and feel yourself become lighter!

- Get comfortable on a floor mat or bed with no environmental distractions such as television, radio, or other noise. Set a timer to go off in 10–15 minutes.
- Focus on something—anything will do—a picture on the wall, the corner of the room, or a ceiling fan. As you do, begin to notice your breathing. Try breathing a little more deeply—but do not fill your lungs to capacity.

- Inhale to the count of one. Exhale to the count of two. Proceed slowly as you count with each breath.

Your goal during the first week is to count to 10 without allowing extraneous thoughts to intrude. When thoughts do enter—and they will—simply begin counting over. Do not be distressed. Eventually you will make it to the count of 10 without interruption. At that point, you will experience a new sense of calm, well-being, and relaxation.

Once you are proficient at this exercise, use it when you feel stress coming on. Positive self-talk is effective for children once they learn the breathing technique. Teach your child to repeat phrases, such as "I can do anything I want," or "I'm looking better all the time," or "This will get easier." These phrases will sink in more after your child has reached a state of relaxation after doing the breathing exercise. Practice these exercises with your child for 10–15 minutes at least two times per week.

ACTIVITY I. MODIFIED YOGA

The instructor will lead a class to music consisting of dynamic stretching movements followed by static stretches as a warm-up. The importance of flexibility will be emphasized. The instructor or a guest instructor will then lead a modified yoga class consisting of safe yoga movements that have been changed to conform to the obese child's needs. A guest instructor, whose routine has been screened for safety, may be utilized for this class.

Key Points: Yoga

Yoga exercises, if performed properly, are beneficial. The instructor should use caution, however, when selecting exercises and should modify the movements where necessary.

ACTIVITY II. RELAX YOUR BACK

The instructor will end the class with the Relax Your Back Series by using the following instructions:

Talking Points: Relax Your Back (Verbal cues for patients or parents and family members)
Read through the following information with your patient or family members to help them to understand the exercise strategy used in the program.

Lie on your back. Relax your head and neck into your hands. Gently press your lower back into the floor. Slowly bring your knees into your chest and squeeze gently. Keep breathing. Keep your upper body relaxed.

Drop one foot to the floor, keeping your knee bent. Squeeze the other knee gently into your chest.

Slowly pull the knee across your body to stretch outer hip. Extend the opposite arm, palm down. Turn your head toward the opposite direction. Slowly return the knee to chest. Repeat with the other leg.

Return both knees, and then the rest of your body, to the starting position.

Slowly slide one arm upward along the floor. Stretch your arms in the direction illustrated. Repeat with other arm.

Place arms behind your head and relax your head and shoulders. Tilt your hips upward as you gently press your lower back into the floor. Tighten and hold in lower abdomen.

Keeping the same lower body position, slowly extend arms overhead. Do not lift the shoulder, neck or head. Keep upper body relaxed. The spine should be completely aligned with floor, and relaxed.

Continue to hold the stomach tight and press your spine gently into the floor. Begin to "walk" the feet out until your back starts to come up. Retilt hips and press spine into floor, holding stomach tight.

Over time, your stomach muscles will become stronger, enabling you to achieve and maintain this position. Keep your back flat and spine gently pressed into the floor. Relax your shoulders and head while keeping stomach tight.

Release the position, allowing back to slowly arch. Relax your abdomen.

Slowly and gently, stretch hands away from feet as shown. Let your rib cage expand, arch back, and stretch your stomach. Relax all muscles. Slowly, return knees to the chest and gently squeeze.

Slowly return to the original stretch position. Drop feet to the floor, keeping knees bent for safety.

Relax all muscles. Slowly return knees to the chest and gently squeeze. Return to starting position.

Roll onto your stomach. Sit back on your heels while extending arms forward, palms down. Keep your face down, head in line with the back. Gently stretch.

LESSON 7, LEVEL 2

Table 6.36   Overview: Lesson 7, Level 2 (Yellow)

Suggested Time: 45–50 minutes	Activities	Materials and Staff Needed
5–10 minutes	Introduction: Fat Metabolism, Steady-State Activities	Parents and patients' educational materials and books (Sothern, von Almen, & Schumacher, 2001) Exercise attire Station markers Treadmill Cycle ergometer Rowing ergometer Rowing machine Stair-climber Music player Stopwatch Staff: Exercise trainer
30–35 minutes	Activity I: Aerobic Circuit with Exercise Equipment	
5–10 minutes	Activity II: Abdominal (stomach) Crunch Challenge	

Objectives
After participation in this lesson the student will be able to: 1. Gain knowledge concerning the effects of varied types of physical activity on fat metabolism. 2. Identify exercises that increase the opportunity to participate in steady-state metabolism. 3. Safely participate in a circuit class using exercise equipment. 4. Identify methods to set individual goals to improve abdominal strength through participation in a timed stomach crunch exercise bout.

INTRODUCTION

The instructor will discuss ways to enhance fat metabolism and the concept of steady-state activities. The class will participate in an aerobic circuit utilizing available exercise equipment. This will be followed by participation in the quarterly abdominal crunch challenge. See lesson 7, level 1 (red), for instructions.

ACTIVITY I. AEROBIC EQUIPMENT AND EXERCISE CIRCUIT

A combination of aerobic equipment and exercise movement stations will be organized so that the patients and their families can participate in a combined circuit. For example, a circuit could be arranged as follows: Station 1, treadmill; Station 2, side jacks; Station 3, cycle ergometer; Station 4, heel backs with arms up; Station 5, rowing ergometer; Station 6, twist; Station 7, stair-climber; and so on. The instructor uses station markers and guides the students from one station to another. Students should spend 2 minutes at each station and be given 30 seconds to change stations. The instructor may choose to use music to motivate the children.

ACTIVITY II. THE QUARTERLY ABDOMINAL CRUNCH CHALLENGE

The instructor will use the personal best scores for each patient achieved during the past 10-week session in lesson 7, level 1 (red). Following the instructions from this class, the abdominal crunch challenge will be repeated. Positive reinforcement will be provided to patients improving the number of crunches they achieve in 5 minutes (personal best). Patients should not be compared with each other, but rather should seek to improve their own individual score.

LESSON 8, LEVEL 2

Table 6.37   Overview: Lesson 8, Level 2 (Yellow)

Suggested time: 45–50 minutes (Total time)	Activities	Materials and staff needed
5–10 minutes	Introduction: Raising Activity Levels	Parents and patients' educational materials and books (Sothern, von Almen, & Schumacher, 2001) Exercise attire Soccer ball Soccer goal and cones Whistle
40–45 minutes	Activity I: Family Team Sports—Aerobic Soccer	
		Staff: Exercise trainer
Objectives After participation in this lesson the student will be able to: 1. Identify ways to organize family events to include exercise activities. 2. Identify safe methods to participate in family field sports. 3. Gain knowledge concerning the proper technique and rules for the game of soccer. 4. Safely participate in a soccer game with friends and family members. 5. Gain knowledge concerning how to pace exercise activities to reduce fatigue by alternating positions on the field.		

INTRODUCTION

The instructor will review methods to increase daily physical activity levels. He or she will then describe how to modify the game of soccer to include new rules that increase opportunity to gain aerobic benefits from participation.

Talking Points: Top 10 Healthy Tips to Increase Physical Activity (Verbal cues for patients or parents and family members)
Read through the following information with your patient or family members to help them to understand the exercise strategy used in the program.

1. Encourage your child to move briskly at every opportunity.
2. Enroll your child in structured dance, sport, or movement classes. Make sure the teachers are qualified and discuss your child's condition with the teacher before enrolling.

3. Create an environment for active play both inside and outside the home.
4. Participate in activities the entire family can enjoy together.
5. Expose your overweight child to as many different kinds of activities as possible in a nonintimidating and nurturing environment.
6. Provide opportunities for your normal weight child to safely climb, run, and jump to help develop muscles strength and bone density.
7. Do not impose adult exercise goals on young children who have immature metabolic systems.
8. Reserve at least one-half day each weekend dedicated to fun, family fitness activities.
9. Do not draw attention to sedentary activities with negative comments. Instead, praise your children when they choose active play.
10. Be a good role model. Parents do not have to be thin, but they must set a good example by participating in healthy physical activities.

ACTIVITY I. AEROBIC SOCCER

In aerobic soccer, there are no boundaries other than those needed for safety reasons. The ball is always in play. Offense and defense players switch places every 10 minutes to enable all members to run up and down the field. Only 5 seconds are allowed to begin play after a goal is made.

The patients and parents will participate in an outdoor soccer game. The warm-up will include a soccer skill review followed by drills for about 5 minutes. Periodic breathing and heart rate checks will illustrate to the kids and parents how soccer raises the metabolic rate, thus encouraging an increase in activity levels and calories burned. Offense and defense positions should alternate every 5 minutes.

To make the soccer game more aerobic or steady-state, and to increase caloric expenditure, try these modifications:

● Announce to the kids and parents that you are playing by *your* rules; only *you* can decide whether the ball is out-of-bounds.
● Allow 3 seconds only for placing the ball back in play from the sideline or the goal. The team loses the ball if they exceed 3 seconds.
● Allow the ball to go outside of the regular boundaries to keep it in play. Only call the ball out-of-bounds when it presents a danger to the kids.

 Key Points: How to Arrange Teams

Teams are selected as follows: All children line up behind the instructor, coach, or parent who will serve as referee for the game. The referee then alternately assigns the children to one of two colors to designate the different teams (e.g., blue and red). This method is efficient and discourages captains and elimination issues, such as being picked last for a team.

LESSON 9, LEVEL 2

Table 6.38   Overview: Lesson 9, Level 2 (Yellow)

Suggested time: 40–45 minutes (Total time)	Activities	Materials and staff needed
5 minutes	Introduction	Parents and patients' educational materials and books (Sothern, von Almen, & Schumacher, 2001) Exercise attire Music player Music
35–40 minutes	Activity I: Guest Instructor: Ballroom or Theme Dancing	
		Staff: Exercise trainer or guest ballroom or theme dance instructor
Objectives		
After participation in this lesson the student will be able to: 1. Recognize safe methods to engage in specialty theme aerobic exercise to music. 2. Identify the benefits of dancing to overall health and well-being. 3. Safely participate in a group dance class to improve aerobic fitness.		

ACTIVITY I. GUEST INSTRUCTOR: BALLROOM DANCING

The instructor will organize a professional ballroom or theme dance instructor to provide instruction to the patients and their families. Options include waltz, swing, tap, salsa, or cha-cha.

LESSON 10, LEVEL 2

Table 6.39   Overview: Lesson 10, Level 2 (Yellow)

Suggested time: 85–100 minutes (Total time)	Activities	Materials and staff needed
10–15 minutes	Introduction: Park Day	Parents and patients' educational materials and books (Sothern, von Almen, & Schumacher, 2001) Exercise attire Music player Luggage cart
75–85 minutes	Activity I: Walking Aerobics	
		Staff: Exercise trainer
Objectives		
After participation in this lesson the student will be able to: 1. Gain knowledge concerning the benefits of group outdoor activities to overall health and well-being. 2. Recognize opportunities to engage in safe methods to participate in physical activities in outdoor settings. 3. Safely participate in activities in a park setting with friends and family members designed to maximize opportunities for movement to promote increased physical activity.		

INTRODUCTION

The instructor will congratulate their patients and family for members for completing the 10-week session. He or she should discuss how to prepare for the follow-up medical tests, which will determine their overall progress. Patients will be informed that rewards will be given out in 2 weeks for attendance and exercise compliance. The instructor will organize a park day as previously described in lesson 10, level 1 (red).

ACTIVITY I. WALKING AEROBICS

The instructor straps a music player to a luggage cart. The patients, parents, and instructor walk the park track while performing aerobic arm moves to the music. Examples of arm moves are arms cross in front, biceps curls, arms overhead, alternate straight arms up and down, monkey arms, bucket arms. All movement is done to the beat of the music.

LESSON 1, LEVEL 3 (GREEN)

Table 6.40   Overview: Lesson 1, Level 3 (Green)

Suggested time: 40–45 minutes (Total time)	Activities	Materials and staff needed
10–15 minutes	Introduction: Increasing Daily Activities: Inside When the Weather Is Bad	Parents and patients' educational materials and books (Sothern, Schumacher, von Almen et al., 2001)
30–35 minutes	Activity I: Musical Balloon Toss, 30-minute Rule Activity II: Balloon Battle Activity III: Imagination Station	Exercise attire CD/iPod player Balloons Large plastic tub filled with indoor physical activity play items Staff: Exercise Trainer
Objectives After participation in this lesson the student will be able to: 1. Gain knowledge concerning the benefits of exercise and increasing daily physical activity to health. 2. Recognize safe methods to engage in exercise inside the home. 3. Identify the benefits to replacing television and computer time with indoor active games. 4. Gain time management skills necessary to include 3–5 minutes of physical activity every 30 minutes at home before and after school and on weekends.		

INTRODUCTION

The instructor will discuss ways to build physical activity into the family's daily routine at home, inside when the weather is poor. He or she will review the following balloon games:

ACTIVITY I. MUSICAL BALLOON TOSS

Ask the parents to purchase a pack of 12 large balloons and have their children try this safe and fun game in their den or living room. Blow the balloons up and gather in the middle of the room with two or more friends. Play one of their favorite songs, and tell the children to try to keep all 12 balloons up in the air for the entire song. Then try another song.

ACTIVITY II. BALLOON BATTLE

Ask the students to blow the balloons up and gather in the middle of the room (requires two or more students). Stretch out a jump rope to create a boundary line. Place the 12 balloons on the floor along the boundary line. Split the students up into two groups and have each group stand on either side of the boundary line. Play a kid-friendly song while the students push the balloons to the other side of the line with only their hands (*kicking is not allowed in this game*). When the song ends, everyone freezes in place and the side with the fewest balloons wins.

THE 30-MINUTE RULE

Research indicates that concentration and work performance begin to decline after 30 minutes of intense mental activity (like studying). Require that your patients take a break for just 5–10 minutes every 30 minutes and then ask them to evaluate whether their performance at school improves. An added benefit is that these small movement periods burn an extra 2000–3000 calories each week.

Companies that make video and computer games spend millions on advertising. Their goal is to see children sit (motionless) before their merchandise all day long. Unfortunately there are children who can do amazing things on the computer, but who never learned to ride a bike or swing a bat. Remember to tell parents that they do not have to wait for holidays to purchase toys, games, and equipment that encourage movement. They should start rewarding their child with fun new things as soon as he or she begins meeting his or her goals. Soon they will have enough "physically active" toys and other items to create imagination stations.

Talking Points: Indoor Activities (Verbal cues for patients or parents and family members)
Read through the following information with your patient or family members to help them to understand the exercise strategy used in the program.

Have you refurbished your house so that your child can stay active during rainy, cold, and snowy months? There are plenty of places to take your child when cabin fever sets in. Sign her up for weekly indoor activities or just go for a one-day visit when the mood strikes.

- Gyms/Fitness Centers: They offer a variety of calorie-burning fun, including gymnastics, tumbling, indoor basketball, wrestling, kick boxing or other martial arts, wall-climbing, track, badminton, volleyball, ping pong, and swimming. Don't forget indoor tennis.
- Dance Studios: Kids are welcome in all kinds of classes including ballet, tap, modern, jazz, hip-hop, line dancing, ballroom dancing, yoga, free movement classes, and other music–dance combination classes.
- Indoor Rinks: Ice skating and roller skating can fill hours of fun on a rainy day.
- Children's Museums: These museums exist in most cities and provide interesting, educational, and fun activities that keep your kid on the move.
- Indoor nature centers or aquariums offer similar movement opportunities.
- Restaurants with Games: They are popping up all over. Choose those that offer the greatest energy burners, including laser tag and other fast-paced activities. Most have salad bars, so plan on light meals.

ACTIVITY III: IMAGINATION STATION

The instructor will demonstrate to the patients and family member how to create an "imagination station," which can be placed in a room in the family home, where areas are set up for the patient to try different activities. He or she will provide a plastic tub filled with costumes, dress-up clothes, and accessories like crowns, wands, toy shields, armor, masks, vests, belts, shoes, hats, grass skirts, scarfs, play jewelry, wigs, and so forth. The patients will be allowed to play together with the item of their choice. Some other ideas for supplies for this activity are as follows:

- Boom box with various dance music CDs
- Microphone, drums, toy musical instruments, stage curtains
- Puppets, marionettes, magician kits, various stuffed animals
- Batons, small flags, pom-poms, streamers, hula-hoops
- Foam mats and wedges, indoor tents, large building blocks or cardboard boxes, bean bag chairs, soft pillows, old blankets, sheets
- Hop-scotch mat, action games like Twister, charades, Simon says, follow the leader
- Paddle balls, indoor ball toss games, bean bags, juggling balls, hacky sack

- Kid-safe dart boards or other target games
- Indoor basketball hoop and soft foam balls
- Jump ropes, skip-it, small kid-safe hand weights, exercise stretch bands

For younger children, try the following:

- Small pull–push toys or plastic wagons
- Toy household cleaning items such as brooms, mops, vacuum cleaners, feather dusters
- Toy kitchen, restaurant, and accessories
- Indoor riding toys

After setting up the imagination station, allow the children and family members to "play" with the items freely. After a few minutes, ask them to take their heart rate. They will be surprised at how vigorous playing with imagination can be. End the session by discussing ways to get active during television commercials and ways to create the "imagination station" at home.

Talking Points: Commercial Boogie and Imagination Station (Verbal cues for patients or parents and family members)
Read through the following information with your patient or family members to help them to understand the exercise strategy used in the program.

When you are gathered in front of the television watching your favorite show, do not forget to stand up and do the "television commercial boogie" whenever the ads come on. You will be amazed at how much moving you will do to the soundtracks of those endless commercials! And be sure to engage in collective booing when junk-food ads fill the screen.
Ask mom and dad to help you create your own "imagination station" in your den, living room, or bedroom. Find a large plastic clothes hamper or tub and put it in the corner. Now, search the house for items that you can use to play indoors. You have 10 minutes. When the time is up, go to your own personal "imagination station" and do your favorite activity with mom and dad.

LESSON 2, LEVEL 3

Table 6.41   Overview: Lesson 2, Level 3 (Green)

Suggested time: 40–50 minutes (Total time)	Activities	Materials and staff needed
10–15 minutes	Introduction: Review Metabolic Systems	Parents and patients' educational materials and books (Sothern, von Almen, & Schumacher, 2001) Exercise attire Music player
30–40 minutes	Activity I: Specialty Aerobics: Salsa/Latin Dance	

Objectives
After participation in this lesson the student will be able to:
1. Identify differences between aerobic versus anaerobic exercise.
2. Gain knowledge concerning the benefits of aerobic exercise to health.
3. Develop pacing skills to monitor exercise performance to increase duration.
4. Identify movement and exercises that will improve cardiorespiratory (aerobic) endurance.
5. Safely participate in a specialty group dance class to improve aerobic fitness.

INTRODUCTION

The instructor will introduce or review the metabolic systems. For instructions, see lesson 2, level 1 (red).

ACTIVITY I. SPECIALTY AEROBICS: SALSA/LATIN DANCE

A guest instructor will teach a Latin or salsa aerobic dance class.

LESSON 3, LEVEL 3

Table 6.42   Overview: Lesson 3, Level 3 (Green)

Suggested time: 90 100 minutes (Total time)	Activities	Materials and staff needed
10–15 minutes	Introduction: Cardiorespiratory Endurance	Parents and patients' educational materials and books (Sothern, von Almen, & Schumacher, 2001)
60–70 minutes	Activity I: The Fit Kit Walking Program	
		Exercise attire Water and containers Cups
		Staff: Exercise trainer or guest ballroom or theme dance instructor

Objectives
After participation in this lesson the student will be able to:
1. Identify safe methods to participate in exercises to improve aerobic endurance.
2. Gain knowledge concerning the benefits of walking as a means to improve aerobic endurance.
3. Gain knowledge and experience in techniques to identify intensity of exercise through heart rate monitoring.
4. Safely participate in a neighborhood or nature walk with classmates, friends, and family members.

INTRODUCTION

The instructor will introduce or review cardiorespiratory fitness. Refer to lesson 3, level 1 (red).

ACTIVITY I. THE FIT KIT WALKING PROGRAM

The instructor will review The Fit Kit Walking Program. The parents and kids will be encouraged to begin the program as a family project.

The Fit Kit Walking Program was designed especially for blue- or green-level kids (red- or yellow-level kids should choose an alternate activity this week, such as biking or swimming). By participating in this program, you will burn lots of calories, train your leg and hip muscles, and improve the efficiency of your heart and lungs. Walking is one of the easiest and most convenient ways you can stay active on a daily basis. There may be times you walk with a friend, whereas at other times you may prefer to walk alone. Either way is fine as long as you keep on truckin'!

Follow these steps to healthy walking:

Step 1: Check Up. Check your shoes, clothes, and walking route.
Shoes—10 Tips for Choosing Walking Shoes
- Select the lightest weight walking shoe available.
- Choose shoes with padding in the tongue, collar, and heel.
- Ensure that the inside is fully lined with light, airy material.
- Select shoes with a leather exterior.
- Do not buy shoes with pointed or tapered toes.

- Choose shoes that have the best shock absorption in the mid-sole and footbed.
- Choose shoes that are flexible. Bend the shoe to determine how flexible it is.
- Check the heel design. It should have a notch that conforms to the Achilles' tendon.
- Select Velcro straps combined with laces to allow a more secure fit.
- Get a new pair of walking shoes about every 6 months. Do not try to save money by wearing them longer. These are your precious feet we are working with!

Clothes

- In the summer, choose loose-fitting, all-cotton tee shirts and tank tops.
- In the winter, dress in layers of warm, soft, loose-fitting clothes, woolen mittens, and a hat.

Walking Route

- Sketch a map of your planned walking route on paper. Make sure to include landmarks, phone locations, water stops, and favorite scenic spots. Post your map on the refrigerator.
- Always tell someone where you will be walking if it is different from your typical route.

Step 2: Form a Plan of Action. Write a 1-week walking schedule and put it into your daily calendar.

Step 3: Get Ready. Choose an appropriate warm-up that includes dynamic stretches (stretch while moving). Do not do any static stretches without warming up first. Wait until after your walking to do static stretches.

Step 4: Put Your Best Foot Forward. Walk slowly at first, swinging your arms naturally. Pick up the pace after a few minutes to a comfortable, moderate level. Remember, if you start to breathe too rapidly, slow down until you are going at the pace that is right for you.

Use the accompanying chart to calculate your walking speed. First try to walk 1 mile (refer to your map) and record how long it took. Then go to the chart. Put one finger on the "1-mile" mark and the other on the time it took you, to the nearest 10 minutes. For example, if it took you 40 minutes to walk 1 mile, you were walking at 1.5 mph.

Distance covered
(in miles): _____

Time it takes
(minutes) _____

Patient Handout: Miles per Hour Chart

Miles walked	Time it took (to the nearest 10 minutes)								
	20	30	40	50	60	70	80	90	100
1	3.0	2.0	1.5	1.2	1.0	.9	.8	.7	.6
2	6.0	4.5	3.0	2.5	2.0	1.8	1.5	1.3	1.2
3	9.0	7.5	4.5	3.8	3.0	2.7	2.3	2.0	1.8
4	12.0	9.0	6.0	5.0	4.0	3.5	3.0	2.2	2.0
5	15.0	11.5	7.5	6.2	5.0	4.5	3.8	3.4	3.0

Step 5: Cool Down and Stretch. Reduce your pace during the last 5–10 minutes of the walk. Finish up with at least one stretch of each major muscle group. See Chapter 4 for proper technique.

Step 6: Keep a Walking Diary. Use the form below to record your experiences.

Patient Handout: My Walking Diary, Week 1

Week 1	Day 1	Day 2	Day 3	Day 4	Day 5	Day 6	Day 7
Date							
Time							
Location							
Terrain							
Weather							
Distance							
Speed							
Conditions							
Comments							

Patient Handout: My Walking Diary, Week 2

Week 2	Day 1	Day 2	Day 3	Day 4	Day 5	Day 6	Day 7
Date							
Time							
Location							
Terrain							
Weather							
Distance							
Speed							
Conditions							
Comments							

Step 7: Weigh the Outcome of Your Walk. Determine how many calories you burned during your walk by using the accompanying chart. First, determine the distance you walked. Then figure out your speed (mph) from the your Miles per Hour Chart on page XX.

Patient Handout: How Many Calories Did I Burn?*

Speed (in mph)	Distance Covered (in miles)				
	1	2	3	4	5
2.0	48–63	96–126	144–189	192–252	240–315
2.5	50–64	100–128	150–192	200–256	250–320
3.0	52–66	104–132	156–198	208–264	260–330
3.5	54–67	108–134	162–201	216–268	270–335
4.0	58–72	116–144	174–216	232–288	290–360
4.5	65–80	130–160	195–240	260–320	325–400
5.0	75–90	150–180	225–270	300–360	375–450

*These figures are based on an average weight of 125–150 pounds. If you weigh more than 150 pounds, you will burn more calories. If you weigh less than 125 pounds, you will burn fewer calories.

Step 8: Take the Next Step. Many people find walking enjoyable once they get into the habit. If this is true for you, consider joining a local club or enter a fun walk or run. Check with your local recreation, church, or school organizations for upcoming opportunities. It is a great way to meet new friends who also love to walk and be active.

And there you have it, the Fit Kit Walking Program!

LESSON 4, LEVEL 3

Table 6.43   Overview: Lesson 4, Level 3 (Green)

Suggested Time: 40–50 minutes (Total time)	Activities	Materials and Staff Needed
5–10 minutes	Introduction: Muscular Strength and Endurance	Parents and patients' educational materials and books (Sothern, von Almen, & Schumacher, 2001) Exercise attire Chair Pull-up bar, if available
35–45 minutes	Activity I: Advanced Resistance Training, Pull Your Own Weight Series	
		Staff: Exercise trainer

Objectives:
After participation in this lesson the student will be able to:
  1. Identify safe methods to participate in exercises to improve muscular strength and endurance.
  2. Gain knowledge concerning the benefits of resistance training to health.
  3. Safely participate in a resistance training routine using his or her own body weight under the supervision of a parent or other adult.
  4. Gain knowledge concerning the specific muscle or muscle group that is responsible for varied types of body movement.

INTRODUCTION

The instructor will discuss muscular strength and endurance facts and review the exercises illustrated in Chapter 4. He or she will lead a class to the Pull Your Own Weight Series using only the child's own body weight. Follow the instructions as prescribed.

Key Points: Muscular Strength and Endurance Facts

Overload
Stress

The body responds to stress in one of two ways, adaption or breakdown. In muscle adaption, this may be referred to as training effect, such as an increase in strength, power, endurance, or speed. Breakdowns result in overuse syndromes and other injuries. The goal of training programs is to obtain as much training effect as possible without sustaining stress injury.

Training Effect

Muscles are the engines of the body. Their performance is improved when stress is applied in excess of their present capacity. This is referred to as overload, which results in a training effect specific to the exercise.

Injury

If stress is excessive, the body's response is a stress injury or overuse syndromes. This may occur as the result of improper technique, too much force, inadequate rest, poor nutrition, or dehydration.

Frequency and Rest

In weight training more demanding workouts require more recovery time. Research supports 2–3 nonconsecutive exercise sessions per week with adequate rest in between.

Specificity of Training
Strength

Strength is defined as the maximum ability of a muscle or group of muscles to apply or resist force. It is a pure and independent factor from endurance and power. Training for strength results in adaption of fibers within the muscles.

Power

Power is defined as performance of work expressed per unit of time. It is dependent on strength because it is the product of strength and speed (POWER = FORCE × VELOCITY). To train for power, exercises must include a rapid speed component specific to the desired goals.

Size

Increases in muscle area size (hypertrophy) are due to three factors:

1. Muscle fiber lengthening and widening and possibly an increase in the number of fibers.
2. Increased vascularization (blood flow and capillary development)
3. Fluid retention (edema) in the muscle area due to stress.

Endurance

Endurance is defined as the ability of a muscle to repeatedly develop near maximal force and to sustain repeated contractions. It is dependent on the level of strength and utilizes mainly aerobic metabolic systems.

Fat Composition

Strength training results in a more lean, less fat body. Skin thickness and fat tissue location is genetic and may inhibit lean appearance.

Technique
Balance

The ultimate goal of weight training is a strong, asymmetrical, and balanced physique. This is achieved by training muscles anteriorly and posteriorly with the same intensity as well as left and right sides. Differences in strength leave the weaker muscles more prone to injury.

Body Part Position
Fixation: Stabilizing unused body parts
Range: Limited by individual differences
Isolation: Dual-angle joint
Secondary: Multidual joint
Primary: Multijoint

One-third to two-third principle of internal rotation
Anatomical positioning of hands and feet

Speed of Movement

Research supports 60 degrees per second or at least 2 seconds for lifting and 2 seconds for lowering. Controlled movement speeds enhance both training safety and training stimulus.

Sets and Repetitions

Research supports 1–3 training sets per exercise; depending on training goals and time availability. Repetitions depend to some degree on muscle fiber type. Research supports 8–12 repetitions.

ACTIVITY I. ADVANCED RESISTANCE TRAINING AND PULL YOUR OWN WEIGHT SERIES

The instructor will discuss advanced resistance training techniques. A circuit class of advanced-level exercises may be organized after technique instruction. (See lesson 4, level 1 (red), for instructions on how to set up.) Patients and family members may participate in the following Pull Your Own Weight Series:

Patient Handout: Pull Your Own Weight Series

Let's say you are out of town visiting relatives or on a family vacation. By now, you love your new, toned, beautiful body and you are aching to do some strengthening exercises.

The exercises below work the major muscle groups, and you do not need a gym or special equipment to do them. Instead you will use your own body weight to tone and strengthen your muscles. Be sure to do them slowly, and be sure to fully extend and contract your muscles to get full strengthening and toning benefit.

Modified Standing Push-Up

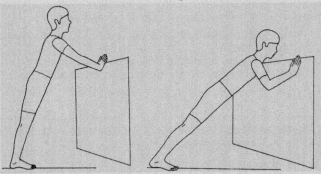

Stand 2–3 feet from a wall, sturdy table, or chair, with your feet together and your hands extended forward. Place your hands on the wall or grasp the table or chair, as you lean your body forward at a 45-degree angle to the floor. Slowly, bend your elbows and lower your chest until it touches the edge of the table or chair. Now, push with your hands, extending your arms, and return to the original position. Keep your head in line with your body. Keep your legs straight and extended throughout the exercise. Repeat 8–12 times.

You are training the chest muscles (pectorals).

Modified Lunge

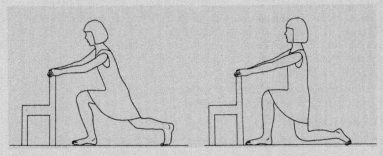

Stand with your feet about 6–8 inches apart and grasp the back of a sturdy chair with both of your hands. Step forward with your right leg approximately 18-36 inches. Keep your head, shoulders, and hips in a straight line. Bend your knees and lower the left knee onto floor. Do not allow the right knee to move in front of your right foot. Push the heel of the right foot into the floor as you lift and return to the starting position. Repeat with your left leg forward. Repeat 8–12 times on each leg.

You are working the buttocks muscles (gluteus), the back of upper leg (hamstrings), and the front upper leg (quads).

Triceps Dip

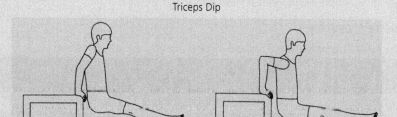

Sit in a sturdy chair with your legs extended straight in front of your body, heels on the floor, toes up and relaxed. Place your hands on either side of your hips, grasping either side of the chair seat. Slowly slide your hips forward slightly in front of the chair, and lower them 6–8 inches. Your elbows will bend as you lower your hips. Then, lift your hips by slowly straightening your elbows (without snapping or locking) and extending your arms to a full, straight position. Repeat this move 8–12 times.
   You are working the back of the upper arm (triceps).

Note: Some of the exercises require spotters. Instruct your patients to have their parents help them at home.

METHODS FOR STIMULATING GREATER MUSCLE DEVELOPMENT

The human body experiences several plateaus in improvement when pursuing any physical activity. Individual genetic factors limit the potential for development of strength and size of muscles. An example of this is that fast-twitch muscles have a greater potential for hypertrophy.

At first the body has a "learning effect" due to nervous system adaptations to strength training. Substantial gains are noticed at this first stage. These gains then level out and it is necessary to use different methods to develop a greater number of muscle fibers.

The key to greater muscle development during a plateau is change.

- Change your training exercises
- Change your training frequency
- Change the relationship between resistance and repetitions
- Increase your training intensity

"Harder" means "smarter"—not necessarily longer. Strength training is limited by the anaerobic respiratory system (30–120 seconds).

High-intensity training includes the following:

- Breakdown training
- Assisted training
- Super-slow training
- Negative training
- One-and-one-quarter training

And if all else fails—

- Get more sleep (quality rest)—at least 7.5 hours per night is necessary.
- Drink more fluids—muscles are 75% water.
- Obtain better nutrition (a well-balanced diet, high in carbohydrates)—increased protein intake promotes dehydration.
- Eat smaller meals more frequently.

Your muscles get stronger after your workout during the rebuilding period. This is when proteins (actin and myosin) are resynthesized and when connective tissue is rebuilt.

Your goal is to exercise the greatest number of muscle fibers per movement and to exercise those fibers in different movement patterns.

LESSON 5, LEVEL 3

Table 6.44   Overview: Lesson 5, Level 3 (Green)

Suggested time: 45–60 minutes (Total time)	Activities	Materials and staff needed
15–20 minutes	Introduction: Planning for Family and Holiday Events	Parents and patients' educational materials and books (Sothern, von Almen, & Schumacher, 2001) Exercise attire Chairs Music player Plastic Easter eggs Paper and pen Physically active toys or games as prizes
15–20 minutes	Activity I: Aerobic Musical Chairs	
15–20 minutes	Activity II: Easter Egg Charades	
		Staff: Exercise trainer

Objectives
After participation in this lesson the student will be able to:
1. Identify ways to organize family events to include exercise activities.
2. Identify safe methods to participate in indoor and outdoor activities with friends and family.
3. Safely participate in outdoor and indoor active holiday games with classmates, friends, and family members.
4. Gain knowledge concerning methods to replace sedentary holiday activities that focus on food with fun physical activities indoors and outdoors.

INTRODUCTION

The instructor will discuss additional ideas to incorporate exercise into family and holiday events. The patients and their families will participate in a game of aerobic musical chairs indoors or Easter egg charades outdoors.

ACTIVITY I. AEROBIC MUSICAL CHAIRS

The kids will participate in a game of musical chairs. A number of chairs one less than the total participants will be placed in a circle, with the seat facing outward. The kids proceed in a circle while music with a good dance beat is played in the background. They perform aerobic-type moves, such as bicep curls, arms overhead, or knees up while they move around the circle of chairs. The music stops abruptly and the kids rush to find a seat. The kid without a chair is excluded from continuing in the circle but must continue to perform the moves to the music and cheer on the remaining participants. This activity continues until only one kid is left and an award is given to him or her. The instructor uses the time to reinforce knowledge about the metabolic systems of the body.

Take Caution: Exercise Safety

Choose activities that are enjoyable but safe. Always try out the equipment beforehand to ensure safety.

ACTIVITY II. EASTER EGG CHARADES

Instead of hiding candy inside those plastic eggs during your next Easter egg hunt, try the following:

- Cut sheets of paper into small pieces (about 3 × 3 inches) so that you have one small piece to insert in each plastic Easter egg.
- Be creative and write down a fun and humorous physical activity note on each piece of paper. Here are some examples: Sing "Here Comes Peter Cottontail" while you hop, Do the twist, give a high-five to all of the members of the class, play air guitar to your favorite song, dance like your favorite rock star, shoot 20 imaginary hoops, recite the alphabet backward while running in place, spell your first and last name with your body, say the "Pledge of Allegiance" while marching in place (Newton et al., 2010; Sothern, Gordon, & von Almen, 2006; Sothern, von Almen, & Schumacher, 2001).
- In one of the eggs, insert a note that says, "You win a prize." Provide a physically active prize, such as jump ropes, balls, sidewalk chalk, outdoor game sets, or water toys, to the class member who gets the egg with this note.

LESSON 6, LEVEL 3

Table 6.45 Overview: Lesson 6, Level 3 (Green)

Suggested time: 45 minutes (Total time)	Activities	Materials and staff needed
10–15 minutes	Introduction: Flex Test	Parents and patients' educational materials and books (Sothern, von Almen, & Schumacher, 2001) Exercise attire Floor mats
30–35 minutes	Activity I: Pilates (guest instructor)	Staff: Exercise trainer or guest Pilates instructor

Objectives
After participation in this lesson the student will be able to: 1. Identify movements that will increase muscular flexibility. 2. Gain knowledge concerning the benefits of muscular flexibility to health. 3. Identify imbalances in the posture that lead to bone and joint problems. 4. Identify movement and exercises that will improve posture and muscular flexibility and reduce the risk of injury. 5. Safely participate in Pilates to improve muscular strength and flexibility with classmates, friends, and family members.

INTRODUCTION

The instructor will again guide the patients and parents through the Flex Test. Refer to lesson 6, level 1 (red).

ACTIVITY I. PILATES (GUEST INSTRUCTOR)

A guest instructor will lead the class in a series of Pilates' movements.

Talking Points: Recipes for a Stress-Free, Active Lifestyle (Verbal cues for patients or parents and family members)
Read through the following information with your patient or family members to help them to understand the exercise strategy used in the program.

Enroll the entire family in a once-per-week karate, modified yoga, or tai chi class.
   At the end of the day, put on some soft, soothing music while preparing a healthy dinner with your child.

Go for a long walk with your child.
Go outside with your child and work in the garden, pick flowers, or watch birds.
Turn on some upbeat music and dance to three songs nonstop with your child.
Turn on music videos and try to learn the latest dance moves with your child.

LESSON 7, LEVEL 3

Table 6.46   Overview: Lesson 7, Level 3 (Green)

Suggested time: 40–50 minutes (Total time)	Activities	Materials and staff needed
10–15 minutes	Introduction: Interval Training and Periodization	Parents and patients' educational materials and books (Sothern, von Almen, & Schumacher, 2001) Parent handbooks Exercise attire Cards or sheets of paper with short- and long-term goals Finish-line markers Whistle
30–35 minutes	Activity I: Be a Goal Getter Activity II: Goal-Getter Relay	
		Staff: Exercise trainer

Objectives
After participation in this lesson the student will be able to:
1. Gain knowledge concerning the benefits of interval training and periodization methods to enhancing fitness and exercise performance.
2. Identify methods to set individual short-term goals that will lead to the achievement of long-term goals.
3. Gain knowledge concerning the benefits of steady-state activities to improving fat metabolism.
4. Safely participate in a relay race with classmates, friends, and family members to gain an understanding of short-term goal setting as a method to reach long-term goals.

INTRODUCTION

The instructor will introduce or review the concept interval training and periodization and setting goals to achieve desired outcomes. The instructor will then lead indoor and outdoor relays using the Be a Goal Getter instructions.

Key Points: Interval Training

Interval training is a workout that draws from a variety of activities interspersed with low-intensity periods followed by repeating the activities. For example: Run very hard for one lap, walk easily for two laps, jog moderately for one lap, run very hard for one lap, and so on. Intensity varies from very high to very low during the workout.

ACTIVITY I. BE A GOAL GETTER
Background
Goal setting has been proven to be an effective method for creating behavior change. It lets students develop a plan that fits their own individual abilities and lifestyles. Instructor guidance is needed to help students develop realistic, attainable goals that will lead to personal success.

Long-term goals take longer to do. Students will need to set a number of short-term goals so that they can reach your long-term goal. Long term goals are something they will want to reach in the future.

Short-term goals are goals that they can do in a short time period like in 1–2 weeks. Short-term goals serve as checkpoints while they are on the road toward a longer goal.

Example 1

A long-term goal might be to be able to do 25 stomach crunches without stopping to rest 4 weeks from now. If they can do five crunches now, then their short-term goal would be to add five more crunches each week until they could do all 25 of them at the end of the 4 weeks. By stepping up their workout a little at a time, they can reach their goals.

Example 2

A long-term goal might be to try out for the swim team next fall. A short-term goal to help reach the long-term goal might be to swim at least five laps without resting in between, for at least 5 days each week for the next 2 weeks.

ACTIVITY II. GOAL-GETTER RELAY (10 MINUTES)

Following are the steps to complete the Goal-Getter Relay:

Step 1. Assign students and family members to two groups. Each group will be given a sheet of paper with a long-term goal and will be instructed to line up in two groups about 10–20 feet apart.

Step 2. On the other side of the exercise area, stacks of 5–10 cards with short-term goals are placed approximately 10–20 feet apart in alignment with the two groups of students and family members. Each stack should have an even distribution of goal cards that are appropriate to the long-term goals and some that are not appropriate.

For example, if the long-term goal is to make the swim team, appropriate short-term goals might be as follows:

- Swim 10 laps every day.
- Practice butterfly kick for 30 minutes three times per week.
- Practice stretching exercise five times per week.

However, inappropriate short-term goals might be as follows:

- Make an appointment to have a manicure.
- Play computer games three times per week for 60 minutes.
- Play a game of chess two times this week with friends.

The object of this activity is for students to find appropriate short-term goals that will help them reach a hypothetical long-term goal.

Step 3. On the signal "go," one student or family member from each group runs to the other side where the short-term goal cards have been placed. They then pull a card from the stack and run back to their group. The group discusses whether the short-term goal is appropriate or not for their long-term goal. If the card has a short-term goal that is appropriate for their long-term goal, they keep the card and the next student in the group then runs to get another card. But, if the card has a short-term goal that is not appropriate for their long-term goal, this individual has to run back to the stack and select another card to bring back to the group. This continues until one of the groups has retrieved all of the appropriate short-term goal cards from their stack.

LESSON 8, LEVEL 3

Table 6.47   Overview: Lesson 8, Level 3 (Green)

Suggested time: 45–50 minutes (Total time)	Activities	Materials and staff needed
5–10 minutes	Introduction: Getting the Most Out of Your Workout	Parents and patients' educational materials and books (Sothern, von Almen, & Schumacher, 2001)
5–10 minutes	Activity I: Getting the Most Out of Your Workout—20 Ways to Burn 20 Calories	
35-40	Activity II: Combined Strength and Aerobic Circuit	Exercise attire Hand weights Ankle weights Resistance bands Jump rope Station markers for strength and aerobic Stopwatch Music player
		Staff: Exercise trainer

Objectives

After participation in this lesson the student will be able to:
1. Gain knowledge concerning individual metabolic rates and the factors that affect this rate.
2. Recognize safe methods to include physical activities into the daily routine to ensure positive impacts on metabolism.
3. Identify the benefits to participating in activities that promote improved aerobic exercise and muscular strength and endurance.
4. Safely participate in a combined strength and aerobic exercise circuit.

INTRODUCTION

The instructor may meet with individual patients to discuss their needs, concerns, and interests. He or she will discuss 20 Ways to Burn 20 Calories as a method for increasing metabolic rates with the parents and kids. The patients and family members will participate in a combined strength and aerobic circuit exercise routine to music.

ACTIVITY I. GETTING THE MOST OUT OF YOUR WORKOUT—20 WAYS TO BURN 20 CALORIES

 Patient Handout: 20 Ways to Burn 20 Calories

1. Do 20 abdominal crunches slowly (4 seconds up, 4 seconds down) before going to sleep. Follow with gentle stretching.
2. Walk upstairs twice.
3. Do 20 toe raises while standing in line (e.g., at the grocery store).
4. Walk briskly to the bus stop and again from the bus to the schoolyard.
5. While standing in front of the television, do 40 side jacks (page XX) with large arm movements.
6. Also while standing in front of the television, do 12 leg squats (page XX) slowly (4 seconds down, 4 seconds up).
7. Walk briskly five times through the school halls.
8. Slowly press your arms above your head 15 times (4 seconds up, 4 seconds down) while sitting in a chair or in front of the television.
9. In that same chair, do 12 double leg extensions slowly (4 seconds up, 4 seconds down).

10. While watching your favorite television show, do sitting stretches for the duration of the show.
11. Walk briskly through the grocery store aisles.
12. March in place for 5 minutes anywhere!
13. Do 15 straight leg lifts (page XX) on each leg and follow with gentle stretching each night before bed.
14. Ride your bike to your friend's house.
15. Skip rope for 5 minutes.
16. Dance to two of your favorite songs without stopping.
17. Help mom or dad with the housework for 10 minutes.
18. Help mom or dad with yard work for 10 minutes.
19. Clean out your closet for 15 minutes.
20. Stand up and do five cheers at your hometown's next football game. They probably will love you for it!

If you do 25 of these activities every day for a full week, you will burn enough calories to lose one pound (3500 calories). Choose the activities that are easy for you to do, and do them several times a day to reach your goal of 25 per day. Now, list the activities you will do for 5–10 minutes that will burn 20 calories.

ACTIVITY II. COMBINED STRENGTH AND AEROBIC CIRCUIT

Using station marker visuals, the patients will alternate between strength exercises and aerobic movement to music. The circuit may be organized in a circle or in two lines with strength in one line and aerobic in the other. The groups alternate between stations. Allow 2 minutes at each exercise station and 30 seconds to change stations.

LESSON 9, LEVEL 3

Table 6.48 Overview: Lesson 9, Level 3 (Green)

Suggested time: 45–50 minutes (Total time)	Activities	Materials and staff needed
5–10 minutes	Introduction: Raising Activity Levels, Family Team Sports	Parents and patients' educational materials and books (Sothern, von Almen, & Schumacher, 2001)
40–45 minutes	Activity I: Aerobic Softball	Exercise attire Baseballs, bats, bases
		Staff: Exercise trainer

Objectives
After participation in this lesson the student will be able to:
1. Gain knowledge concerning methods to increase moderate to vigorous physical activity during field sports.
2. Identify the benefits of aerobic exercise to overall health and well-being.
3. Safely participate in softball game outdoors with classmates, friends, and family members.

INTRODUCTION

The instructor will inform the patients and their families that today's activity, aerobic softball, will alter the rules of softball to encourage movement at all times. For example, aerobic softball requires that all team members walk or run the bases when a run is scored and perform 10 jumping jacks or side jacks when the batter gets a strike.

ACTIVITY I. AEROBIC SOFTBALL

The group will participate in team sports outdoors. The aerobic softball game follows regulation rules; however, the participants are instructed that when one of the teams scores a point, they must all walk or run the bases. Likewise, when the team up to bat makes a run, they must all walk or run the bases. To keep the kids even more active, you also may add 10 side jacks for each catch in the field or when a batter makes it to first base. Periodically check breathing and heart rate.

> **Key Points:** Organizing Teams
>
> When organizing teams try this method: Tell the kids and parents to make a "train" behind you. Then assign every other participant to a different name of an animal. For example: Tiger team, Jaguar team, Tiger team, and so on. Assign the Tiger team to the outfield and the Jaguar team to home plate.

LESSON 10, LEVEL 3

Table 6.49   Overview: Lesson 10, Level 3 (Green)

Suggested time: 75–100 minutes (Total time)	Activities	Materials and staff needed
15–20 minutes	Introduction and Set-up	Parents and patients' educational materials and books (Sothern, von Almen, & Schumacher, 2001)
60–80 minutes	Activity I: PEP Step Contest: Fun Walk or Run in the Park	Exercise attire Registration table Time slips Number markers for runners Stopwatch Water containers Ice, cups Ribbons, medals Staff: Exercise trainer and two additional staff or volunteers to assist

Objectives
After participation in this lesson the student will be able to:
1. Gain knowledge concerning the benefits of group physical activities to overall health and well-being.
2. Recognize opportunities to engage in safe methods to participate in physical activities in an outdoor setting.
3. Safely participate in Fun Walk or Run event with friends and family members in their community.

INTRODUCTION

The instructor will congratulate their patients and family members completing the 10-week session. He or she should discuss how to prepare for the follow-up medical tests, which will determine their overall progress. Patients will be informed that rewards will be given out in 2 weeks for attendance and exercise compliance. Patients and their family members will participate in a Fun Walk or Run in the park.

ACTIVITY I. PEP STEP CONTEST—FUN WALK OR RUN IN THE PARK

The instructor will organize a Fun Walk or Run for the patients and parents. Use different categories: under 12 walk, under 12 run, over 12 walk, over 12 run, adult (18) walk, adult (18) run. Set up water stations every 0.5–1 mile. Award ribbons and announce winners in a newsletter. Also, a group may be organized to participate in an existing walk or run event in the area.

This event can become an annual race open to other members of the community. Tee shirts might be given out and the event might serve as a fund-raising effort. The race times of the participants should be recorded in the patient files for future reference and to underscore improvements in performance.

LESSON 1, LEVEL 4 (BLUE)

Table 6.50   Overview: Lesson 1, Level 4 (Blue)

Suggested time: 110–120 minutes (Total time)	Activities	Materials and staff needed
15–20 minutes	Introduction: Increasing Daily Activities—Exercising on the Road	Parents and patients' educational materials and books (Sothern, von Almen, & Schumacher, 2001)
95–100 minutes	Activity I: Roller or Inline Skating Field Trip or Annual Party	Exercise attire Low-calorie snacks Diet soft drinks Roller or inline skates for each participant Staff: Exercise trainer

Objectives
After participation in this lesson the student will be able to:
1. Gain knowledge concerning the benefits of exercise and increasing daily physical activity to health.
2. Recognize safe methods to engage in physically active field trips.
3. Safely participate in roller or inline skating with classmates, friends, and family members.

INTRODUCTION

The instructor will discuss ways to ensure that the patient stays physically active when he or she travels for family vacations. He or she will demonstrate how families can be flexible while still making wise choices. The patient will need the cooperative efforts of the entire family to make your trip a healthy one.

Talking Points: Keeping Fit on the Trip (Verbal cues for patients or parents and family members)
Read through the following information with your patient or family members to help them to understand the exercise strategy used in the program.

You may not be able to take your local swimming pool, tennis court, or baseball team with you on your travels, but you can still provide plenty of opportunities for your child to exercise and stay active. In fact, sometimes traveling inspires even more activity, because there are so many new things to do and wonderful sights to see.

If the drive to your destination is lengthy, stop every few hours at town parks, playgrounds, or restaurants with play areas. Allow your children to romp around as long as time permits. Join in and stretch out the kinks. Start a game of tag, bring along a ball and kick it around, or simply lead your family in some good Stretch-and-Flex exercises. The idea is to keep up the habit of family activity, even though you may not be following your typical routine.

Once you arrive at your hotel or other destination, ask whether they have a gym on the premises. If so, check the equipment before allowing your child to work out, making certain it is safe and secure. Most kids love the hotel pool, if there is one. Parks and skating rinks are good alternatives to gyms, and most towns offer at least some other forms of child-friendly recreation. If the hotel management has few suggestions and you are stumped, call the local chamber of commerce or visitor's center and ask what is available, where it is, and what it costs.

In summer months when many families travel, it is easy to spend hours strolling through zoos, splashing in pools, and exploring parks. Consider a day trip to the mountains for a long, leisurely hike, some rowing in a fishing boat, climbing trees, or skipping rocks on a lake.

Winter months offer plenty of activities, too. If your family does not ski, consider ice skating, snowshoeing, sledding, and even building snowmen. Children's museums provide hours of indoor activities. Or, go to the local mall and walk briskly from one end to the other.

Remind your child that natural consequences also come into play if he chooses not to exercise while on vacation. He will begin to feel sluggish, and it will be harder for him to resume his routine once he is back home. If he remains active by playing or doing his stretches and aerobic workout, he will have more energy on the trip and will be able to resume his routine at home with ease.

Active families deserve trips that encourage fun and learning. These days, complete vacation packages are available in which kids can learn to sail, ski, swim, hike, play tennis or golf, or even excavate dinosaur bones—you name it, it's out there! Aside from keeping your kids fit and teaching them new skills, these resorts often include child care for those times when you and your spouse want a little time away. Contact a travel agent to learn more.

ACTIVITY I. ROLLER OR INLINE SKATING FIELD TRIP

The instructor will organize an off-site event at a local skating rink. Bring healthy snacks and diet drinks. Encourage the kids to invite friends and extended family.

Key Points: Field Trips

If it is possible to reserve the skating rink so that only program participants and family attend, you will have a safer and more encouraging atmosphere. Many of the participants may not have skated before and may need assistance or a special area to practice.

Other field trip options include the following:

- Aquarium
- Boating or fishing
- Children's museum
- Fun run race or outdoor cycling event
- Gymnastics or tumbling center
- Horseback riding
- Indoor rock climbing
- Kayaking or rowing
- Miniature golf
- Nature hike
- Sledding or cross-country skiing
- Snorkeling, sailing, or waterskiing
- Waterslide park
- Zoo or nature park

LESSON 2, LEVEL 4

Table 6.51   Overview: Lesson 2, Level 4 (Blue)

Suggested time: 40–45 minutes (Total time)	Activities	Materials and staff needed
5–10 minutes	Introduction: Aerobic Versus Anaerobic Exercise	Parents and patients' educational materials and books (Sothern, von Almen, & Schumacher, 2001)
35–40 minutes	Activity I: Beach Party Aerobics with Beach Balls	Exercise attire Beach balls Volleyball net Music player Music Staff: Exercise trainer

Objectives
After participation in this lesson the student will be able to:
1. Identify differences between aerobic versus anaerobic exercise.
2. Gain knowledge concerning the benefits of aerobic exercise to health.
3. Develop pacing skills to monitor exercise performance in order to increase duration.
4. Safely participate in a beach volleyball activity to music with classmates, friends, and family members.

INTRODUCTION
The instructor will review the differences between aerobic and anaerobic exercise. Then he or she will lead the class in an aerobic dancing session to beach party 1960s music using beach balls. Other activity options using beach balls include balloon battle (see lesson 1, level 3 [green]) or beach ball volleyball.

ACTIVITY I. BEACH PARTY AEROBICS
The instructor will lead the class in an aerobics class to beach party 1960s music using beach balls. Different movements and class patterns, such as a circle, make this activity enjoyable. The instructor should use his or her imagination and let the kids create the movements as well.

LESSON 3, LEVEL 4

Table 6.52   Overview: Lesson 3, Level 4 (Blue)

Suggested time: 40–50 minutes (Total time)	Activities	Materials and staff needed
5–10 minutes	Introduction: Cardiorespiratory endurance	Parents and patients' educational materials and books (Sothern, von Almen, & Schumacher, 2001)
35–45 minutes	Activity I: Aerobic Equipment, Triathlon	Exercise attire Treadmill Cycle ergometer Rowing ergometer Stopwatch Record sheets Awards: ribbons, medals, other Staff: Exercise trainer and additional staff or volunteers to assist

Objectives
After participation in this lesson the student will be able to:
1. Identify safe methods to participate in exercises to improve aerobic endurance.
2. Gain knowledge concerning the benefits of aerobic endurance training to health.
3. Gain knowledge and experience in performing exercise on varied aerobic equipment.
4. Safely participate in an activity utilizing varied aerobic exercise machines with classmates, friends, and family members.

INTRODUCTION

The instructor will review cardiorespiratory fitness and the benefits of engaging in cardiorespiratory (aerobic) exercise. See lesson 3, level 1 (red).

ACTIVITY I. AEROBIC EQUIPMENT TRIATHLON

The patients will participate in an aerobic equipment triathlon as follows: A distance goal is set for each apparatus (e.g., 1 mile or 2 miles). The participant begins, for example, on the treadmill and walks or runs as fast as he or she can for the distance established. The time is recorded. Then he or she immediately runs to the cycle ergometer and proceeds in the same manner. Finally, he or she performs on a rowing ergometer or stair-climber. At each piece of equipment, the time is recorded and then a total time is recorded. First, second, and third place awards are given for the fastest total times and individual event times. If you have a large number of patients, this event can take place over several class periods.

LESSON 4, LEVEL 4

Table 6.53   Overview: Lesson 4, Level 4 (Blue)

Suggested time: 40–45 minutes (Total time)	Activities	Materials and staff needed
5–10 minutes	Introduction: Muscular Strength and Endurance	Parents and patients' educational materials and books (Sothern, von Almen, & Schumacher, 2001)
35–40 minutes	Activity I: Band-Aid for Out-of-Shape Muscles	Exercise attire Resistance bands Music player Staff: Exercise trainer

Objectives
After participation in this lesson the student will be able to:
1. Identify safe methods to participate in exercises to improve muscular strength and endurance.
2. Gain knowledge concerning the benefits of resistance training to health.
3. Safely participate in a strength training circuit using stretch bands that provide resistance under the supervision of a parent or other adult.
4. Gain knowledge concerning the specific muscle or muscle group that is responsible for varied types of body movement.

INTRODUCTION

The instructor will review muscular strength and endurance concepts. See lesson 4, level 1 (red). He or she will then guide the kids and parents through the Band-Aid for Out-of-Shape Muscles Series.

ACTIVITY I. BAND-AID FOR OUT-OF-SHAPE MUSCLES

A resistance band will be used to perform the exercises. A stretch band is a large rubber band, of sorts. It usually is made of soft latex, and is about 3–4 feet long. The routine may be done to music.

Parent Handout: Band-Aid for Out-of-Shape Muscles

Once you are used to the great feeling of toned muscles, it is hard to go back to that loose, flabby feeling. But sometimes, it is hard to get to the gym, and you probably do not have the space for big, heavy weights in your room. And what about when you are traveling?

Here are some exercises to do using a stretch band. When you pull on the band, it resists your weight much like those fancy weight-room machines do. But, unlike weights, you can easily store it under your bed, on a shelf, or in your suitcase.

These exercises work just like training with weights. Do them exactly as instructed, as the technique is specific and safe. If you do the exercises incorrectly, you may hurt a muscle or joint.

The following exercises should be performed 8–12 times, once, but preferably twice, a week. Read the instructions aloud to your child until she knows them by memory.

Exercise for Stretch Band 1: Shoulder Raise, Sitting

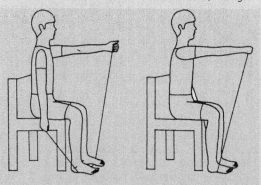

Sit in a sturdy chair with your feet flat on the floor. Place the middle of the band under both of your feet. Grasp one end of the band in each hand.

Keep your left hand straight down alongside your hip while you lift the right hand straight up, pulling the band for 2–4 seconds. Make sure your right elbow is slightly bent.

Pull the band until your hand is even with your shoulder and hold for one second. As you pull, keep your upper body still. Slowly lower your right hand for two to four seconds, until it is alongside your hip.

Now, repeat with your left hand. Do 8–12 repetitions of this exercise. You are training the shoulder muscles (deltoids).

Common errors your child may make include bending the elbows too much or keeping elbows too straight, moving the upper body, or lifting hands too high.

Exercise for Stretch Band 2: Standing Squat 'N' Pull

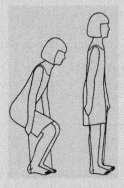

Stand with your feet pointing forward, about 18 inches apart. Place the middle of the band under both of your feet. Grasp one end of the band in each hand while bending your knees, pushing your hips back, and dropping your chest forward. Your knees should not be in front of your feet. Keep your head in line with your body and your heels on the floor.

Slowly, over 2–4 seconds, extend your hips forward and come up to a standing position while pulling the band. Keep your elbows straight throughout the entire movement. Great.

Now lower over 2–4 seconds, return to the starting position and do it again.

Do this exercise 8–12 times. You are training the upper leg muscles (quadriceps) and the buttocks muscles (gluteus).

Exercise for Stretch Band 3: Reverse Butterfly

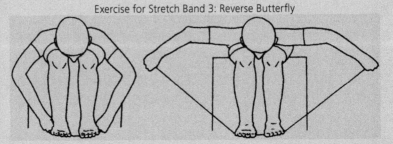

Sit in a sturdy chair with your feet flat on the floor. Place the middle of the band under both of your feet. Grasp one end of the band in each hand.

Bend forward until your chest rests on your lap. Keep your head in line with your body and point your face downward. Slowly pull the ends of the band out to the sides and up while keeping your elbows slightly bent. Keep pulling for 2–4 seconds. Great job!

Now, squeeze your shoulder blades together as you stretch the band and feel a slight tension in your upper back and shoulder. Hold for 1 second. Good.

Now, gently release the band over 2–4 seconds, returning to the starting position.

Do 8–12 repetitions of this exercise. You are training the upper back muscles (rhomboids) and the rear shoulder muscles (deltoids).

Common errors your child may make include keeping elbows too bent or too straight, arching the neck, and pulling the band too close to the body.

LESSON 5, LEVEL 4

Table 6.54   Overview: Lesson 5, Level 4 (Blue)

Suggested time: 60–80 minutes (Total time)	Activities	Materials and staff needed
10–15 minutes	Introduction: Indoor and Outdoor Family Fun	Parents and patients' educational materials and books (Sothern, von Almen, & Schumacher, 2001)
50–70 minutes	Activity I: Family Field Sports: The Family Hike (if it rains, play laser tag or go roller/inline skating indoors)	Exercise attire Healthy snacks Water and containers Ice Staff: Exercise trainer

Objectives
After participation in this lesson the student will be able to:
1. Identify ways to organize family events to include exercise activities.
2. Identify safe methods to participate in family field sports or a family hike.
3. Gain knowledge concerning the proper technique and rules for outdoor field games.
4. Safely participate in a family field sport or hike with classmates, friends, and family members.
5. Gain knowledge concerning how to select alternate indoor physical activities when the weather prohibits participation in outdoor physical activities.

INTRODUCTION

The instructor will review indoor and outdoor family fun and organize a field trip to a nearby outdoor nature park or reserve.

ACTIVITY I. FAMILY HIKE

Patients and their family members will participate in a family hike. (If it rains, adjust the activity to either laser tag or indoor roller or inline skating.) Families should be instructed to bring a healthy snack and plenty of water.

LESSON 6, LEVEL 4

Table 6.55   Overview: Lesson 6, Level 4 (Blue)

Suggested time: 45–55 minutes (Total time)	Activities	Materials and staff needed
15–20 minutes	Introduction: Flex Test	Parents and patients' educational materials and books (Sothern, von Almen, & Schumacher, 2001)
30–40 minutes	Activity I: Interactive Martial Arts Demonstration	Exercise attire Floor mats Staff: Exercise trainer or guest martial arts instructor

Objectives
After participation in this lesson the student will be able to:
1. Identify movements that will increase muscular flexibility.
2. Gain knowledge concerning the benefits of muscular flexibility to health.
3. Identify imbalances in the posture that lead to bone and joint problems.
4. Identify movement and exercises that will improve posture and muscular flexibility and reduce the risk of injury.
5. Safely participate in martial arts activities to improve muscular flexibility and strength with classmates, friends, and families.

INTRODUCTION

The kids and parents will again be guided through the Flex Test. See lesson 6, level 1 (red), for instructions and directions.

ACTIVITY I. INTERACTIVE MARTIAL ARTS DEMONSTRATION

A martial arts instructor will perform an interactive demonstration of martial arts (e.g., karate, self-defense).

> **!**
>
> **Take Caution:** Exercise Safety
>
> The instructor should preview the martial arts class beforehand to determine whether it is appropriate for children. Concerns include proper warm-up, knee positions in the drills, and cooling down.

LESSON 7, LEVEL 4

Table 6.56 Overview: Lesson 7, Level 4 (Blue)

Suggested time: 35–50 minutes (Total time)	Activities	Materials and staff needed
25–30 minutes	Activity I: Exercise and Health, Team Sports (basketball)	Parents and patients' educational materials and books (Sothern, von Almen, & Schumacher, 2001) Exercise attire Basketballs Goals Whistle Stopwatch
5–10 minutes	Activity II: Crunch Challenge	Staff: Exercise trainer

Objectives
After participation in this lesson the student will be able to:
1. Gain knowledge concerning the importance of aerobic fitness and abdominal (core) strength to overall health.
2. Safely participate in a game of basketball with classmates, friends, and family members to improve aerobic endurance.
3. Identify methods to set individual goals to improve abdominal strength through participation in a timed stomach crunch exercise bout.

ACTIVITY I. BASKETBALL GAME

The kids will participate in a basketball game. Refer to lesson 10, level 1 (red), for instructions on how to select teams. An adult assistant or guest instructor will need to referee and supervise the activity.

ACTIVITY II. CRUNCH CHALLENGE

The instructor will guide the kids through the abdominal crunch challenge (see Lesson 7, Level 1).

LESSON 8, LEVEL 4

Table 6.57 Overview: Lesson 8, Level 4 (Blue)

Suggested time: 40–50 minutes (Total time)	Activities	Materials and Staff Needed
5–10 minutes	Introduction: Exercise Techniques	Parents and patients' educational materials and books (Sothern, von Almen, & Schumacher, 2001) Exercise attire Tennis balls (1 per pair) Tennis racquets (1 per student)
35–40 minutes	Activity I: Tennis Lesson and Drills	Staff: Exercise trainer

Objectives
After participation in this lesson the student will be able to:
1. Gain knowledge concerning the importance of proper exercise technique to the performance of recreational and competitive sports and activities.
2. Gain skills necessary to successfully participate in the game of tennis.
3. Safely participate in a tennis match with classmates, friends, and family members.

ACTIVITY I. DOUBLES TENNIS

The instructor will discuss the importance of proper exercise technique. The instructor will divide the kids into two groups. While one group participates in a doubles tennis game (depending on the number of courts available), the others meet with the instructor for an individual session. Parents may serve as referees.

LESSON 9, LEVEL 4

Table 6.58   Overview: Lesson 9, Level 4 (Blue)

Suggested time: 35–45 minutes	Activities	Materials and staff needed
30–35 minutes	Activity I: Guest Speaker (professional athlete)	Parents and patients' educational materials and books (Sothern, von Almen, & Schumacher, 2001) Podium Microphone Chairs arranged auditorium style
		Staff: Exercise trainer and guest speaker

Objectives
After participation in this lesson the student will be able to:
1. Gain knowledge concerning safe and effective participation in sports and recreational activities that promote the attainment of muscular power.
2. Recognize the value of proper exercise training to successfully participate in sports.

ACTIVITY I. POWER SPORTS DEMONSTRATION
The instructor will organize a Power Sports Demonstration by a guest speaker (professional athlete, athletic trainer, or coach).

LESSON 10, LEVEL 4

Table 6.59   Overview: Lesson 10, Level 4 (Blue)

Suggested time: 95–105 minutes (Total time)	Activities	Materials needed
10–15 minutes	Introduction and Set-up	Parents and patients' educational materials and books (Sothern, von Almen, & Schumacher, 2001)
85–90 minutes	Activity I: Family Field Sports, Field Day (annual)	Exercise attire Colored wrist bands, tape, or cloth Jump ropes Cabbage baseball, bats, bases, home plate Soccer balls, goals Clipboards, whistles, stopwatches Volleyball, net Soccer balls Soccer goal markers Footballs Football goal markers Boundary markers (cones) Score sheets, ribbons, awards Soccer balls (2)
		Staff: Exercise trainers and additional staff or volunteers to assist

Objectives
After participation in this lesson the student will be able to:
1. Gain knowledge concerning the benefits of group sports activities to overall health and well-being.
2. Recognize opportunities to engage in safe methods to participate in physical activities in an outdoor setting.
3. Safely participate in a field day event with friends and family members designed to maximize opportunities for movement to promote increased physical activity.

INTRODUCTION

The instructor will organize a Family Field Day for their patients and family members.

ACTIVITY I. FAMILY FIELD DAY

Patients, friends, and family members will be assigned at random to one of four teams (red, yellow, green, blue) upon arrival to the playing area. A colored wrist band will be stapled around the right wrist as each person comes in. Team equality is not guaranteed by this method, and it is not possible to accommodate requests to place friends or family members on the same team. The day proceeds as follows: red and yellow teams play soccer or flag football; green and blue teams play volleyball or softball; then the teams rotate to another event. Relays (e.g., jump rope, over and under) can be used at the end to serve as final point-gaining events or tiebreakers. Refer to the schedule and instructions that follow. A 15- to 20-minute time limit is allowed for each event. When time is called, the team with the most points receives a total point award. Then the teams rotate to the next event. Ribbons or buttons can be given as awards.

Key Points: Family Field Day

This event requires increased staff support or parent assistance. An adult referee should be stationed at each event to record point. One master score person should tally all results.

OFFICIAL RULES

- Coin toss will determine which team serves, bats, etc., first.
- All play begins at the sound of the whistle.
- All play ends at the sound of the whistle.
- Points accumulated within the designated time will be credited to the individual team.
- All scores are worth 1 point (i.e., baseball run = 1, volleyball point = 1, soccer goal = 1, football goal = 1).
- Jump-rope relay is scored as follows:
  - First place = 3 points
  - Second place = 2 points
  - Third place = 1 point
- Scores will be tallied at the end of the jump rope relay and awards will be given immediately thereafter.
- All calls by the officials are *final.*

SCHEDULE OF EVENTS

Table 6.60   Field Day Schedule

Time	Event	Teams	Officials
4:55–5:00	Coin toss	All	
5:00–5:15	Softball, Volleyball	Red versus Yellow, Blue versus Green	
5:15–5:20	Coin toss	All	
5:20–5:35	Softball, Volleyball	Green versus Blue, Red versus Yellow	
5:35–5:45	Field set-up, Coin toss	All	
5:45–6:00	Soccer, Ultimate Frisbee™	Red versus Blue, Green versus Yellow	
6:00–6:05	Coin toss	All	
6:05–6:20	Soccer	Green versus Yellow, Red versus Blue	
6:20–6:30	Jump-Rope Relay	All four teams	
6:30	Awards	All	

Table 6.61   Official Score Sheet—Spring Kickoff Sports Day

Team	Event	Total event	Total points
Red	Softball		
	Volleyball		
	Soccer		
	Ultimate Frisbee™		
	Jump-Rope Relay		
Yellow	Softball		
	Volleyball		
	Soccer		
	Ultimate Frisbee™		
	Jump-Rope Relay		
Green	Softball		
	Volleyball		
	Soccer		
	Ultimate Frisbee™		
	Jump-Rope Relay		
Blue	Softball		
	Volleyball		
	Soccer		
	Ultimate Frisbee™		
	Jump-Rope Relay		

REFERENCES

Alpert, B. S. (1999). Exercise in hypertensive children and adolescents: Any harm done? *Pediatric Cardiology*, 20, 66–69.

Alpert, B. S. (2000). Exercise as a therapy to control hypertension in children. *International Journal of Sports Medicine*, 21(Suppl 2), S94–S97.

American Lung Association. (2007). *Asthma-friendly schools initiative toolkit.* Retrieved from http://www.lung.org/lung-disease/asthma/creating-asthma-friendly-environments/asthma-in-schools/asthma-friendly-schools-initiative/asthma-friendly-schools-initiative-toolkit.html.

Arshi, M., Cardinal, J., Hill, R. J., Davies, P. S., Wainwright, C. (2010). Asthma and insulin resistance in children. *Respirology*, 15(5), 779–784.

Balagopal, P. B., Gidding, S. S., Buckloh, L. M., Yarandi, H. N., Sylvester, J. E., George, D. E., et al. (2010). Changes in circulating satiety hormones in obese children: A randomized controlled physical activity-based intervention study. *Obesity (Silver Spring, Md.)*, 18(9), 1747–1753.

Bandura, A. (1986). *Social Foundations of Thoughts and Actions: A Social Cognitive Theory.* Englewood Cliffs, NJ: Prentice-Hall.

Baraldi, E., de Jongste, J.C. (2002). Measurement of exhaled nitric oxide in children. *European Respiratory Journal*, 20, 223–237.

Barbeau, P., Johnson, M. H., Howe, C. A., Allison, J., Davis, C. L., Gutin, B., et al. (2007). Ten months of exercise improves general and visceral adiposity, bone, and fitness in black girls. *Obesity (Silver Spring, Md.)*, 15(8), 2077–2085.

Barlow, S. E., Trowbridge, F. L., Klish, W. J., Dietz, W. H. (2002). Treatment of child and adolescent obesity: Reports from pediatricians, pediatric nurse practitioners, and registered dietitians. *Pediatrics*, 110(1 Pt 2), 229–235.

Bar-Or, O., Rowland, T. W. (2004). *Pediatric Exercise Medicine: From Physiologic Principles to Health Care Application*. Champaign, IL: Human Kinetics.

Bastard, J. P., Jardel, C., Bruckert, E., Blondy, P., Capeau, J., Laville, M., Vidal, H., Hainque, B. (2000). Elevated levels of interleukin 6 are reduced in serum and subcutaneous adipose tissue of obese women after weight loss. *Journal of Clinical Endocrinology and Metabolism*, 85, 3338–3342.

Behm, D., Faigenbaum, A., Falk, B., Klentrou, P. (2008). Canadian Society for Exercise Physiology position paper: resistance training in children in children and adolescents. *Applied Physiology, Nutrition and Metabolism*, 33, 547–561.

Ben Ounis, O., Elloumi, M., Makni, E., Zouhal, H., Amri, M., Tabka, Z., et al. (2010). Exercise improves the ApoB/ApoA-I ratio, a marker of the metabolic syndrome in obese children. *Acta Paediatrica*, 99(11), 1679–1685.

Benson, A. C., Torode, M. E., Fiatarone Singh, M. A. (2007). A rationale and method for high-intensity progressive resistance training with children and adolescents. *Contemporary Clinical Trials*, 28(4), 442–450.

Beuther, D. A., Sutherland, E. R. (2007). Overweight, obesity, and incident asthma: A meta-analysis of prospective epidemiologic studies. *American Journal of Respiratory and Critical Care Medicine*, 175, 661–666.

Bey, L., Hamilton, M. T. (2003). Suppression of skeletal muscle lipoprotein lipase activity during physical inactivity: A molecular reason to maintain daily low-intensity activity. *Journal of Physiology*, 551(Pt 2), 673–682.

Bovet, P., Auguste, R., Burdette, H. (2007). Strong inverse association between physical fitness and overweight in adolescents: a large school-based survey. *International Journal of Behavioral Nutrition and Physical Activity*, 4(1), 24.

Brambilla, P., Pozzobon, G., Pietrobelli, A. (2011). Physical activity as the main therapeutic tool for metabolic syndrome in childhood. *International Journal of Obesity*, 35(1), 16–28.

Brandou, F., Savy-Pacaux, A. M., Marie, J., Bauloz, M., Maret-Fleuret, I., Borrocoso, S., et al. (2005). Impact of high- and low-intensity targeted exercise training on the type of substrate utilization in obese boys submitted to a hypocaloric diet. *Diabetes Metabolism*, 31(4 Pt 1), 327–335.

Busse, W. W., Lemanske, R. F., Jr. (2001). Asthma. *New England Journal of Medicine*, 344, 350–362.

Byrne, H. K., Wilmore, J. H. (2001). The relationship of mode and intensity of training on resting metabolic rate in women. *International Journal of Sport Nutrition and Exercise Metabolism*, 11(1), 1–14.

Carlisle, L., Gordon, S., Sothern, M. (2005). Can obesity prevention work for our children? *Journal of the Louisiana State Medical Society*, 157, S34–S41.

Carroll, C. L., Bhandari, A., Zucker, A. R., Schramm, C. M. (2006). Childhood obesity increases duration of therapy during severe asthma exacerbations. *Pediatric Critical Care Medicine*, 7, 527–531.

Cliff, D. P., Okely, A. D., Morgan, P. J., Jones, J. R., Steele, J. R., Baur, L. A. (2012). Proficiency deficiency: Mastery of fundamental movement skills and skill components in overweight and obese children. *Obesity (Silver Spring, Md.)*, 20(5), 1024–1033.

Considine, R. V., Sinha, M. K., Heiman, M. L., Kriauciunas, A., Stephens, T. W., Nyce, M. R., Ohannesian, J. P., Marco, C. C., McKee, L. J., Bauer, T. L. (1996). Serum immunoreactive-leptin concentrations in normal-weight and obese humans. *New England Journal of Medicine*, 334, 292–295.

Cook, D. G., Mendall, M. A., Whincup, P. H., Carey, I. M., Ballam, L., Morris, J. E., Miller, G. J., Strachan, D. P. (2000). C-reactive protein concentration in children: relationship to adiposity and other cardiovascular risk factors. *Atherosclerosis*, 149, 139–150.

Corcoran, M. P., Lamon-Fava, S., Fielding, R. A. (2007). Skeletal muscle lipid deposition and insulin resistance: effect of dietary fatty acids and exercise. *American Journal of Clinical Nutrition*, 85(3), 662–677.

Daniels S., Arnett, D., Eckel, R., Gidding, S. S., Hayman, L. L., Kumanyika, S., et al. (2005). Overweight in children and adolescents: Pathophysiology, consequences, prevention, and treatment. *Circulation*, 111(15), 1999–2012.

Daniels, S. R., Jacobson, M. S., McCrindle, B. W., Eckel, R. H., Sanner, B. M. (2009). American Heart Association childhood obesity research summit: Executive summary. *Circulation*, 119(15), 2114–2123.

Dao, H. H., Frelut, M. L., Peres, G., Bourgeois, P., Navarro, J. (2004). Effects of a multidisciplinary weight loss intervention on anaerobic and aerobic aptitudes in severely obese adolescents. *International Journal of Obesity and Related Metabolic Disorders*, 28(7), 870–878.

Davis, J. N., Gyllenhammer, L. E., Vanni, A. A., Meija, M., Tung, A., Schroeder, E. T., Spruijt-Metz, D., Goran, M. I. (2011). Startup circuit training program reduces metabolic risk in Latino adolescents. *Medicine and Science in Sports and Exercise*, 43(11), 2195–2203.

Davis, C., Pollock, N., Waller, J., Allison, J., Dennis, B., Bassali, R. I., Melendez, A., Boyle, C., Gower, B. (2012). Exercise dose and diabetes risk in overweight and obese children. *JAMA*, 308(11), 1103–1112.

D'Hondt, E., Deforche, B., Gentier, I., De Bourdeaudhuij, I., Vaeyens, R., Philippaerts, R., Lenoir, M. (2013). A longitudinal analysis of gross motor coordination in overweight and obese children versus normal-weight peers. *International Journal of Obesity*, 237(1), 61–67. doi: 10.1038/ijo.2012.55. [Epub 2012 Apr 17]

Drinkard, B., Roberts, M. D., Ranzenhofer, L. M., Han, J. C., Yanoff, L. B., Merke, D. P., et al. (2007). Oxygen-uptake efficiency slope as a determinant of fitness in overweight adolescents. *Medicine and Science in Sports and Exercise*, 39(10), 1811–1816.

Eisenmann, J.; for the Subcommittee on Assessment in Pediatric Obesity Management Programs, National Association of Children's Hospital and Related Institutions. (2011). Assessment of obese children and adolescents: A survey of pediatric obesity-management programs. *Pediatrics*, 128(Suppl 2), S51–S52.

Erickson, S. J., Robinson, T. N., Haydel, K. F., Killen, J. D. (2000). Are overweight children unhappy? Body mass index, depressive symptoms, and overweight concerns in elementary school children. *Archives of Pediatric and Adolescent Medicine*, 154(9), 931–935.

Evans, W., Finkelstein, E., Kamerow, D., Renaud, J. (2005) Public perceptions of childhood obesity. *American Journal of Preventive Medicine*, 28, 26–32.

Faigenbaum, A. D., Kraemer, W. J., Blimkie, C. J., Jeffreys, I., Micheli, L. J., Nitka, M., Rowland, T. W. (2009). Youth resistance training: updated position statement paper from the national strength and conditioning association. *Journal of Strength and Conditioning Research*, 23(5 Suppl), S60–S79.

Faigenbaum, A., Myer, G. (2010). Pediatric resistance training: Benefits, concerns, and program design considerations. *Current Sports Medicine Reports*, 9(3), 161–168.

Freedman, D. S., Khan, L. K., Dietz, W. H., Srinivasan, S. R., Berenson, G. S. (2001). Relationship of childhood obesity to coronary heart disease risk factors in adulthood: The Bogalusa Heart Study. *Pediatrics*, 108, 712–718.

Gold, D. R., Rotnitzky, A., Damokosh, A. I., Ware, J. H., Speizer, F. E., Ferris, B. G., Jr., Dockery, D. W. (1993). Race and gender differences in respiratory illness prevalence and their relationship to environmental exposures in children 7 to 14 years of age. *American Review of Respiratory Disease*, 148, 10–18.

Goldberg, B. (1995). *Sports and Exercise for Children with Chronic Health Conditions*. Champaign, IL: Human Kinetics.

Gonzalez, C. A. (2006). Nutrition and cancer: the current epidemiological evidence. *British Journal of Nutrition*, 96(Suppl 1), S42–S45.

Goran, M., Fields, D. A., Hunter, G. R., Herd, S. L., Weinsier, R. L. (2000). Total body fat does not influence maximal aerobic capacity. *International Journal of Obesity and Related Metabolic Disorders*, 24(7), 841–848.

Gray, J. S., Spear Filigno, S., Santos, M., Ward, W. L., Davis, A. M. (2012). The status of billing and reimbursement in pediatric obesity treatment programs. *Journal of Behavioral Health Services and Research*. [Epub ahead of print]

Hadley, J. (2007). Insurance coverage, medical care use, and short-term health changes following an unintentional injury or the onset of a chronic condition. *JAMA*, 297(10), 1073–1084.

Hassink, S. G., Zapalla, F., Falini, L., Datto, G. (2008). Exercise and the obese child. *Progress in Pediatric Cardiology*, 25(2), 153–157.

Hurley, B. F., Hagberg, J. M. (1998). Optimizing health in older persons: Aerobic or strength training? *Exercise and Sport Sciences Reviews*, 26, 61–89.

International Study of Asthma and Allergies in Childhood Steering Committee. (1998). Worldwide variation in prevalence of symptoms of asthma, allergic rhinoconjunctivitis, and atopic eczema. *Lancet*, 351, 1225–1232.

Irving, D., Cook, J., Young, M., Menz, H. (2007). Obesity and pronated foot type may increase the risk of chronic plantar heel pain: A matched case-control study. *BMC Musculoskeletal Disorders*, 8, 41.

Ivy, J. L., Zderic, T. W., Fogt, D. L. (1999). Prevention and treatment of non-insulin-dependent diabetes mellitus. *Exercise and Sport Sciences Reviews*, 27, 1–35.

Jacobson, M. (2006). Medical complications and comorbidities of pediatric obesity. In M. Sothern, S. Gordon, T. K. von Almen (Eds.), *Handbook of Pediatric Obesity: Clinical Management* (pp. 31–39). Boca Raton, FL: Taylor & Francis.

Janssen, J., LeBlanc, A. G. (2010). Systematic review of the health benefits of physical activity and fitness in school-aged children and youth. *International Journal of Behavioral Nutrition and Physical Activity*, 7, 40.

Jatakanon, A., Uasuf, C., Maziak, W., Lim, S., Chung, K. F., Barnes, P. J. (1999). Neutrophilic inflammation in severe persistent asthma. *American Journal of Respiratory and Critical Care Medicine*, 160, 1532–1539.

Kahle, E. B., Zipf, W. B., Lamb, D. R., Horswill, C. A., Ward, K. M. (1996). Association between mild, routine exercise and improved insulin dynamics and glucose control in obese adolescents. *International Journal of Sports Medicine*, 17(1), 1–6.

Kang, H. S., Gutin, B., Barbeau, P., Owens, S., Lemmon, C. R., Allison, J., Litaker, M. S. Le, N. A. (2002). Physical training improves insulin resistance syndrome markers in obese adolescents. *Medicine and Science in Sports and Exercise*, 34(12), 1920–1927.

Kaufman, K., Brodine, S., Shaffer, R., Johnson, C. Cullison, T. (1999). The effect of foot structure and range of motion on musculoskeletal overuse injuries. *American Journal of Sports Medicine, 27*, 585–593.

Kelley, D. E., Goodpaster, B., Wing, R. R., Simoneau, J. A. (1999). Skeletal muscle fatty acid metabolism in association with insulin resistance, obesity, and weight loss. *American Journal of Physiology*, 277(6 Pt 1), E1130–E1141.

Kitzmann, K. M., Dalton, W. T., III, Stanley, C. M., Beech, B. M., Reeves, T. P., Buscemi, J., et al. (2010). Lifestyle interventions for youth who are overweight: A meta-analytic review. *Health Psychology*, 29(1), 91–101.

Koenig, S. M. (2001). Pulmonary complications of obesity. *American Journal of Medical Sciences*, 321, 249–279.

Kramer, C. K., von Muhlen, D., Gross, J. L., Laughlin, G. A., Barrett-Connor, E. (2009). Blood pressure and fasting plasma glucose rather than metabolic syndrome predict coronary artery calcium progression. *Diabetes Care*, 32, 141–146.

Krebs, N., Sothern, M. (2006). Diagnosis, medical testing, monitoring and follow-up. In M. Sothern S. Gordon, T. K. von Almen (Eds.), *Handbook of Pediatric Obesity: Clinical Management* (pp. 79–94). Boca Raton, FL: Taylor & Francis.

LeMura, L. M., Maziekas, M. T. (2002). Factors that alter body fat, body mass, and fat-free mass in pediatric obesity. *Medicine and Science in Sports and Exercise*, 34(3), 487–496.

Loftin, M., Heusel, L., Bonis, M., Sothern, M. (2005). Oxygen uptake kinetics and oxygen deficit in obese and normal weight adolescent females. *Journal of Sports Science and Medicine*, 4, 430–436.

Loftin, M., Sothern, M., Trosclair, L., O'Hanlon, A., Miller, J., Udall, J. (2001). Scaling VO(2) peak in obese and non-obese girls. *Obesity Research*, 9(5), 290–296.

Loftin, M., Sothern, M., VanVrancken, C., Udall, J. (2003). Low heart rate peak in obese female youth. *Clinical Pediatrics*, 42(6), 505–510.

Loftin, M., Sothern, M., Warren, B., Udall, J. (2004). Comparison of VO_2 peak during treadmill and bicycle ergometry in severely overweight youth. *Journal of Sports Science and Medicine*, 3, 254–260.

Losekam, S., Goetzky, B., Kraeling, S., Rief, W., Hilbert, A. (2010). Physical activity in normal-weight and overweight youth: associations with weight teasing and self-efficacy. *Obesity Facts*, 3(4), 239–244.

Lowry, R., Lee S., Galuska, D., Fulton, J., Barrios, L., Kann, L. (2007). *Journal of Physical Activity and Health*, 4(3), 325–342.

Luder, E., Melnik, T.A., DiMaio, M. (1998). Association of being overweight with greater asthma symptoms in inner city black and Hispanic children. *Journal of Pediatrics*, 132, 699–703.

Mark, A. E., Janssen, I. (2008). Dose-response relation between physical activity and blood pressure in youth. *Medicine and Science in Sports and Exercise*, 40, 1007–1012.

McCambridge, T. M., Benjamin, H. J., Brenner, J. S., Cappetta, C. T., Demorest, R. A., Gregory, A. J. (2010). Athletic participation by children and adolescents who have systemic hypertension. *Pediatrics*, 125(6), 1287–1294.

McGavock, J., Sellers, E., Dean, H. (2007). Physical activity for the prevention and management of youth-onset type 2 diabetes mellitus: focus on cardiovascular complications. *Diabetes and Vascular Disease Research*, 4(4), 305–310.

Metcalf, J. A., Roberts, S. O. (1993). Strength training and the immature athlete: An overview. *Pediatric Nursing*, 19, 325–332.

Milteer, R. M., Ginsburg, K. R., Council on Communications and Media, Committee on Psychosocial Aspects of Child and Family Health. (2012). The importance of play in promoting healthy child development and maintaining strong parent-child bond: Focus on children in poverty. *Pediatrics*, 129(1), e204–e213.

Moen, M., Tol, J., Weir A., Steunebrink, M., De Winter, T. (2009). Medial tibial stress syndrome: A critical review. *Sports Medicine*, 39, 523–546.

Murray, R., Ramstetter, C., Council on School Health Executive Committee. (2013). The crucial role of recess in school. *American Academy of Pediatrics*, 131(1), 183–188.

Nassis, G. P., Papantakou, K., Skenderi, K., Triandafillopoulou, M., Kavouras, S. A., Yannakoulia, M., Chrousos, G. P., Sidossis, L. S. (2005). Aerobic exercise training improves insulin sensitivity without changes in body weight, body fat, adiponectin, and inflammatory markers in overweight and obese girls. *Metabolism*, 54, 1472–1479.

National High Blood Pressure Education Program, Working Group on High Blood Pressure in Children and Adolescents. (2004). The fourth report on the diagnosis, evaluation, and treatment of high blood pressure in children and adolescents. *Pediatrics*, 114, 555–576.

Newton, R. L., Han, H., Anton, S., Martin, C. K., Stewart, T. M., Lewis, L., Champagne, C., Sothern, M., Ryan, D. H., Williamson, D. A. (2010). An environmental excess weight gain prevention program in African American students: A pilot study. *American Journal of Health Promotion*, 24, 340–343.

Niess, A. M., Simon, P. (2007) Response and adaptation of skeletal muscle to exercise—the role of reactive oxygen species. *Frontiers in Bioscience*, 12, 4826–4838.

Norman, A. C., Drinkard, B., McDuffie, J. R., Ghorbani, S., Yanoff, L. B., Yanovski, J. A. (2005). Influence of excess adiposity on exercise fitness and performance in overweight children and adolescents. *Pediatrics*, 115, e690–e696.

Okely, A. D., Booth, M. L., Chey, T. (2004). Relationships between body composition and fundamental movement skills among children and adolescents. *Research Quarterly for Exercise and Sport*, 75(3), 238–247.

Owens, S. (2006). Exercise and physical activity: Exercise training programs and metabolic health. In M. Sothern, S. Gordon, T. K. von Almen (Eds.), *Handbook of Pediatric Obesity: Clinical Management* (pp. 189–198). Boca Raton, FL: Taylor & Francis.

Owens, S., Gutin, B. (1999) Exercise testing of the child with obesity. *Pediatric Cardiology*, 20, 79–83.

Philpott, J. F., Houghton, K., Luke, A. (2010). Physical activity recommendations for children with specific chronic health condition: Juvenile arthritis, hemophilia, asthma, and cystic fibrosis. *Clinical Journal of Sports Medicine*, 20(3), 167–172.

Prochaska, J. O., Redding, C. A., Evers, K. E. (2002). The transtheoretical model and stages of change. In K. Glanz, B. K. Rimer, F. M. Lewis (Eds.), *Health Behavior and Health Education* (pp. 97–122). San Francisco, CA: Jossey-Bass.

Radak, Z., Chung, H. Y., Goto, S. (2008). Systemic adaptation to oxidative challenge induced by regular exercise. *Free Radical Biology and Medicine*, 44, 153–159.

Riddell, M. C., Iscoe, K. E. (2006). Physical activity, sport, and pediatric diabetes. *Pediatric Diabetes*, 7(1), 60–70.

Riddiford-Harland, D. L., Steele, J. R., Baur, L. A. (2006). Upper and lower limb functionality: Are these compromised in obese children? *International Journal of Pediatric Obesity*, 1(1), 42–49.

Rodriguez, M. A., Winkleby, M. A., Ahn, D., Sundquist, J., Kraemer, H. C. (2002). Identification of population subgroups of children and adolescents with high asthma prevalence: Findings from the Third National Health and Nutrition Examination Survey. *Archives of Pediatrics and Adolescent Medicine*, 156, 269–275.

Rosenzweig, J. L., Ferrannini, E., Grundy, S. M., Haffner, S. M., Heine, R. J., Horton, E. S., Kawamori, R. (2008). Primary prevention of cardiovascular disease and type 2 diabetes in patients at metabolic risk: An endocrine society clinical practice guideline. *Journal of Clinical Endocrinology and Metabolism*, 93(10), 3671–3689.

Rowland, T., Loftin, M. (2006). Exercise testing. In M. Sothern, S. Gordon, T. K. von Almen (Eds.), *Handbook of Pediatric Obesity: Clinical Management* (pp. 113–117). Boca Raton, FL: Taylor & Francis.

Ruzic, L., Sporis, G., Matkovic, B. R. (2008). High volume-low intensity exercise camp and glycemic control in diabetic children. *Journal of Pediatrics and Child Health*, 44(3), 122–128.

Salvy, S. J., Bowker, J. C., Germeroth, L., Barkley, J. (2012). Influence of peers and friends on overweight/obese youths' physical activity. *Exercise and Sport Sciences Reviews*, 40(3), 127–132.

Schmitz, K. H., Jacobs, D. R., Jr., Hong, C. P., Steinberger, J., Moran, A., Sinaiko, A. R. (2002). Association of physical activity with insulin sensitivity in children. *International Journal of Obesity and Related Metabolic Disorders*, 26(10), 1310–1316.

Schultz, S., Browning, R., Schutz, Y., Maffeis, C., Hills, A. (2011). Childhood obesity and walking guidelines and challenges. *International Journal of Pediatric Obesity*, 6, 332–341.

Schultz, S., Hills, A., Sitler, M., Hillstrom, H. (2010). Body size and walking cadence affect hip power in children's gait. *Gait Posture*, 32, 248–252.

Schultz, S., Sitler, M., Tierney, R., Hillstrom, H., Song, J. (2009). Effects of pediatric obesity on joint kinematic and kinetics during two walking cadences. *Archives of Physical Medicine and Rehabilitation*, 90(12), 2146–2154.

Schwimmer, J. D., Burwinkle, T. M., Varni, J. W. (2003). Health-related quality of life of severely obese children and adolescents. *JAMA*, 289(14), 1813–1819.

Shaheen, S. O., Sterne, J. A., Montgomery, S. M., Azima, H. (1999). Birth weight, body mass index and asthma in young adults. *Thorax*, 54, 396–402.

Shaibi, G. Q., Ball, G. D., Cruz, M. L., Weigensberg, M. J., Salem, G. J., Goran, M. I. (2006). Cardiovascular fitness and physical activity in children with and without impaired glucose tolerance. *International Journal of Obesity (London)*, 30(1), 45–49.

Shaibi, G. Q., Michaliszyn, S. B., Fritschi, C., Quinn, L., Faulkner, M. S. (2009). Type 2 diabetes in youth: A phenotype of poor cardiorespiratory fitness and low physical activity. *International Journal of Pediatric Obesity*, 4(4), 332–337.

Silverstein, J., Klingensmith, G., Copeland, K., Plotnick, L., Kaufman, F., Laffel, L., et al. (2005). Care of children and adolescents with type 1 diabetes: A statement of the American Diabetes Association. *Diabetes Care*, 28(1), 186–212.

Simpson, L. A., Cooper, J. (2009). Paying for obesity: A changing landscape. *Pediatrics*, 123(Suppl 5), S301–S307.

Sinha, R., Fisch, G., Teaque, B., Tamborlane, W. V., Banyas, B., Allen, K., Savote, M., Rieger, V., Taksali, S., Barbette, G., Sherwin, R. S., Caprio, S. (2002). Prevalence of impaired glucose intolerance among children and adolescents with marked obesity. *New England Journal of Medicine*, 346(22), 802–810.

Sothern, M. (2002). Encouraging outdoor physical activity in overweight elementary school children. In K. Wellhousen, *Outdoor Play Every Day: Innovative Play Concepts for Early Childhood*. Albany, NY: Delmar Publishers.

Sothern, M. (2001). Exercise as a modality in the treatment of childhood obesity. *Pediatric Clinics of North America*, 48(4), 995–1015.

Sothern, M. (2004). Obesity prevention in children: Physical activity and nutrition. *Nutrition*, 20(7-8), 704–708.

Sothern, M. (1998). Physiologic function during weight-bearing exercise in obese children: Implications for clinical prescription and curriculum design. Dissertation Abstracts International, doctoral dissertation, University of New Orleans, New Orleans, LA.

Sothern, M. (2006). The business of pediatric weight management. In M. Sothern, S. Gordon, T. K. von Almen (Eds.), *Handbook of Pediatric Obesity: Clinical Management* (pp. 9–28). Boca Raton, FL: Taylor & Francis.

Sothern, M., Gordon, S. (2005). Family-based weight management in the pediatric health care setting. *Obesity Management*, 1(5), 197–202.

Sothern, M., Gordon, S. (2003). Prevention of obesity in young children: A critical challenge for the medical professional. *Clinical Pediatrics*, 42(2), 101–111.

Sothern, M., Gordon, S., von Almen, T. K. (Eds.). (2006). *Handbook of Pediatric Obesity: Clinical Management*. Boca Raton, FL: Taylor & Francis.

Sothern, M., Hunter, S., Suskind, R., Brown, R., Udall, J., Blecker, U. (1999). Motivating the obese child to move: The role of structured exercise in pediatric weight management. *Southern Medical Journal*, 92(6), 577–584.

Sothern, M., Loftin, M., Blecker, M., Suskind R., Udall, J. (1999a). Health benefits of physical activity in children and adolescents: Implications for chronic disease prevention. *European Journal of Pediatrics*, 158, 271–274.

Sothern, M., Loftin, M., Blecker, M., Suskind R., Udall, J. (1999b). Physiologic function and childhood obesity. *International Journal of Pediatrics*, 14(3), 1–5.

Sothern, M., Loftin, M., Blecker, U., Suskind, R., Udall, J. (2000). The impact of significant weight loss on maximal oxygen uptake in obese children and adolescents. *Journal of Investigative Medicine*, 48(6), 411–416.

Sothern, M., Loftin, M., Suskind, R., Udall, J. (1999). The impact of significant weight loss on resting energy expenditure in obese youth. *Journal of Investigative Medicine*, 47(5), 222–226.

Sothern, M., Loftin, J., Udall, J. N., Suskind, R. M., Ewing, T., Tang, S. C., Blecker, U. (1999). Inclusion of resistance exercise in a multi-disciplinary outpatient treatment program for preadolescent obese children. *Southern Medical Journal*, 92(6), 585–592.

Sothern, M. S., Loftin, J. M., Udall, J. N., Suskind, R. M., Ewing, T. L., Tang, S. C., Blecker, U. (2000). Safety, feasibility, and efficacy of a resistance training program in preadolescent obese children. *American Journal of the Medical Sciences*, 319(6), 370–375.

Sothern, M., Schumacher, H., von Almen, T. K., Carlisle, L., Udall, J. (2002). Committed to Kids: an integrated, four level team approach to weight management in adolescents. *Journal of the American Dietetic Association*, 102(3), S81–S85.

Sothern, M., Udall, J. Suskind, R., Vargas, A., Blecker, U. (2000). Weight loss and growth velocity in obese children after very low calorie diet, exercise and behavior modification. *Acta Paediatrica*, 89(9), 1036–1043.

Sothern, M., VanVrancken-Tompkins, C., Brooks, C., Thélin, C. (2006). Increasing physical activity in overweight youth in clinical settings. In M. Sothern, S. Gordon, T. K. von Almen (Eds.), *Handbook of Pediatric Obesity: Clinical Management* (pp. 173–188). Boca Raton, FL: Taylor & Francis.

Sothern, M., von Almen, T. K., Schumacher, H. (2001). *Trim Kids: The Proven Plan That Has Helped Thousands of Children Achieve a Healthier Weight.* New York, NY: Harper Collins.

Sothern, M., von Almen, K., Schumacher, R. D., Suskind, R., Blecker, U. A. (1999). Multidisciplinary approach to the treatment of childhood obesity. *Delaware Medical Journal*, 71(6), 255–261.

Sothern, M., von Almen, T., Schumacher, H., Zelman, M., Farris, R., Carlisle, L., Udall, J., Suskind, R. (1993). An effective multi-disciplinary approach to weight reduction in youth. In C. Williams, S. Kimm (Eds.), *Annals of the New York Academy of Sciences: Prevention and Treatment of Childhood Obesity* (pp. 292–294). New York, NY: New York Academy of Sciences.

Stratton, G., Jones, M., Fox, K. R., Tolfrey, K., Harris, J., Maffulli, N., Lee, M., Frostick, S. P., REACH Group. (2004). BASES position statement on guidelines for resistance exercise in young people. *Journal of Sports Sciences*, 22(4), 383–390.

Strong, W. B., Malina, R. M., Blimkie, C. J., Daniels, S. R., Dishman, R. K., Gutin, B., et al. (2005). Evidence-based physical activity for school-age youth. *Journal of Pediatrics*, 146(6), 732–737.

Stunkard, A. J. (1996). Current views on obesity. *American Journal of Medicine*, 100, 230–236.

Suskind, R., Sothern, M., Farris, R., von Almen, T., Schumacher, H., Loftin, M., Escobar, O., Vargas, A., Brown, R., Udall, J. (1993). Recent advances in the treatment of childhood obesity. In C. Williams, S. Kimm (Eds.), *Annals of the New York Academy of Sciences: Prevention and Treatment of Childhood Obesity* (pp. 181–199). New York, NY: New York Academy of Sciences.

Suskind, R., Sothern, M., von Almen, K., Schumacher, H., Schultz, S., DeLeon, E., et al. (1996). Review of recent advances in the treatment of childhood obesity. In A. Angel, H. Anderson, C. Bouchard, D. Lau, L. Leiter, R. Mendelson (Eds.), *Progress in Obesity Research* (pp. 733–738). London: John Libbey.

Talanian, J. L., Galloway, S. D., Heigenhauser, G. J., Bonen, A., Spriet, L. L. (2007). Two weeks of high-intensity aerobic interval training increases the capacity for fat oxidation during exercise in women. *Journal of Applied Physiology, 102*(4), 1439–1447.

Taylor, E., Theim, K., Mirch, M., Ghorbani, S., Tanofsky-Kraff, M., Adler-Wailes, D., et al. (2006). Orthopedic complications of overweight in children and adolescents. *Pediatrics, 117*, 2167–2174.

Thomas, A. S., Greene, L. F., Ard, J. D., Oster, R. A., Darnell, B. E., Gower, B. A. (2009). Physical activity may facilitate diabetes prevention in adolescents. *Diabetes Care, 32*, 9–13.

Thomas, E. L., Hamilton, G., Patel, N., O'Dwyer, R., Dore, C. J., Goldin, R. D., et al. (2005). Hepatic triglyceride content and its relation to body adiposity: A magnetic resonance imaging and proton magnetic resonance spectroscopy study. *Gut, 54*(1), 122–127.

Tonkonogi, M., Krook, A., Walsh, B., Sahlin, K. (2000). Endurance training increases stimulation of uncoupling of skeletal muscle mitochondria in humans by non-esterified fatty acids: An uncoupling-protein-mediated effect? *Biochemical Journal, 351*(Pt 3), 805–810.

Treuth, M. S., Figueroa-Colon, R., Hunter, G. R., Weinsier, R. L, Butte, N. F., Goran, M. I. (1998). Energy expenditure and physical fitness in overweight vs. non-overweight prepubertal girls. *International Journal of Obesity and Related Metabolic Disorders, 22*(5), 440–447.

Trick, J. (1990). Effective management of a hospital-based health promotion program: keys to success. *American Journal of Health Promotion, 4*, 317–319.

Udall, J., Sothern, M. (2004). Obesity in childhood and adolescence. In L. Martin (Ed.), *Obesity Surgery*. Toronto, Ontario, Canada: McGraw Hill.

U.S. Centers for Disease Control and Prevention. (2012). Overweight and obesity: Consequences. Retrieved June 9, 2012, from http://www.cdc.gov/obesity/childhood/basics.html.

U.S. Department of Health and Human Services. (2008). Physical activity guidelines for Americans. Retrieved June 25, 2009, from http://www.health.gov/paguidelines.

U.S. Preventive Services Task Force. (2010). Screening for obesity in children and adolescents: U.S. Preventive Services Task Force recommendation statement. *Pediatrics, 125*(2), 361–367.

VanVrancken-Tompkins, C. L., Sothern, M.S. (2006). Preventing obesity in children birth to five years. In *Encyclopedia on Early Childhood Development*. Montreal, Quebec, Canada: Centre of Excellence for Early Childhood Development. Retrieved from http://www.excellenceearlychildhood.ca/liste_theme.asp?lang=EN&act=32.

VanVrancken-Tompkins, C., Sothern, M., Bar-Or, O. (2006). Strengths and weaknesses in the response of the obese child to exercise. In M. Sothern, S. Gordon, T. K. von Almen (Eds.), *Handbook of Pediatric Obesity: Clinical Management* (pp. 67–75). Boca Raton, FL: Taylor & Francis.

Visser, M. (2001). Higher levels of inflammation in obese children. *Nutrition, 17*, 480–481.

Visser, M., Bouter, L. M., McQuillan, G. M., Wener, M. H., Harris, T. B. (1999). Elevated C-reactive protein levels in overweight and obese adults. *JAMA, 282*, 2131–2135.

Visser, M., Bouter, L. M., McQuillan, G. M., Wener, M. H., Harris, T. B. (2001). Low-grade systemic inflammation in overweight children. *Pediatrics*, 107(1), E13.

von Almen, T. K., Sothern, M., Schumacher, H. (2006). Inter-disciplinary, interactive, group instruction. In M. Sothern, S. Gordon, T. K. von Almen (Eds.), *Handbook of Pediatric Obesity: Clinical Management* (pp. 235–269). Boca Raton, FL: Taylor & Francis.

Wilmore, J. H., Costill, D. L. (1994). *Physiology of Sport and Exercise*. Champaign, IL: Human Kinetics.

Yu, C. C., Sung, R. Y., So, R. C., Lui, K. C., Lau, W., Lam, P. K., et al. (2005). Effects of strength training on body composition and bone mineral content in children who are obese. *Journal of Strength and Conditioning Research*, 19(3), 667–672.

Yudkin, J. S., Kumari, M., Humphries, S. E., Mohamed-Ali, V. (2000). Inflammation, obesity, stress and coronary heart disease: is interleukin-6 the link? *Atherosclerosis*, 148, 209–214.

Zabaleta, J., Velasco-Gonzalez, C., Estrada, J., Ravussin, E., Pelligrino, N., Mohler, M. C., et al. (2013). Inverse correlation of serum inflammatory markers with metabolic parameters in healthy, Black and White prepubertal youth. *International Journal of Obesity*. doi:10.1038/ijo.2013.220. [Epub ahead of print]

Zorba, E., Cengiz, T., Karacabey, K. (2011). Exercise training improves body composition, blood lipid profile and serum insulin levels in obese children. *Journal of Sports Medicine and Physical Fitness*, 51(4), 664–669.

Chapter 7

MONITORING PROGRESS

THE IMPORTANCE OF REGULAR MEDICAL
SELF-MONITORING

The objective of implementing regular medical and self-monitoring into a pediatric weight management program is to ensure that the intervention is safe and effective. It is important to establish baseline information regarding the child's medical condition and performance before providing recommendations to increase physical activity or incorporate a structured exercise routine (Gordon & Sothern, 2006). This is particularly important for overweight children. This goal may be accomplished by evaluating the program's impact on physiologic, metabolic, biochemical, and psychosocial parameters. We have shown in several clinical observations that the approach detailed in this book promotes enhanced physical fitness (Sothern, 2001; Sothern, Loftin, & Blecker, 2000), increased physical activity levels (PALs) (Reed et al., 2001), decreased total body weight (Sothern et al., 1999; Sothern et al., 2000; Sothern, Suskind, Vargas, & Blecker, 2000; Sothern et al., 2002), decreased body mass index (BMI) (Sothern, 2001; Sothern et al., 1999; Sothern et al., 2000), decreased body adiposity (Olivier et al., 2002; Sothern et al., 1999; Sothern et al., 2000; Sothern et al., 2000), maintenance of lean body mass (Olivier et al., 2002), maintenance of resting energy expenditure (Sothern et al., 1999), improved lipid profiles (Brown et al., 2000; Sothern et al., 2000), maintenance of biochemical status (Sothern et al., 2000; Suskind et al., 2000; von Almen, Figueroa-Colon, & Suskind, 1991), and improved psychosocial parameters (von Almen et al., 1991). Likewise, a multitude of other investigations have documented similar short-term (Barbeau et al., 2007; Ben Ounis et al., 2010; Dao et al., 2004; Savoye et al., 2007; Shaibi et al., 2006; Sothern et al., 2006; Yu et al., 2005) and long-term (American Dietetic Association, 2006; Kitzmann et al., 2010; U.S. Preventive Services Task Force Recommendation Statement, 2010) outcomes after implementation of similar multidisciplinary, group, and family-based pediatric weight management programs.

TRACKING OBESITY IN CHILDREN

According to the U.S. Surgeon General, physicians are the best source for the diagnosis of pediatric obesity. Doctors and other health care professionals are the best source in determining whether a child or adolescent's weight is healthy, and they can help rule out rare medical problems as the cause of unhealthy weight (Gordon & Sothern, 2006). BMI can be calculated from measurements of height and weight. Health professionals often use a BMI "growth chart" to help them assess whether a child or adolescent is overweight (Eisenmann, for the Subcommittee on Assessment in Pediatric Obesity Management Programs, National Association of Children's Hospital and Related Institutions, 2011; Ganley et al., 2011) (Table 7.1). A physician also will consider a child or adolescent's age and growth patterns to determine whether his or her weight is healthy (Barlow, 2007; Krebs et al., 2007). Only providers trained in pediatric medicine possess the level of expertise required to provide an accurate assessment of pediatric obesity. Regardless, studies indicate that pediatric health care providers diagnosed overweight in less than one-half of overweight children (Carlisle, Gordon, & Sothern, 2005; O'Brien, Holubkov, & Reis, 2004).

Physicians also provide guidance to parents so that they may best understand the definition of overweight or at risk for overweight in children. Then, with the parents' input, they can decide on the best plan of action for the overweight child. Research suggests that at this point about 75% of physicians will refer patients initially to registered dieticians (Barlow et al., 2002) and only about 20% of patients to weight management programs. In a recent survey of pediatric obesity–weight management programs, Eisenmann and colleagues (2011) reported that most programs followed the 2007 Expert Committee assessment recommendations

Table 7.1 Body Mass Index Charts

Boys: 5–17 years of age				
Age	Level 1: Red Severe obesity (>120% of 95th BMI or absolute BMI >35 kg/m²)	Level 2: Yellow Clinical obesity (more than 95th percentile BMI)	Level 3: Green Overweight (more than 85th percentile BMI)	Level 4: Blue Healthy weight (50–85th percentile BMI)
<5 years	See your pediatrician	See your pediatrician	See your pediatrician	See your pediatrician
5 years	>19	>18	>17	16–17
6 years	>19	>18	>17	15–17
7 years	>20	>19	>17	16–17
8 years	>21	>20	>18	16–18
9 years	>22	>21	>19	16–19
10 years	>24	>22	>19	17–18
11 years	>25	>23	>20	17–20
12 years	>26	>24	>21	18–21
13 years	>27	>25	>22	19–22
14 years	>28	>26	>23	19–23
15 years	>29	>27	>23	20–23
16 years	>29	>28	>24	21–24
17 years	>30	>28	>25	21–25
Girls: 5–17 years of age				
Age	Level 1: Red Severe obesity (>120% of 95th BMI or absolute BMI >35 kg/m²)	Level 2: Yellow Clinical obesity (more than 95th percentile BMI)	Level 3: Green Overweight (more than 85th percentile BMI)	Level 4: Blue Healthy weight (50–85th percentile BMI)
<5 years	See your pediatrician	See your pediatrician	See your pediatrician	See your pediatrician
5 years	>19	>18	>17	15–17
6 years	>20	>19	>17	15–17
7 years	>21	>20	>18	16–18
8 years	>22	>21	>18	16–18
9 years	>23	>22	>19	16–19
10 years	>25	>23	>20	17–20
11 years	>26	>24	>21	18–21
12 years	>27	>25	>22	18–22
13 years	>28	>26	>23	19–23
14 years	>29	>27	>23	19–23
15 years	>30	>28	>24	20–24
16 years	>31	>29	>25	21–25
17 years	>32	>30	>25	21–25

Sources: Adapted from Centers for Disease Control and Prevention. (2010). *Growth Charts*. Retrieved from http://www.cdc.gov/growthcharts; Kelly, A. S., Barlow, S. E., Rao, G., et al., *Circulation*, 128(15), 1689–1712, 2013; Sothern, M. S., Von Almen, T. K., Schumacher, H., *Trim Kids: The Proven Plan That Has Helped Thousands of Children Achieve a Healthier Weight*, HarperCollins, New York, NY, 2001.
Note: BMI scores are rounded to the nearest 1.0.

(Barlow, 2007), which included using the U.S. Centers for Disease Control and Prevention (CDC, 2010) BMI reference values to determine weight status or obesity level.

Table 7.2 Diagnosing Overweight and Risk for Overweight (Initial Medical Evaluation)

Family/medical history and physical exam
Anthropometric measures
Weight and height
Calculate body mass index (BMI)
Laboratory evaluation (>95th BMI)
Chem 20; CBC w/diff; lipid profile; thyroid profile
Maturation level (Tanner stage)

PERFORMING THE INITIAL MEDICAL EVALUATION

An initial medical history and physical examination (Table 7.2) is recommended before enrollment into the treatment program. This medical information is reviewed with the parent(s) and child before entry into the program. Assessment and discussion of the child's growth chart and current weight status occurs at this time. To determine the child's goal weight, the physician observes on the BMI growth chart what weight would match the child's height percentile (CDC, 2010). This is the child's ideal body weight. The child's goal weight is this weight plus an additional 20%.

ORDERING AND INTERPRETING LABORATORY BLOOD WORK

The pediatrician orders an initial battery of blood work (Table 7.2) that includes a complete blood count (Chem 20; CBC w/diff), metabolic panel, and lipid profile. These laboratory tests are repeated 3 months into the program and at the end of the program. Other tests may be ordered after the initial medical evaluation as needed.

PROVIDING ONGOING MEDICAL SUPERVISION

In group interventions a pediatrician may choose to attend some or all of the intervention sessions, especially during the first 3 months of the program. He may elect to weigh the children and check vital signs while discussing their progress and answering questions. This helps to ensure medical safety throughout the course of the program (Table 7.3). However, a nurse or other trained health care professional, such as an exercise professional or registered

Table 7.3 Medical Supervision

Quarterly anthropometric measurements—
• Document and follow height and growth • Bioelectrical impedance, body mass index, circumferences, skinfolds
Physician is available by phone or beeper during the week.
Active weekly participation by the physician— • Get to know the children personally. • Present for questions from kids and family. • Participate in activities with kids.

Table 7.4 Normal and Overweight Children ≤6 Years with Parental Obesity

Regular visits with the pediatrician to monitor growth and development
Parent training and fitness education
Limit access to television, video, and computer
Increased opportunities for unstructured physical activity (free play) • Create an environment inside the home that promotes active play. • Create an environment outside the home that promotes play.

dietician, may oversee the weigh-in and vital sign-monitoring period of the session. Whether the physician attends the sessions routinely or not, he or she should be available by phone to address questions or problems that arise during the intervention program. In overweight and normal-weight children with parental obesity, frequent monitoring, reduced television viewing, and increased opportunities for unstructured active play are recommended by the physician because these children are at increased risk for developing obesity (Table 7.4).

Weight Record and Vital Signs								
Patient Name:								
Date	Week	Height (cm)	Weight (kg)	Weight (lbs)	Weekly Loss/Gain	Loss to Date	BP	RHR

Note: BP = blood pressure; RHR = resting heart rate.

Both short-term (weekly) and longer (every 3 months) monitoring procedures are recommended. Weekly procedures include checking or collecting diet and exercise self-monitoring forms and booklets, checking goal sheets, symptoms monitoring and reporting, recording attendance, and distributing incentives and awards for goals achieved. Sample forms can be found in the next few pages of this chapter.

Initial Group Check-In Form

Hello, my name is _____.

I am _____ years old. I attend _____ school and am in _____ grade.

Some things I do really well (or am proud of) include

_____

_____

Some things I would like to do to be healthier include

_____

_____

Weekly Group Check-In Form

Hello, my name is _____.

This week I (check one below)

_____ Lost _____ pounds

_____ Gained _____ pounds

_____ Stayed the same.

Since beginning the program I have (check one below)

_____ Lost _____ pounds

_____ Gained _____ pounds

_____ Stayed the same

My accomplishments for the week are

_____

_____

_____

My questions or challenges this week are

_____

_____

_____

Commitment Rating Form

How badly do you want to lead a healthier lifestyle?

Parents and Children: Rate yourself on the scale below from 0–100. Circle the number that describes how you feel right now.

0		25		50		75		100
Not		∧				∧		Very
At All		Little		Somewhat		Lot		Much

Do you think you will feel the same way in 6 months? YES or NO

Do you think you will feel the same way 1 year from now? YES or NO

Short-Term and Long-Term Goals Form

Short-Term Goals

My short-term goals are

_____

_____

_____

Examples: walk a half mile without resting, ride my bike 3 days this week

Long-Term Goals

My long-term goals are

_____

_____

_____

Examples: walk a 10K race, try out for the basketball team

Once the initial evaluation is performed, participants are assigned to Levels 1 (Red), 2 (Yellow), 3 (Green), or 4 (Blue) based on their initial BMI percentile, fitness and PAL, and medical condition. Table 7.5 details the various levels.

These levels are also used to determine a recommended term of treatment. Children in level 1 are encouraged to attend the program for 1–2 years. Those in level 2 should participate in the program for at least 1 year and, children in level 3 are given a 6- to 12-month term of treatment. Detailed protocols of these measures are found in Chapter 8: Measuring Health and Fitness Outcomes.

Weekly Goal-Setting and Action-Planning Form

My goal this week is to

_____

_____

_____

_____

1. Does it say what you WILL do (NOT what you WON'T do this week)?
2. Do you have control over it?
3. Is it easy to do?

Steps and reminders (include who, when, where, or how)

_____

_____

_____

My reward for accomplishing my goal is

_____

Table 7.5 Select the Level That Best Corresponds to the Greatest Number of Selected Categories

Color code	Weight level	Physical activity level	Cardiorespiratory fitness level	Muscular strength and endurance	Flexibility	Comorbidity (e.g., asthma, hypertension, diabetes)
Red	Level 1: Severe obesity (>120% of 95th BMI or absolute BMI >35 kg/m²)	Sedentary	Unfit	Poor	Poor	Uncontrolled or severe
Yellow	Level 2: Obesity (>95–<99th percentile BMI)	Moderately active	Moderately fit	Average	Average	Controlled or moderate
Green	Level 3: Overweight (>85–<99th percentile BMI)	Active	Fit	Good	Good	Well-controlled or mild
Blue	Level 4: Healthy weight (>5–<85th percentile BMI)	Very active	Very fit	Excellent	Excellent	No comorbidities

EVALUATING LONG-TERM PROGRESS

At the beginning of treatment for pediatric obesity and every 3 months afterward, it is recommended that patients undergo a comprehensive evaluation. A sample test preparation letter and evaluation checklist are provided below. The results of the evaluations may be distributed to the children and parents and discussed with the family as necessary. Sample

---

Test Preparation Letter

<insert name and address of institution>

Dear Parent,

Your child is required to have a blood test prior to _____.

He or she will not be allowed to begin the program until this test has been completed.

The laboratory is located at_____.

Their hours of operation are _____.

To make an appointment call _____.

Instructions before the test:

Fasting is required (no food) 12 hours beforehand. We suggest scheduling an early morning appointment so that the fasting may be done overnight. Drinking water is fine.

Should you have any further questions regarding this test, please contact the weight management program office at _____.

Thank you.

Sincerely,

Program Director

Evaluation Checklist

Patient name: _____

Date: _____

☐ Measurements
☐ Height
☐ Weight
☐ Blood pressure
☐ Resting heart rate
☐ BIA/DEXA
☐ Skinfolds
☐ Circumferences
☐ Photograph
☐ Questionnaires and Forms
☐ Physical Activity Record
☐ Laboratory forms (blood work: baseline, 3, 6, and 12 months)
☐ Consent or HIPAA waiver form (if applicable)

Note: BIA = bioelectrical impedance; DEXA = dual-energy x-ray absorptiometry, HIPAA = Health Insurance Portability and Accountability Act.

evaluation forms can be found in the next few pages of this chapter. In some cases, the health care professional may refer the family to a staff psychologist, if available, or other appropriate mental health professional. A registered dietician or exercise professional should be available to assist with interpretation and to answer questions as well. These evaluations consist of the following 10 items.

GROWTH AND DEVELOPMENT

The measurement of height or stature is a major indicator of growth and development, bone length, and general body size. The recommended technique for height measurement includes the use of a vertical board with an attached metric rule and horizontal headboard, collectively known as a stadiometer. The standard measure of weight should be recorded using a calibrated electronic scale. The kilograms should be recorded in the patient's chart. For both height and weight measures, the patient should remove shoes and heavy clothing or objects before the measurement.

BODY MASS INDEX AND CDC PERCENTILES

BMI is a calculated number that adjusts weight for height using the following formula:

$$BMI = Weight\ (kilograms)/Height\ (meters^2)$$

In adults, a BMI value greater than or equal to 25 but less than 30 is considered overweight, and a BMI value greater than or equal to 30 defines obesity or severe overweight (Hubbard, 2000). These BMI cutoffs are not appropriate for classifying children's weight status. The CDC (2010) has defined overweight as a BMI between greater than the 85th percentile and less than the 95th percentile for age. Children are considered obese if the BMI is greater than the 95th percentile for age. In growing children, BMI initially declines during infancy and early childhood and then increases with age (Ganley et al., 2011). Because of these changes in BMI with growth, age-specific criteria are needed (Barlow, 2007; Krebs et al., 2007). Gender-specific criteria also are needed due to differences in body composition and timing of growth patterns in adolescence for boys and girls). Revised growth charts with smoothed age and sex-specific BMI percentile curves were developed by the National Center for Health Statistics for children ages 2–17 years old (CDC, 2010).

It is recommended that children with a BMI greater than the 85th percentile be further evaluated for complications associated with overweight and for recent excessive weight gain. Assessments should include the evaluation of potential genetic, endocrine, or psychological syndromes (Arslanian, 2002; Barlow, 2007; Barlow & Dietz, 1998; Brown et al., 2000; Caprio, 2002; Krebs et al., 2007; Zannolli et al., 1993). Family medical, diet, and physical activity history should be obtained to identify primary risk factors for overweight, such as parental obesity, sedentary behaviors, early feeding practices, metabolic or hormonal stress, socioeconomic factors, and ethnicity (Arslanian, 2002; Barlow, 2007; Birch & Davison, 2001; Dietz, 1994; Dietz & Gortmaker, 2001; Dowda et al., 2001; Eisenmann et al., 2011; Fogelholm et al., 1999; Hill & Throwbridge, 1989; Krebs et al., 2007; Law et al., 1992; Micic, 2001; Steinbeck, 2001).

WAIST CIRCUMFERENCE

An additional method of assessing body composition is the measurement of girth of various body sections (Lohman, Roche, & Martorell, 1988). A metal or fiberglass measuring tape with a metric scale is used to measure the circumference of the waist or hip. The waist circumference is a useful indicator for determining reduction in abdominal fat weight after treatment (Ganley et al., 2011). The routine use of circumference measurements, especially waist circumference, is not recommended for clinical settings (Barlow, 2007); however, in a recent survey, 83% of pediatric weight management programs reported using this measure as an estimate of abdominal adiposity (Eisenmann et al., 2011). Concerns included a lack of specific guidelines and difficulty in determining the precise measurement locations, among others. If this option is considered, health care providers should adhere precisely to the instructions contained in detailed protocols and ensure that staff are well-trained.

BLOOD PRESSURE AND HEART RATE

Resting blood pressure measurement is taken as a measure of the force of the heart's pumping action. Hypertension in children and adolescents continues to be defined as systolic BP (SBP) or diastolic BP (DBP) that is, on repeated measurement, in the 95th percentile. BP between the 90th and 95th percentile in childhood had been designated "high normal." To be consistent, pediatric hypertension often is observed in overweight children especially those with severe conditions. According to the Seventh Report of the Joint National Committee on the Prevention, Detection, Evaluation, and Treatment of High Blood Pressure (Chobanian et al., 2003), this level of BP will now be termed "prehypertensive" and is an indication for lifestyle modifications (Chobanian et al., 2003; Fujita & Midori Awazu, 2012; Krebs et al., 2007).

LABORATORY BLOOD WORK

Biochemical markers, total cholesterol, triglycerides, high-density lipoproteins, and low-density lipoproteins should be examined by drawing 10–20 cubic centimeters (cc) of whole blood in a certified laboratory. Children should be required to fast for 12 hours before the test. In addition, health care providers may consider obtaining blood samples to determine insulin and glucose levels.

BODY COMPOSITION ANALYSIS: ESTIMATE OF THE PERCENTAGE OF BODY FAT

Skinfold analysis measures the thickness of a double fold of skin and subcutaneous adipose tissue at various body locations (Roche, Heymsfield, & Lohman, 1996). The use of skinfold calipers is a widely used method for determining obesity as it provides more detail concerning the distribution of fat than what is provided by the BMI measure (Ganley et al., 2011). Recent guidelines for evaluating body composition do not include the use of skinfolds for several reasons, including a lack of reference data and criteria or cut points and concern for measurement error (Barlow, 2007). The advantage of this method is that it is relatively inexpensive and nonevasive, although there is concern that the measure may induce psychological discomfort (Eisenmann et al., 2011). In addition, very little space is needed. Therefore, although not ideal, skinfolds do provide an option for assessing body composition in nonclinical settings as long as trained health care providers are utilized (Table 7.6). Specific descriptions of the measurement of skinfold thickness and various equations have been developed in the prediction of body composition (Bray et al., 2002; Cameron et al., 2004; Durnin & Womersley, 1974; Goran et al., 1996; Gutin et al., 1996; Jackson & Pollock, 1978; Lohman, 1981; Lohman et al., 1988; Sloan, 1967). A two-site formula was developed by Slaughter et al. (1988) and later validated in a study by Janz et al. (1993). The formula includes specific equations for overweight youth, which are shown to be highly correlated with both underwater weighing and dual-energy x-ray absorptiometry (DEXA) measurements (Boye et al., 2002).

Table 7.6 Childhood Obesity Treatment Quarterly Evaluation

Body composition • Dual-energy x-ray absorptiometry • Skin folds • Bioelectrical impedance
Dietary history
Physical activity rating
Psychological measures • Self-esteem • Depression • Self-efficacy

Bioelectrical impedance (BIA) may be used to measure the density of lean and adipose tissue in relation to hydration (Bray et al., 2002; Fors et al., 2002; Goran et al., 1996; Gutin et al., 1996). Studies have demonstrated that total body water (TBW) and electrical impedance are related (Eisenkolbl, Kartasurya, & Widhalm, 2001; Hoffer, Meador, & Simpson, 1969). Further studies also report the utility and reliability of body impedance measurements in the assessment of total body fat (Casanova Roman et al., 2004; Fors et al., 2002). Both BIA and skinfolds provide a reasonably accurate, time-, and cost-effective method of assessing body fat in overweight children (Bray et al., 2002; Cameron et al., 2004; Goran et al., 1996). Care should be taken, however, to select a formula specific to the age, race, and gender of the child as accuracy varies by study (Boye et al., 2002; Loftin et al., 2007; Morrison et al., 2001; Parker et al., 2003).

Talking Points: Body Composition (Verbal cues for patients or parents and family members)
Read through the following information with your patient or parent to help him or her to understand the measurements used in the program.

Our bodies are made up of many different tissues. Body composition refers to the percentage of your body weight composed of fat and the percentage of body weight composed of lean tissue and bone. Fat is a soft tissue primarily found underneath your skin. The rest of our tissues—muscles and bones—are classified as lean body mass. Exercise burns fat tissue and helps to maintain or improve lean muscle tissue. Your body composition changes after you begin exercising regularly and by engaging in different types of exercise. Your doctor helped you recognize what percentage of body fat you had before you started the program. You will check again with the doctor in another 3 months to see how your percentage of body fat and classification has changed.

More accurate methods of determining body composition are available, but typically they are reserved for severe overweight conditions or research studies. These include underwater weight and DEXA. For many years, underwater or hydrostatic weighing was termed the "gold standard" for measurement of body fat (Roche et al., 1996). The use of underwater weighing is based on Archimedes' principle. Simply stated, Archimedes reasoned that an object submerged in water is buoyed up by a counterforce equaling the weight of the displaced water. An object "loses weight in water." Therefore, if an object weighs 50 kilograms (kg) in air and 3 kg when submerged, the loss of weight in water (47 kg) equals the weight of displaced water. We then can calculate the volume of water displaced because the density of water at any temperature is known. More recently, DEXA has been used to determine percentage of fat (%fat), lean body mass (LBM), and bone mineral density accurately and safely in children and adolescents (Bray et al., 2002; Goran et al., 1996; Gutin et al., 1996; Ogle, Allen, & Humphries, 1995; Shypailo et al., 2008; Steinberger et al., 2005). DEXA utilizes an x-ray source to generate photons to scan subjects (Pietrobelli et al., 1996). Bone-mineral content measurements previously calibrated against secondary standards with ashed bone sections are used to help calculate fat free mass (Friedl et al., 1992; Mazess et al., 1990). Percentage of fat and fat-free body can be predicted with accuracy by observing the ratio of absorbance of the different-energy-level photons, which are linearly related to the percentage of fat in the soft tissues of the body (Nguyen et al., 1996). The coefficient of variation of fat-free tissue measurement has been calculated at 2%, which is comparable to that obtained by hydrodensitometry (Ellis et al., 1994).

PHYSICAL ACTIVITY LEVEL
The measurement of an individual's physical activity level (PAL; Table 7.7) provides important clues regarding behaviors that may be contributing to the overweight condition (Gordon & Sothern, 2006). Sedentary behaviors are highly associated with childhood obesity. Accurate laboratory procedures can be used to determine PAL. These include accelerometry, total

Pediatric Weight Management Quarterly Evaluation Form

<insert name of institution>

LOCATION: _____

NAME	SEX			D.O.B.		DATE OF EXAM	
GROUP	RACE			AGE		VISIT	
MEASURE	1	2		3		AVERAGE	EXAMINER
WEIGHT (kg)							
HEIGHT (cm)							
BODY MASS INDEX				%		LEVEL OF OBESITY	
MEASURE	1	2		3		AVERAGE	EXAMINER
MIDARM CIRC. (cm)							
WAIST CIRC. (cm)							
HIP CIRC. (cm)							
MID-THIGH (mm)							
TRICEPS (mm)							
SUBSCAPULAR (mm)							
MEDIAL CALF (mm)							
HEAD (cm)							
BIA RESISTANCE (if applicable)						RESTING HEART RATE (bpm)	
BLOOD PRESSURE (mm Hg)							
NUMBER OF CLASSES ATTENDED	NUMBER OF CLASSES CONDUCTED			PHOTOGRAPH CONSENT		Yes	No

energy expenditure by doubly labeled water, VO_2 portable equipment, heart-rate monitoring by telemetry, time lapse or video photography, and others (Bar-Or & Rowland, 2004). The use of such methods is not feasible or cost-effective in primary care settings. Likewise, direct observation techniques, such as System for Observing Fitness Instruction Time (SOFIT), System for Observing Play and Recreation in Communities (SOPARC; McKenzie et al., 2010), and System for Observing Play and Leisure Activity in Youth (SOPLAY; McKenzie et al., 2000), are impractical in clinical settings. Several self-report questionnaires have been validated in youth 10 years or older and are shown to be good predictors of PAL (Corder et al., 2008, 2009; Table 7.7).

PHYSICAL FITNESS
Maximal oxygen uptake (VO_2max) is an indicator of physical fitness level in both adult and youth populations (Astrand et al., 1986; Casaburi et al., 1989; McArdle & Magel, 1970; Mitchell & Blomqvist, 1971; Rowell, Taylor, & Wang, 1964). The maximal oxygen uptake

Pediatric Weight Management Evaluation Results Form

<insert name of institution>

Pediatric Weight Management Program Evaluation Results

Name: _____   Age: _____

Today's Date: _____   Level: _____

Group: _____

Your child's weight is _____ lbs.

Your child's height is _____ ft. _____ in.

1. Your child's Body Mass Index is _____. This value is based on the U.S. Centers for Disease Control and Prevention, *Pediatric Growth Charts* (http://www.cdc.gov/ growthcharts).

Your child is in level _____ of the program.

Based on your child's present height, his/her goal weight is _____. This value will increase as your child grows.

Your child is made up of _____ percent body fat. The healthy range for girls (ages 7–17 years) is 17–32%, and for boys (ages 7–17 years) is 10–25%. This means that your child has _____ lbs of fat and _____ lbs of muscle, bone, and water combined.

Your child's cholesterol level is _____. The healthy level for children 7–17 years is 140–170.

Your child's triglyceride level is _____. The healthy triglyceride range for children 7–17 years is 10–140.

Your child's LDL (low-density lipoprotein, the "bad" cholesterol) is _____. The healthy range for children ages 7–17 years is <130.

Your child's HDL (high-density lipoprotein, the "good" cholesterol) is _____. The HDL healthy range for children ages 7–17 years is 35–65.

Your child's circumference measurements are_____ in. (waist) and_____ in. (hips).

Table 7.7 Physical Activity Rating

Accelerometry
• Intensity-weighted minutes of physical activity
• Records acceleration and deceleration of movement
• Objective measure that provides activity counts and intensity
Heart rate monitoring
• Uses heart rate values to determine amount and intensity of physical activity
Self-report questionnaires
• Godin Leisure Time, 7-day recall, Self-Administered Physical Activity Checklist (SAPAC)
Direct observation
• System for Observing Fitness Instruction Time (SOFIT)
• System for Observing Play and Leisure Activity in Youth (SOPLAY)
• System for Observing Play and Recreation in Communities (SOPARC)

Table 7.8 Metabolic Testing

Maximal oxygen uptake (VO_2max) • Graded treadmill test • Indirect calorimetry • Heart rate and blood pressure
Resting metabolic rate (RMR or REE) • Indirect calorimetry hood system
Respiratory quotient (RQ or RER) • Ratio of oxygen to carbon dioxide • Indicates fuel source (oxidation)
Total energy expenditure • Stable isotopes (doubly labeled water)

indicates the functional capacity of the heart, lungs, and skeletal muscle and generally is assumed to be the single best indicator of physical fitness (Astrand et al., 1986; Table 7.8). The VO_2max is determined by exercising a subject and determining O_2 intake and O_2 and CO_2 concentrations in expired air. All VO_2max tests should be supervised by trained and certified exercise physiologists and/or physicians. Assessing cardiopulmonary fitness in the pediatric population has become the focus of recent research in pediatric medicine and exercise science (American College of Sports Medicine, 2011; Bar-Or et al., 1998; Greiwe et al., 1995; Rowland et al., 2003; Rowland, Koenigs, & Miller, 2003), Cardiovascular responses to exercise stress can be evaluated by obtaining a value for: (1) submaximal steady-state or (2) peak or max exercise value (peak or max VO_2). Maximal oxygen consumption (VO_2max) has been used as an indicator of health-related physical fitness (Astrand & Saltin, 1961). The criteria for achieving a peak VO_2 response in the pediatric population may not be similar to that of adults (Rowland et al., 1999). Obtaining a plateau in oxygen consumption in children often can be difficult. Several protocols, however, have been used and validated for pediatric exercise testing (Loftin et al., 2001, 2003, 2004, 2005; Sothern, 2001; Sothern et al., 2000). A sample fitness evaluation form can be found below.

Exercise and Fitness Evaluation			
Date: _____ Location: _____			
Name: _____			
Date of Birth:	Age:	Sex:	Tanner Stage:
Group:	Site:	Tested by:	
Cardiorespiratory Condition			
Resting Heart Rate (RHR, bpm):		Resting Blood Pressure (RBP, mm Hg):	
Maximum Estimated Heart Rate (HR, bpm: 220 − age): _____			
Target Heart Rate (THR): 220 − age(_____) − RHR(_____) × (_____)*% + RHR(_____) = *Levels 1 (Red), 2 (Yellow), and 3 (Green) = 55–65%; Level 4 (Blue) = 65–75%			

Aerobic Capacity (Submaximal Cycle Ergometry)	
Seat height:	Predicted max heart rate (bpm):
80% predicted max HR (bpm):	Seconds, 30 beats:
Workloads	Heart Rates
1st workload:	2nd min:
kg	3rd min:
watts	4th min:
2nd workload:	2nd min:
kg	3rd min:
watts	4th min:
3rd workload:	2nd min:
kg	3rd min:
watts	4th min:
4th workload:	2nd min:
kg	3rd min:
watts	4th min:
Activity code: Estimated VO$_2$:	Sub max VO$_2$:
Flexibility Muscular	Strength and Endurance
Trunk flexion:	Bench press:
_____ in	_____ lb _____ kg
_____ cm	_____ reps
FLEX CHECK results:	
Body Composition	

Weight (kg):	Height (cm):	Body Mass Index (BMI):
Percent Fat:		Fat Body Weight (FBW, kg):
Goal Weight:		Lean Body Weight (LBW, kg):

Growth and development are affected by many complex factors. Various outcome measures could reflect innate physiological factors rather than reflect our proposed intervention outcome. To assess the effects of nonmodifiable factors—such as age and gender on measurement of growth (e.g., weight, height)—and body composition (LBM; %fat), sexual maturity rating may be determined using methods from Falkner and Tanner (Falkner, 1979) on all subjects at fixed intervals (baseline, 10 weeks, 6 months, and 12 months). Sexual maturity ratings (Tanner staging) should be performed during the physical examination by a physician who is trained specifically in pediatric or adolescent medicine. Alternatively, a self-report tool is available that allows the patient to self-examine their level of maturation (Carskadon & Acebo, 1993).

Quarterly Evaluation Results Form

<insert name of institution>

Pediatric Weight Management Program Quarterly Evaluation Results

Name: _____   Age: _____

Today's Date: _____   Level/Color: _____

Group: _____   Quarterly Evaluation: _____

3 MONTHS AGO . . .	NOW . . .
Your child's weight was _____lbs.	Your child's weight is now _____lbs. Your child lost _____lbs. in the last _____ months!
Your child's height was ____ft. ____in.	Your child's height is now ____ft.____in. Your child grew _____in. in the past _____ months!
Your child's BMI was _____.	Your child's BMI is now _____.
Your child was in level _____, the _____ color.	Your child graduated to level _____, the _____ color.
Based on your child's past height, his/her goal weight was _____lbs.	Your child's new goal weight is _____lbs. This will increase as your child grows.
Your child's percent body fat was _____%.	Your child's percent body fat is _____%. Your child reduced his/her percent body fat by _____%.
Based on the body composition measure, your child had _____lbs of fat, and _____lbs of muscle, bone, and water.	Your child has _____lbs of fat, and _____ lbs of muscle, bone, and water. He/she lost _____lbs of fat.
Your child's cholesterol level was _____.	Your child's cholesterol level is _____.
	The normal level for children 7–17 years is <170.
Your child's triglyceride level was _____.	Your child's triglyceride level is _____.
	The normal range for children 7–17 years is _____.
Your child's LDL level was _____.	Your child's LDL level is _____.
This is the "bad" cholesterol (low-density lipoprotein).	The normal range for children 7–17 years is _____.
Your child's HDL level was _____.	Your child's HDL level is _____.
This is the "good" cholesterol (high-density lipoprotein).	The normal range for children 7–17 years is _____.
Your child's waist and hip measures were _____in. (waist) _____in. (hip)	Your child's waist and hip measure are _____in. (waist) _____in. (hip)
	He/she lost _____in. in the waist and _____in. in the hip.

American College of Sports Medicine. (2011). Position stand: Quantity and quality of exercise for developing and maintaining cardiorespiratory, musculoskeletal, and neuromotor fitness in apparently healthy adults: Guidance for prescribing exercise. *Medicine and Science in Sports and Exercise*, 43(7), 1334–1359.

American Dietetic Association. (2006). Position of the American Dietetic Association: Individual-, family-, school-, and community-based interventions for pediatric overweight. (2006). *Journal of the American Dietetic Association*, 106(6), 925–945.

Arslanian, S. A. (2002). Metabolic differences between Caucasian and African-American children and the relationship to type 2 diabetes mellitus. *Journal of Pediatric Endocrinology and Metabolism*, 15 (Suppl 1), 509–517.

Astrand, P. O., Hultman, E., Juhlin-Dannfelt, A., Reynolds, G. (1986). Disposal of lactate during and after strenuous exercise in humans. *Journal of Applied Physiology*, 61(1), 338–343.

Astrand, P. O., Saltin, B. (1961). Maximal oxygen uptake and heart rate in various types of muscular activity. *Journal of Applied Physiology*, 16, 977–981.

Barbeau, P., Johnson, M. H., Howe, C. A., Allison, J., Davis, C. L., Gutin, B., et al. (2007). Ten months of exercise improves general and visceral adiposity, bone, and fitness in black girls. *Obesity (Silver Spring, Md.)*, 15(8), 2077–2085.

Barlow, S. (2007). Expert committee recommendations regarding the prevention, assessment and treatment of child and adolescent overweight and obesity: Summary report. *Pediatrics*, 120(Suppl 4), S164–S192.

Barlow, S. E., Dietz, W. H. (1998). Obesity evaluation and treatment: Expert committee recommendations. The Maternal and Child Health Bureau, Health Resources and Services Administration and the Department of Health and Human Services. *Pediatrics*, 102(3), E29.

Barlow, S. E., Trowbridge, F. L., Klish, W. J., Dietz, W. H. (2002). Treatment of child and adolescent obesity: Reports from pediatricians, pediatric nurse practitioners, and registered dietitians. *Pediatrics*, 110(1 Pt 2), 229–235.

Bar-Or, O., Foreyt, J., Bouchard, C., Brownell, K., Dietz, W., Ravussin, E., et al. (1998). Physical activity, genetic and nutritional considerations in childhood weight management. *Medicine and Science in Sports and Exercise*, 30(1), 2–10.

Bar-Or, O., Rowland, T. W. (2004). *Pediatric Exercise Medicine: From Physiologic Principles to Health Care Application*. Champaign, IL: Human Kinetics.

Ben Ounis, O., Elloumi, M., Makni, E., Zouhal, H., Amri, M., Tabka, Z., et al. (2010). Exercise improves the ApoB/ApoA-I ratio, a marker of the metabolic syndrome in obese children. *Acta Paediatrica*, 99(11), 1679–1685.

Birch, L. L., Davison, K. K. (2001). Family environmental factors influencing the developing behavioral controls of food intake and childhood overweight. *Pediatric Clinics of North America*, 48(4), 893–907.

Boye, K. R., Dimitriou, T., Manz, F., Schoenau, E., Neu, C., Wudy, S., Remer, T. (2002). Anthropometric assessment of muscularity during growth: Estimating fat-free mass with 2 skinfold-thickness measurements is superior to measuring midupper arm muscle area in healthy prepubertal children. *American Journal of Clinical Nutrition*, 76(3), 628–632.

Bray, G. A., DeLaney, J. P., Volaufova, D. W., Harsha, D. W., Champaign, C. (2002). Prediction of body fat in 12-y-old African American and white children: Evaluation of methods. *American Journal of Clinical Nutrition*, 76, 980–990.

Brown, R., Sothern, M., Suskind, R., Udall, J., Blecker, U. (2000). Racial differences in the lipid profiles of obese children and adolescents before and after significant weight loss. *Clinical Pediatrics*, 39(7), 427–431.

Cameron, N., Griffiths, P. L., Wright, M. M., Blencowe, C., Davis, N. C., Pettifor, J. M. Norris, S. A. (2004). Regression equations to estimate percentage body fat in African prepubertal children aged 9 y. *American Journal of Clinical Nutrition*, 80, 70–75.

Caprio, S. (2002). Insulin resistance in childhood obesity. *Journal of Pediatric Endocrinology and Metabolism*, 15(Suppl 1), 487–492.

Carlisle, L. K., Gordon, S. T., Sothern, M. S. (2005). Can obesity prevention work for our children? *Journal of the Louisiana State Medical Society*, 157(Spec No. 1), S34–S41.

Carskadon, M. A., Acebo, C. (1993). A self-administered rating scale for pubertal development. *Journal of Adolescent Health*, 14(3), 190–195.

Casaburi, R., Spitzer, S., Haskell, R., Wasserman, K. (1989). Effect of altering heart rate on oxygen uptake at exercise onset. *Chest*, 95(1), 6–12.

Casanova Roman, M., Rodriguez Ruiz, I., Rico de Cos, S., Casanova Bellido, M. (2004). [Body composition analysis using bioelectrical and anthropometric parameters]. *Anales de Pediatria (Barcelona)*, 61(1), 23–31.

Centers for Disease Control and Prevention. (2010). Growth charts. Retrieved from http://www.cdc.gov/growthcharts.

Chobanian, A. V., Bakris, G. L., Black, H. R., Cushman, W. C., Green, L. A., Izzo, J. L., Jr, et al. (2003). The seventh report of the joint national committee on prevention, detection, evaluation, and treatment of high blood pressure: The JNC 7 report. *JAMA*, 289(19), 2560–2572.

Corder, K., Ekelund, U., Steele, R. M., Wareham, N. J., Brage, S. (2008). Assessment of physical activity in youth. *Journal of Applied Physiology*, 105(3), 977–987.

Corder, K., van Sluijs, E. M., Wright, A., Whincup, P., Wareham, N. J., Ekelund, U. (2009). Is it possible to assess free-living physical activity and energy expenditure in young people by self-report? *American Journal of Clinical Nutrition*, 89(3), 862–870.

Dietz, W. H. (1994). Critical periods in childhood for the development of obesity. *American Journal of Clinical Nutrition*, 59(5), 955–959.

Dietz, W. H., Gortmaker, S. L. (2001). Preventing obesity in children and adolescents. *Annual Review of Public Health*, 22, 337–353. doi:10.1146/annurev.publhealth.22.1.337

Dowda, M., Ainsworth, B. E., Addy, C. L., Saunders, R., Riner, W. (2001). Environmental influences, physical activity, and weight status in 8- to 16-year-olds. *Archives of Pediatrics and Adolescent Medicine*, 155(6), 711–717.

Durnin, J. V., Womersley, J. (1974). Body fat assessed from total body density and its estimation from skinfold thickness: Measurements on 481 men and women aged from 16 to 72 years. *British Journal of Nutrition*, 32(1), 77–97.

Eisenkolbl, J., Kartasurya, M., Widhalm, K. (2001). Underestimation of percentage fat mass measured by bioelectrical impedance analysis compared to dual energy X-ray absorptiometry method in obese children. *European Journal of Clinical Nutrition*, 55(6), 423–429.

Eisenmann, J., for the Subcommittee on Assessment in Pediatric Obesity Management Programs, National Association of Children's Hospital and Related Institutions. (2011). Assessment of obese children and adolescents: A survey of pediatric obesity-management programs. *Pediatrics*, 128(Suppl 2), S51–S58.

Ellis, K. J., Shypailo, R. J., Pratt, J. A., Pond, W. G. (1994). Accuracy of dual-energy x-ray absorptiometry for body-composition measurements in children. *American Journal of Clinical Nutrition*, 60, 660–665.

Falkner, F., Tanner, J. M. (1979). *Human Growth*. London: Bailliere Tindall.

Fogelholm, M., Nuutinen, O., Pasanen, M., Myohanen, E., Saatela, T. (1999). Parent-child relationship of physical activity patterns and obesity. *International Journal of Obesity and Related Metabolic Disorders*, 23(12), 1262–1268.

Fors, H., Gelander, L., Bjarnason, R., Albertsson-Wikland, K., Bosaeus, I. (2002). Body composition, as assessed by bioelectrical impedance spectroscopy and dual-energy X-ray absorptiometry, in a healthy pediatric population. *Acta Paediatrica*, 91(7), 755–760.

Friedl, K. E., DeLuca, J. P., Marchitelli, L. J., Vogel, J. A. (1992). Reliability of body-fat estimations from a four-compartment model by using density, body water, and bone mineral measurements. *American Journal of Clinical Nutrition*, 55(4), 764–770.

Fujita, H., Midori, S., Awazu, M. (2012). Ambulatory blood pressure in prehypertensive children and adolescents. *Pediatric Nephrology*, 27(8), 1361–1367.

Ganley, K., Paterno, M., Miles, C., Stout, J., Brawner, P., Girolami, G., Warran, M. (2011). Health-related fitness in children and adolescents. *Pediatric Physical Therapy*, 23(3), 208–220.

Goran, M. I., Driscoll, P., Johnson, R., Nagy, T. R., Hunter, G. (1996). Cross-calibration of body-composition techniques against dual-energy X-ray absorptiometry in young children. *American Journal of Clinical Nutrition*, 63(3), 299–305.

Gordon, S., Sothern, M. (2006). The role of the physician. In M. Sothern, T. K. von Almen, S. Gordon (Eds.), *Handbook of Pediatric Obesity: Clinical Management* (pp. 41–52). Boca Raton, FL: Taylor & Francis.

Gortmaker, S. L., Peterson, K., Wiecha, J., Sobol, A. M., Dixit, S., Fox, M. K., Laird, N. (1999). Reducing obesity via a school-based interdisciplinary intervention among youth: Planet health. *Archives of Pediatrics and Adolescent Medicine*, 153(4), 409–418.

Greiwe, J. S., Kaminsky, L. A., Whaley, M. H., Dwyer, G. B. (1995). Evaluation of the ACSM submaximal ergometer test for estimating VO_2max. *Medicine and Science in Sports and Exercise*, 27(9), 1315–1320.

Gutin, B., Litaker, M., Islam, S., Manos, T., Smith, C., Treiber, F. (1996). Body-composition measurement in 9–11-y-old children by dual-energy X-ray absorptiometry, skinfold-thickness measurements, and bioimpedance analysis. *American Journal of Clinical Nutrition*, 63(3), 287–292.

Hill, J., Throwbridge, F. (1989). The causes and health consequences of obesity in children and adolescents. *Pediatrics*, 101, 497–575.

Hoffer, E. C., Meador, C. K., Simpson, D. C. (1969). Correlation of whole-body impedance with total body water volume. *Journal of Applied Physiology*, 27(4), 531–534.

Hubbard, V. S. (2000). Defining overweight and obesity: What are the issues? *American Journal of Clinical Nutrition*, 72(5), 1067–1068.

Jackson, A. S., Pollock, M. L. (1978). Generalized equations for predicting body density of men. British *Journal of Nutrition*, 40(3), 497–504.

Kelly, A. S., Barlow, S. E., Rao, G., Inge, T. H., Hayman, L. L., Steinberger, J., et al. (2013). Severe obesity in children and adolescents: Identification, associated health risks, and treatment approaches–A scientific statement from the American Heart Association. *Circulation*, 128(15), 1689–1712.

Kitzmann, K. M., Dalton, W. T., III, Stanley, C. M., Beech, B. M., Reeves, T. P., Buscemi, J., et al. (2010). Lifestyle interventions for youth who are overweight: A meta-analytic review. *Health Psychology*, 29(1), 91–101.

Krebs, N., Himes, J., Jacobson, D., Nicklas, T., Guilday, P., Styne, D. (2007). Assessment of child and adolescent overweight and obesity. *Pediatrics*, 120(Suppl 4), S193–S228.

Law, C. M., Barker, D. J., Osmond, C., Fall, C. H., Simmonds, S. J. (1992). Early growth and abdominal fatness in adult life. *Journal of Epidemiology and Community Health,* 46(3), 184–186.

Loftin, M., Heusel, L., Bonis, M., Sothern, M. (2005). Oxygen uptake kinetics and oxygen deficit in obese and normal weight adolescent females. *Journal of Sports Science and Medicine,* 4, 430–436.

Loftin, M., Nichols, J., Going, S., Sothern, M., Schmitz, K., Ring, K., Tuuri, G., Stevens, J. (2007). Comparison of the validity of anthropometric and bioelectric impedance equations to assess body composition in adolescent girls. *International Journal of Body Composition Research,* 5(1), 1 8.

Loftin, M., Sothern, M., Trosclair, L., O'Hanlon, A., Miller, J., Udall, J. (2001). Scaling VO(2) peak in obese and non-obese girls. *Obesity Research,* 9(5), 290–296.

Loftin, M., Sothern, M., VanVrancken, C., Udall, J. (2003). Low heart hate peak in obese female youth. *Clinical Pediatrics,* 42(6), 505–510.

Loftin, M., Sothern, M., Warren, B., Udall, J. (2004). Comparison of VO2 peak during tread-mill and bicycle ergometry in severely overweight youth. *Journal of Sports Science and Medicine,* 3, 254–260.

Lohman, T. G. (1981). Skinfolds and body density and their relation to body fatness: A review. *Human Biology,* 53(2), 181–225.

Lohman, T. G., Roche, A. A., Martorell, R. (Eds.). (1988). *Anthropometric Standardization Reference Manual.* Champaign, IL: Human Kinetics.

Mazess, R. B., Barden, H. S., Bisek, J. P., Hanson, J. (1990). Dual-energy x-ray absorptiometry for total-body and regional bone-mineral and soft-tissue composition. *American Journal of Clinical Nutrition,* 51(6), 1106–1112.

McArdle, W. D., Magel, J. R. (1970). Physical work capacity and maximum oxygen uptake in treadmill and bicycle exercise. *Medicine and Science in Sports and Exercise,* 2(3), 118–123.

Micic, D. (2001). Obesity in children and adolescents—a new epidemic? Consequences in adult life. *Journal of Pediatric Endocrinology and Metabolism,* 14(Suppl 5), 1345–1352; discussion 1365.

Mitchell, J. H., Blomqvist, G. (1971). Maximal oxygen uptake. *New England Journal of Medicine,* 284(18), 1018–10122.

Morrison, J. A., Guo, S. S., Specker, B., Chumlea, W. C., Yanovski, S. Z., Yanovski, J. A. (2001). Assessing the body composition of 6–17-year-old black and white girls in field studies. *American Journal of Human Biology,* 13(2), 249–254.

Motl, R. W., Dishman, R. K., Dowda, M., Pate, R. R. (2004). Factorial validity and invariance of a self-report measure of physical activity among adolescent girls. *Research Quarterly for Exercise and Sport,* 75(3), 259–271.

Nguyen, V. T., Larson, D. E., Johnson, R. K., Goran, M. I. (1996). Fat intake and adiposity in children of lean and obese parents. *American Journal of Clinical Nutrition,* 63(4), 507–513.

O'Brien, S. H., Holubkov, R., Reis, E. C. (2004). Identification, evaluation, and management of obesity in an academic primary care center. *Pediatrics,* 114(2), e154–e159.

Ogle, G. D., Allen, J. R., Humphries, I. R. (1995). Body-composition assessment by dual-energy x-ray absorptiometry in subjects aged 4–26 y. *American Journal of Clinical Nutrition,* 61, 746–753.

Parker, L., Reilly, J. J., Slater, C., Wells, J. C., Pitsiladis, Y. (2003). Validity of six field and labora-tory methods for measurement of body composition in boys. *Obesity Research,* 11(7), 852–858.

Pickering, T., Clemow, L., Davidson, K., Gerin, W. (2003). Behavioral cardiology—has its time finally arrived? *Mount Sinai Journal of Medicine*, 70(2), 101–112.

Pietrobelli, A., Formica, C, Wang, Z., Heymsfield, S. (1996). Dual-energy X-ray absorptiometry body composition model: Review of physical concepts. *American Journal of Physiology*, 271, E941–E951.

Price, J. H., Desmond, S. M., Ruppert, E. S., Stelzer, C. M. (1989). Pediatricians' perceptions and practices regarding childhood obesity. *American Journal of Preventive Medicine*, 5(2), 95–103.

Rippe, J. M., Hess, S. (1998). The role of physical activity in the prevention and management of obesity. *Journal of the American Dietetic Association*, 98(10 Suppl 2), S31–S38.

Roche, A. F., Heymsfield, S. B., Lohman, T. G. (Eds.). (1996). *Human Body Composition*. Champaign, IL: Human Kinetics.

Rowell, L. B., Taylor, H. L., Wang, Y. (1964). Limitations to prediction of maximal oxygen intake. *Journal of Applied Physiology*, 19, 919–927.

Rowland, T., Bhargava, R., Parslow, D., Heptulla, R. A. (2003). Cardiac response to progressive cycle exercise in moderately obese adolescent females. *Journal of Adolescent Health*, 32(6), 422–427.

Rowland, T., Kline, G., Goff, D., Martel, L., Ferrone, L. (1999). One-mile run performance and cardiovascular fitness in children. *Archives of Pediatrics and Adolescent Medicine*, 153(8), 845–849.

Rowland, T., Koenigs, L., Miller, N. (2003). Myocardial performance during maximal exercise in adolescents with anorexia nervosa. *Journal of Sports Medicine and Physical Fitness*, 43(2), 202–208.

Slaughter, M. H., Lohman, T. G., Boileau, R. A., Horswill, C. A., Stillman, R. J., Van Loan, M. D., Bemben, D. A. (1988). Skinfold equations for estimation of body fatness in children and youth. *Human Biology*, 60(5), 709–723.

Sloan, A. W. (1967). Estimation of body fat in young men. *Journal of Applied Physiology*, 23(3), 311–315.

Sothern, M. S. (2001). Exercise as a modality in the treatment of childhood obesity. *Pediatric Clinics of North America*, 48(4), 995–1015.

Sothern, M. S., Despinasse, B., Brown, R., Suskind, R. M., Udall, J., Blecker, U. (2000). Lipid profiles of obese children and adolescents before and after significant weight loss: Differences according to sex. *Southern Medical Journal*, 93(3), 278–82.

Sothern, M. S., Hunter, S., Suskind, R. M., Brown, R., Udall, J., Blecker, U. (1999). Motivating the obese child to move: The role of structured exercise in pediatric weight management. *Southern Medical Journal*, 92(6), 577–584.

Sothern, M. S., Loftin, M., Blecker, Suskind, R., Udall, J. (2000). Impact of significant weight loss on maximal oxygen uptake in obese children and adolescents. *Journal of Investigative Medicine*, 48(6), 411–416.

Sothern, M. S., Loftin, J. M., Udall, J. N., Suskind, R. M., Ewing, T. L., Tang, S. C., Blecker, U. (2000). Safety, feasibility, and efficacy of a resistance training program in preadolescent obese children. *American Journal of the Medical Sciences*, 319(6), 370–375.

Sothern, M., Schumacher, H., von Almen, T., Carlisle, L., Udall, J. (2002). Committed to kids: An integrated, four level team approach to weight management in adolescents. *Journal of the American Dietetic Association*, 102(Suppl 3), S81–S85.

Sothern, M., Udall, J., Jr., Suskind, R. M., Vargas, A., Blecker, U. (2000). Weight loss and growth velocity in obese children after very low calorie diet, exercise, and behavior modification. *Acta Paediatrica*, 89(9), 1036–1043.

Sothern, M., von Almen, T. K., Schumacher, H. (2001). *Trim Kids: The Proven Plan That Has Helped Thousands of Children Achieve a Healthier Weight*. New York, NY: Harper Collins.

Steinbeck, K. S. (2001). The importance of physical activity in the prevention of overweight and obesity in childhood: A review and an opinion. *Obesity Reviews*, 2(2), 117–130.

U.S. Preventive Services Task Force. (2010). Screening for obesity in children and adolescents: U.S. Preventive Services Task Force recommendation statement. *Pediatrics*, 125(2), 361–367.

Yu, C. C., Sung, R. Y., So, R. C., Lui, K. C., Lau, W., Lam, P. K., et al. (2005). Effects of strength training on body composition and bone mineral content in children who are obese. *Journal of Strength and Conditioning Research*, 19(3), 667–672.

Zannolli, R., Rebeggiani, A., Chiarelli, F., Morgese, G. (1993). Hyperinsulinism as a marker in obese children. *American Journal of Diseases of Children*, 147(8), 837–841.

Chapter 8

MEASURING HEALTH AND FITNESS OUTCOMES

Accurate and reliable assessment of outcomes related to the prevention and management of obesity in children and adolescents is essential to achieving the recommended goals of improving physical health through the attainment of permanent healthy lifestyle behaviors (Barlow et al., 2007; Eisenmann et al., 2011; Krebs et al., 2007; Table 8.1). Measurements obtained before and after participation in an exercise program are necessary to determine whether selected modalities, volumes, and intensities were adequate and appropriate to meeting the goals of achieving a healthier weight and improvement of body composition and related metabolic parameters (Krebs & Sothern, 2006; Sothern, 2006). This chapter includes appropriate and reliable protocols for measuring outcomes before and after participation in exercise interventions.

ANTHROPOMETRICS AND BODY COMPOSITION

MEASUREMENT OF HEIGHT

The measurement of height or stature is a major indicator of bone length and general body size. The recommended technique for height measurement includes the use of a vertical board with an attached metric rule and horizontal headboard, collectively known as a stadiometer (Eisenmann et al., 2011; Table 8.1).

A calibrated stadiometer (e.g., Holtain, Ltd., United Kingdom, Dyfed) should be used to obtain the height in centimeters of each individual. The individual will remove his or her shoes and step onto the floor platform facing in an outward direction with the heels together. The heel, scapula, and buttocks will remain in contact with the back of the stadiometer during the measure with the arms hanging naturally along the side of the body. The head is positioned in a horizontal plane. The clinician will move the headboard onto the most superior aspect of the individual's head. This procedure is repeated two additional times. If the two measurements were greater than 0.5 centimeters apart, a third measurement is taken. The average height to the nearest 10th of a centimeter (0.1 cm) should be calculated on a data statistical form. The reliability of this instrument was established previously with intermeasurer differences for large samples as follows: M = 2.4 mm (SD = 2.1 mm) at 5–10 years: M = 2.0 mm (SD = 1.9 mm) at 10–15 years; M = 2.3 mm (SD = 2.4 mm) at 15–20 years (Chumlea & Roche, 1979).

MEASUREMENT OF WEIGHT

An electronically calibrated scale (e.g., Indiana Scale, Terre Haute, Indiana, or Detecto-USA, Webb City, Missouri) should be used to obtain the weight in kilograms of each individual (Eisenmann et al., 2011; Table 8.1). The individual will remove his or her shoes and step on the scale. The individual will remain as still as possible. The individual's weight in kilograms is recorded once the digital reading is constant. The individual will remain on the scale until the weight is recorded. The process is repeated two additional times. The average weight in kilograms of each measure is calculated and recorded on the data statistical form. The reliability of this instrument was established previously with intermeasurer differences as follows: M = 1.2 g (SD = 3.2g) at 5–10; m = 1.5 g (SD = 3.6 g) at 10–15 years; 1.7 g (SD = 3.8 g) at 15–20 years (Chumlea & Roche, 1979). The National Center for Health statistics reported intermeasurer and intrameasurer technical errors were about 1.2 kg with pairs of measures 2 weeks apart (Hamill, Drizd, & Johnson 1979; Lohman, Roche, & Martorell, 1988).

WEIGHT STATUS AND ESTIMATE OF BODY COMPOSITION

Body mass index (BMI) is a standard height–weight ratio for expressing body mass of an individual (Bray, 1987). Height and weight are converted to body mass index (kg/m^2). Body mass index (BMI) is calculated as weight (kg)/height (m)^2. This procedure is shown to be

Table 8.1 Recommendations for Best-Practice Assessment of the Obese Patient

Calculate decimal age from observation date and birth date.
Provide anthropometric training for clinical personnel.
Measure height and weight on hard surface using calibrated equipment.
Record BMI (including past BMI pattern).
Calculate BMI percentile according to CDC BMI growth chart.
Determine body composition by BIA or air-displacement plethysmography (skinfolds should not be assessed in the obese patient).
Track resting metabolic rate via prediction equation or calorimetry.
Inquire about parental obesity and family medical history.
Evaluate weight-related problems.
Assess diet and physical activity.
Assess eating behavior to examine the following—
Self-efficacy and readiness to change
Frequency of eating outside the home at restaurants or fast-food establishments
Excessive consumption of sweetened beverages
Consumption of excessive portion sizes for age
Excessive consumption of 100% fruit juice
Breakfast consumption (frequency and quality)
Excessive consumption of foods high in energy density
Low consumption of fruits and vegetables
Meal frequency and snacking patterns (including quality)
Conduct physical activity assessment to determine the following—
Self-efficacy and readiness to change
Reliable and valid self-report physical activity instruments
Environment and social support and barriers to physical activity
Whether the child is meeting recommendations of at least 60 minutes of moderate physical activity per day
Level of sedentary behavior, which should include hours of behavior using television, video games, and computer, and comparison to a baseline of less than 2 hours per day
Routine activity patterns, such as walking to school or performing yard work
Assess practical resources and barriers (e.g., neighborhood parks, grocery stores, recreation centers, and neighborhood children with whom to play can all support a healthier lifestyle).
Inquire about family cultural values, ethnicity, religion, and education background.

Source: From Eisenmann, J. C., for the Subcommittee on Assessment in Pediatric Obesity Management Programs, National Association of Children's Hospital and Related Institutions, *Pediatrics*, 128, S51, 2011. With permission.

valid in pediatric populations and is currently the recommended tool for screening children and adolescents for obesity (Barlow, 2007; Krebs et al., 2007; Praphul, Bryan, & Howat, 2012).

In growing children, BMI initially declines during infancy and early childhood and then increases with age (Ganley et al., 2011); therefore, BMI values should be converted to BMI z-scores based on norms for age and gender derived from the 2003 National Health and Nutrition Examination Survey (NHANES) database (Centers for Disease Control and Prevention [CDC], 2006; Eisenmann et al., 2011; Table 8.1). Therefore, height and weight measurements with age in months and sex are used to calculate BMI z-scores using the CDC's program for calculating BMI percentiles and z-scores (CDC, 2010).

The "2007 Expert Committee Recommendations Regarding the Prevention, Assessment, and Treatment of Child and Adolescent Overweight and Obesity: Summary" report emphasized the importance of using BMI adjusted for age and gender to ensure validity of childhood overweight and obesity studies (Krebs et al., 2007). Children and adolescents whose BMI score falls between the 5th and 85th percentile on the CDC growth charts are considered to be at a healthy weight (Ganley et al., 2011). The following chart details the various levels of overweight and obesity in children and adolescents and provides color-coded levels, which can be used to tailor exercise recommendations to each individual child (see Chapter 6).

Select the Level That Best Corresponds to the Greatest Number of Selected Categories						
Color Code	Weight Level	Physical Activity Level	Cardiorespiratory Fitness Level	Muscular Strength and Endurance	Flexibility	Comorbidity, (e.g., Asthma, Hypertension, Diabetes)
Red	Level 1: Severe Obesity (>120% of 95th BMI or absolute BMI >35 kg/m²)	Sedentary	Unfit	Poor	Poor	Uncontrolled or severe
Yellow	Level 2: Obesity (>95–<99th percentile BMI)	Moderately active	Moderately fit	Average	Average	Controlled or moderate
Green	Level 3: Overweight (>85–<99th percentile BMI)	Active	Fit	Good	Good	Well – controlled or mild
Blue	Level 4: Healthy Weight (>5–<85th percentile BMI)	Very active	Very fit	Excellent	Excellent	No comorbidities

The BMI is considered a reasonable estimation of body composition; however, this measure does not distinguish between lean and fat tissue.

CIRCUMFERENCE MEASUREMENTS

An additional method of assessing body composition is the measurement of girth of various body sections (Lohman et al., 1988). From the sum of the measurements, percent body fat is determined from equations, tables, or nomograms. More important, the waist circumference, in particular, is an indicator of abdominal (central or visceral) adiposity in children and adolescents (Ganley et al., 2011). Furthermore, pediatric waist circumference percentiles, which are age, sex, and ethnicity specific, are available for children and adolescents (Cook, Auinger, & Huang, 2009) and preschool-age children, 3–5 years of age (Taylor et al., 2008). Despite these options, the routine use of circumference measurements, especially waist circumference, is not recommended for clinical settings (Barlow, 2007); however, in a recent survey, 83% of pediatric weight management programs reported using this measure as an estimate of abdominal adiposity (Eisenmann et al., 2011). Concerns included a lack of specific guidelines and difficulty in determining the precise measurement locations, among others. Therefore, health care providers considering this option should adhere precisely to the instructions contained in detailed protocols. Likewise, they should ensure that staff members are well trained before implementation of waist circumference measurements.

Equipment needed:

- Metal or fiberglass measuring tape
- Metric scale

Several various sections of the body are measured based on gender. The standard areas measured in males are the shoulders, chest, waist, biceps, thigh, and calf. In females, the standard areas are shoulders, bust, waist, abdomen, hips, thigh, calf, and biceps. Regardless of sites to be measured, the general rules are as follows:

1. Both the clinician and subject are in a standing position.
2. Unless noted otherwise, clinician is positioned in front of subject.
3. When applying tape to the site, no air space should be between the subjects' skin and the tape. Conversely, the tape should not be pulled tightly.
4. The tape always should be positioned in a horizontal plane to the subject.
5. The tape should be read to the closest 0.25 inch.
6. Clinician should have strong knowledge of anatomy to locate areas to be measured.

The sites mentioned above are located and measured as follows:

FOR MALE SUBJECTS

Shoulders: Subject stands erect with weight evenly distributed between both feet. Shoulders should be back and arms hang freely at sides. The clinician positions tape over the largest area of the deltoids below the acromion.

Chest: Subject will stand erect with feet shoulder-width apart. The subject abducts arms slightly so that the tape can be positioned around chest. The clinician locates the fourth costosternal joint and the measurement is taken at this level.

Waist: The measurement of girth at the waistline also provides an estimation of abdominal fat. Individuals will wear light clothing for this measurement. They are asked to stand erect and in an upright position with abdomen relaxed, arms at sides, and feet together. Measures are made at the end of normal expiration at the umbilicus (Fernandez et al., 2004). The measurements are recorded to the nearest 0.1 cm. This process is repeated and the average of each of the two circumferences is used in analysis (a third measurement is obtained if the first two measurements are greater than 0.5 cm apart). Figure 8.1 provides a graphic representation of the measurement site for waist circumference.

Biceps: Subject stands erect with arms relaxed at sides. Clinician locates the most muscular aspect of the bicep and tape is positioned.

Thigh: (Mid-thigh) For most accurate results, clinician will measure the midpoint between the inguinal crease and the proximal border of the patella. This measurement is made when the subject's knee is flexed to 90 degrees. This site is marked and the tape is placed here once the subject returns to an erect, standing position.

Calf: Subject stands with weight evenly distributed on both feet. Clinician locates maximum circumference of the gastrocnemius (calf) muscle and positions tape for measurement.

FOR FEMALE SUBJECTS

Shoulders: See instructions for male subjects.

Bust: Subject stands erect with arms relaxed at sides. Measurement is made across the chest, at the nipple line.

Waist: See instructions for male subjects.

Abdomen: Subject stands with arms by the sides and feet together. The clinician places tape at the level of the greatest anterior extension of the abdomen. The level usually will be at the navel.

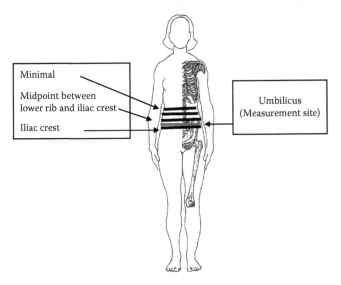

Figure 8.1 Measurement site for waist circumference.

Hips: Subject stands erect with arms at sides and feet together. The tape is positioned at the maximum circumference of the buttocks.

Thigh: See instructions for male subjects.

Calf: See instructions for male subjects.

Biceps: See instructions for male subjects.

SKINFOLD ANALYSIS

Skinfold analysis measures the thickness of a double fold of skin and subcutaneous adipose tissue at various body locations (Roche, Heymsfield, & Lohman, 1996). The use of skinfold calipers is a widely used method for determining obesity as it provides more detail concerning the distribution of fat than what is provided by the BMI measure (Ganley et al., 2011). Recent guidelines for evaluating body composition, however, do not include the use of skinfolds for several reasons, including a lack of reference data and criteria or cut points and concern for measurement error (Barlow, 2007). The advantage of this method is that it is relatively inexpensive and nonevasive, although there is concern that the measure may induce psychological discomfort (Eisenmann et al., 2011; Table 8.1). In addition, very little space is needed. Therefore, although not ideal, skinfold analysis does provide an option for assessing body composition in nonclinical settings as long as trained health care providers are utilized. Specific descriptions of the measurement of skinfold thickness and various equations have been developed in the prediction of body composition (Bray et al., 2002; Cameron et al., 2004; Durnin, de Bruin, & Feunekes, 1997; Durnin & Womersley, 1974; Goran et al., 1996; Gutin et al., 1996; Jackson & Pollock, 1978; Lohman, 1981; Lohman et al., 1988; Sloan, 1967). A two-site formula was developed by Slaughter et al. (1988) and later validated in a study by Janz et al. (1993). The formula includes specific equations for overweight youth shown to be highly correlated with both underwater weighing and DEXA measurements (Boye et al., 2002).

The following equipment is needed to take skinfold measurements:

- Skinfold caliper
- Tape measure
- Black felt pen

The general rules for taking skinfolds are as follows:

1. All measurements should be taken on the right side of the body for uniformity with most U.S. research efforts.

2. Sites to be measured should be marked for best accuracy until clinician is sufficiently skilled.

3. Clinicians should feel the sites to familiarize themselves with the subject and area.

4. Subject should not have exercised immediately prior to measurement. Shifts in body fluid to skin will inflate normal skinfold values.

5. Clinician should take a minimum of two measurements at each site, spacing each measure at least 15 seconds apart.

6. Calipers should be accurately calibrated before measurement.

7. Caliper dial should be read approximately 4 seconds after pressure from hand on caliper jaw has been released.

8. Thumb and index finger pressure should be maintained throughout each measurement.

Several sites have been designated and standardized for use by clinicians. For purposes of this investigation, two sites (triceps and subscapular) are used. Instructions for skinfold measurements at these sites are as follows:

Measurement of skinfolds: A skinfold caliper (Harpenden), tape measure, and black felt pen are utilized to measure triceps and subscapular skinfold thickness. All measurements are taken on the right side of the body. All sites are marked with a black felt pen for accuracy after the anatomic location of the measurement has been verified by a trained technician. The subject will refrain from exercise at least 2 hours prior to the test. A minimum of three measurements are taken at each site at least 15 seconds apart. The calipers are calibrated prior to each measurement. The caliper dial is read approximately 4 seconds after pressure from the hand on the caliper is released.

Triceps skinfold: A vertical skinfold on the posterior midline of the upper arm is examined. With the subject's right elbow flexed at 90 degrees, the clinician will measure the distance between the lateral projection of the acromion process of the scapula and the inferior border of the olecranon process of the elbow. The site then will be marked with the black felt pen at the midpoint on the lateral side of the arm. With the subject's arm relaxed at his or her side, the clinician will stand behind the subject and grasp the skinfold site with the thumb and index finger approximately 0.5 inch above the mark. The calipers then will be applied at the mark.

Subscapular skinfold: A diagonal skinfold is obtained just below the lowest angle of the scapula. The clinician will feel for the bottom of the scapula to locate the site. The site is marked and the skinfold is grasped with thumb and index finger about 0.5 inch above the mark. The skinfold will then be taken on a 45-degree diagonal line toward the right side of the subject's body.

Estimation of body fat from the sum of the two skinfolds then is made using a nomogram or quadratic equation. The levels of chemical immaturity in female and male youths is addressed when applying percentage of body fat (%fat) computational formulas (Slaughter et al., 1988). The formulas utilized are designed for females and males 8–18 years of age and were shown previously to be more accurate than preexisting methods (Forbes, 1991; Jackson et al., 1988). Considering bone density, as well as water and bone mineral content, the equations produced an R^2 coefficient of determination of 77% and a standard error of the estimate of 3.9%. This new application may positively affect the results by tailoring the %fat estimate to the age, race, and gender of the subjects. The formula addresses male–female differences in adults through the use of unique constants (Slaughter et al., 1988).

BIOELECTRICAL IMPEDANCE

Bioelectrical impedance (BIA) has been validated as a measure of body fat and lean body mass (LBM). BIA may be used to measure the density of lean and adipose tissue in relation to hydration (Bray et al., 2002; Goran et al., 1996; Gutin et al., 1996). Studies have shown total body water (TBW) and electrical impedance to be related (Eisenkolbl, Kartasurya, & Widhalm, 2001). Further studies also report the utility and reliability of body impedance measurements in the assessment of total body fat (Casanova Roman et al., 2004). Assessment by BIA provides a reasonably accurate and a time- and cost-effective method of assessing body fat in overweight children (Bray et al., 2002; Cameron et al., 2004; Eisenmann et al., 2011; Goran et al., 1996; Table 8.1). Care should be taken to select a formula specific to the age, race, and gender of the child as accuracy varies by study (Boye et al., 2002; Loftin et al., 2007; Parker et al., 2003).

MEASUREMENT OF DIFFERENTIAL PHOTON ABSORPTION USING DUAL-ENERGY X-RAY ABSORPTIOMETRY

Dual-energy x-ray absorptiometry (DEXA) can be used to determine %fat, LBM, and bone mineral density (BMD) accurately and safely in children and adolescents (Shypailo, Butte, & Ellis, 2008; Steinberger et al., 2005). DEXA utilizes an x-ray source to generate photons to scan individuals. Bone mineral content measurements previously calibrated against secondary standards with ashed bone sections are used to help calculate fat-free mass. Percentage of fat mass and fat-free mass can be predicted with accuracy by observing the ratio of absorbency of the different-energy-level photons, which are related linearly to the %fat in the soft tissues of the body. The coefficient of variation of fat-free tissue measurement has been calculated at 2%, which is comparable to that obtained by hydrodensitometry (Ellis et al., 1994; Friedl et al., 1992; Mazess et al., 1990).

Individuals receive total body scans with the DEXA apparatus (e.g., Hologics QRX 2000). This machine is approved by the Food and Drug Administration as a market device used for scanning the anterior–posterior and lateral spine, femur, total body, and forearm to determine BMD. The speed of the scan is determined by the size of the individual. Larger individuals are programmed in the slow-speed mode; smaller individuals are programmed in the fast-speed mode. The individuals are instructed to remove all metal and jewelry as well as their shoes before they are positioned correctly on the scan table, lying down on their back with their arms to their side. The DEXA will measure x-rays as they are transmitted through the individual's body. The individuals are exposed to ionizing radiation, but there is no discomfort during the measurement. When using the DEXA, the dose of radiation is 0.02–0.03 millirem for each total body scan (Hologics). This exposure is less than the 125 mR per year, which is the amount individuals receive from nonmedical background radiation (Lunar). The low dose of radiation will not adversely affect the bone or surrounding tissue. Except in pregnant or nursing mothers, use of the DEXA has no side effects. The entire process causes little discomfort and is a totally noninvasive step-by-step process.

CENTRAL ADIPOSITY: ABDOMINAL (VISCERAL) FAT

Novel pediatric specific measurement tools have been developed to evaluate abdominal fat using magnetic resonance imaging (MRI). Scans are taken at the lumbar (L4) level, aligned with the umbilicus. The testing is performed with a 0.5 Tesla superconducting unit (MRT-50 A, Toshiba, Tokyo). A trained technician acquires spin-echo (SE) T1-weighted (TR = 500; TE = 20) images. The manual trackball technique is used to define adipose tissue. The MRI fat signal between the skin and abdominal muscle walls and intra-abdominal adipose tissue area—along with signals from intraperitoneal, mesenteric, and omental depots—are used to calculate subcutaneous adipose tissue area (Brambilla et al., 1999).

ECTOPIC FAT IN SKELETAL MUSCLE AND LIVER USING PROTON MAGNETIC RESONANCE SPECTROSCOPY

Intrahepatic lipid may be measured on a commercially available clinical 1.5 T whole-body imaging and spectroscopy system (Signa XL Horizon 2001 MRI Unit, General Electric, Medical Systems, Milwaukee, Wisconsin) located in the radiation department of most hospitals, using the PRESS (point resolved spectroscopy) technique (Larson-Meyer et al., 2010). Children are positioned in a prone, feet-first orientation (i.e., on their belly, feet first going into the magnet). An external amplitude reference phantom is created using a test tube filled with a known volume of peanut oil and is positioned vertically across the child's tailbone and secured with surgical tape. This placement helps ensure that the phantom is placed close to the homogeneous spot of the magnet. A single water-suppressed PRESS voxel (~$3 \times 3 \times 3$ cm³, echo time [TE] = 40 ms, repetition time [TR] = 1500 ms) then is collected using the commercially provided 1H-body coil using standard GE PRESS acquisitions in an area of the middle right lobe that is visually free from heavy vascularization as determined from T1-weighted axial images (25 slices, 8 mm thick, 2 mm separation) and not located too close to the surface subcutaneous fat. The larger voxel size allows for collection of a lower number of averages and a shorter scan time. Children are informed when the scan begins and are asked to remain still and take shallow breaths during the procedure. An investigator may practice shallow breathing with the children before positioning the magnet and also stress the importance of remaining motionless during the acquisition. A single non-water-suppressed PRESS voxel then is collected from the phantom (~$3 \times 1.5 \times 1.5$ cm³ voxel, TE = 40 ms, TR = 1500 ms, 64 scans). To keep the children entertained during the 20-minute procedure and to reduce the discomfort associated with the loud noises, children may listen to personal music or audio books via child-size headphones. Peak positions and areas of interest, including the methylene (CH2; frequency = 1.4) and methyl group (CH3; frequency = 1.0) fatty-acid-chain resonances then are determined by time domain fitting using Java-Based Magnetic Resonance User Interface (jMRUI) 19 by a single investigator. The residual water peak is removed using a Hankel–Lanczos singular value decomposition (HLSVD) algorithm, and lipid resonances are fit using single Lorentzian line shapes and referenced to the oil (phantom) resonance. The CH2 resonance relative to the phantom (expressed as a percentage) is used as intrahepatic lipid (IHL; Larson-Meyer et al., 2010).

MEASUREMENT OF RESTING BLOOD PRESSURE

Two types of methods are used to assess systolic and diastolic blood pressure in children: manual or automated, and both are utilized equally in clinical settings (Eisenmann et al., 2011). Automated assessments typically utilize a Dynamap® system. Two readings are taken and averaged. If the two values differ by more than 5 mm Hg, an additional reading is obtained. A small cuff is used for younger children. The individual should be instructed to abstain from eating and heavy exercise for at least 2 hours before the test. Individuals also should be instructed not to ingest caffeine within 30 minutes before blood pressure measurements. During the assessment, the individual should be seated comfortably, with the arm slightly flexed, palm up, and the entire forearm supported at heart level on a smooth surface.

MEASUREMENT OF RESTING HEART RATE

A stethoscope and watch with second hand or digital readout in seconds are utilized to measure resting heart rate. The individual will sit quietly for at least 5 minutes before the test. The heart rate is taken by auscultation. The stethoscope is placed to the left of the sternum just above the level of the nipple. The heartbeats are counted for 30 seconds and then multiplied by two. This will give total beats per minute. An average of three separate readings are noted.

LABORATORY BLOOD WORK

Biochemical markers, total cholesterol, triglycerides, high-density lipoproteins, and low-density lipoproteins (LDL) are examined in a certified laboratory. Individuals are required to fast for 12 hours before the test.

BLOOD COLLECTION AND PROCESSING

Venous blood should be collected in the morning after a 12-hour fast with the individual seated. Blood is collected in tubes containing 1.5 mg/mL ethylenediaminetetraacetic acid (EDTA) for procedures requiring plasma, in tubes with no additives for serum measures, and in citrate tubes for homeostasis endpoints (Sothern, Despeney, et al., 2000).

CHEMISTRY AND LIPID MEASURES

All routine chemistry and lipid analyses may be performed on a Beckman Synchron CX5 automated chemistry analyzer, and the LDL cholesterol is calculated using the Friedewald equation. The coefficient of variation for these assays is less than 2%, and the laboratory is required to participate in the CDC ongoing lipid standardization program.

MEASURES OF PHYSICAL ACTIVITY LEVEL AND FITNESS

The measurement of the patient's physical activity level (PAL) provides important clues regarding behaviors that may be contributing to the overweight condition (Eisenmann et al., 2011; Gordon & Sothern, 2006; Table 8.1). Sedentary behaviors are highly associated with childhood obesity. Both objective and subjective methods are available to determine physical activity.

MEASUREMENT OF PHYSICAL ACTIVITY BY ACCELEROMETER

Physical activity may be measured objectively by the GT1M ActiGraph uniaxial accelerometer or the ActiGraph A model GT3X (Manufacturing Technologies Inc. Health Systems, ActiGraph, Fort Walton Beach, Florida). The ActiGraph accelerometer is a small, electromechanical device that records acceleration and deceleration of movement. The ActiGraph records these accelerations and decelerations as activity counts and provides data for different intensities of physical activity (Kwon et al., 2011). The accelerometer is worn by the individual during waking hours for a minimum of 3 days (72 hours) and a maximum of 7

Patient Handout: Accelerometer Instructions

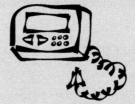

- Please wear the accelerometer for a minimum of 3 full days, but you may keep it on for as long as 7 days. The accelerometer should be worn for at least 2 weekdays (Monday through Friday) and 1 weekend day (Saturday or Sunday).
- Do not take a shower, bath, or go swimming with the accelerometer.
- You may take the accelerometer off to sleep at night (or you can leave it on, whatever is more comfortable for you).
- The accelerometer should be worn around the waist either under or over clothes and can be as tight or as loose as you want.
- The accelerometer already has been programmed to begin recording so you do not need to turn it on or off.
- When your child is finished wearing the accelerometer, please bring it with you to your next visit or return it by mail if provided with an envelope.

If you have any questions, please call _____.

days (168 hours) (Newton et al., 2011). Accelerometers should be initialized to begin collecting data at 5:00 A.M. on the day after they are distributed. Data are collected and stored in 30-second intervals. Individuals are directed to wear accelerometers on the provided elastic belt around the waist, to the right side of their body. Individuals are given the accelerometer upon arrival and asked to remove the accelerometer only when bathing, swimming, or sleeping.

Accelerometer data are reduced using methods previously described (Catellier et al., 2005; Newton et al., 2011; Treuth et al., 2004). Missing accelerometry data within a student's 3- to 7-day record is replaced via imputation. The count threshold (counts·30 sec^{-1}) for moderate to vigorous physical activity is set at 1500 counts·30 sec^{-1} based on previous studies (Treuth et al., 2004). Moderate to vigorous physical activity (MVPA) is measured on the randomly selected days of observation. The ActiGraph provides physical activity measurements, such as activity counts, energy expenditure, steps taken, activity intensity levels, metabolic equivalent (MET), and more. Daily MET-weighted minutes of MVPA are calculated by summing METS for MVPA over the entire day so that 1 MET-minute represents one metabolic equivalent of energy expended for 1 minute.

Key Points: Accelerometers (ActiGraph® GT3X+ -15) Directions
The GT3X+ allows you to choose the length of the epoch and the number of axes.
Accelerometers can be charged individually on a computer or en masse using the charger on a computer or through an outlet. Fully charged accelerometers will last about 2–3 weeks before additional charging is required.
Accelerometers will blink when connected to the charger for charging until fully charged. Once fully charged, the light will remain on and remain constant while it is still connected to the charger. When the accelerometer is detached, the light will go out.
When an accelerometer is charged and programmed to begin measurements, it will blink until the start time. Once it begins measurements, the light will go out. Once it has completed taking its measurements, the light will stay out.
The accelerometers can be initiated individually or en masse on a computer using the charger with the rectifier disconnected.
Downloading files must be done individually.
Both initiating (programming) accelerometers and downloading files from an accelerometer requires the use of the Actilife® Program on the laptop.

Downloaded accelerometry data are condensed into time spent in MVPA during the chosen time period using previously validated cut points and a data reduction program (Dowda et al., 1997; Wills & Salmon, 2004). Individuals are asked to keep a self-report record of the days and times that the accelerometers are worn.

Other objective measurement tools for determining physical activity level include pedometers, SenseWear Pro armband (http://www.sensewear.com), and heart rate monitors (Eisenmann et al., 2011).

SYSTEM FOR OBSERVING FITNESS INSTRUCTION TIME

Percent of time spent in MVPA may be obtained through direct observation using System for Observing Fitness Instruction Time (SOFIT), which provides simultaneous records of individual activity levels, the lesson context in which they occurred, and teacher behavior. Physical activity levels are recorded for randomly selected individuals, whereas lesson context and teacher behavior are coded every 20 seconds throughout the entire lesson. Lesson context refers to how the lesson time is being allocated at the observation moment and includes time for class management, knowledge, physical fitness, skill drills, game play, and free play.

Patient Handout: Accelerometry Self-Report Record

Name: _____

Please use this worksheet to record what times the study participant wakes up in the morning and goes to sleep each night while wearing the accelerometer.

Today is _____. I went to sleep last night at _____ P.M.
This morning I woke up at _____ A.M.

Today is _____. I went to sleep last night at _____ P.M.
This morning I woke up at _____ A.M.

Today is _____. I went to sleep last night at _____ P.M.
This morning I woke up at _____ A.M.

Today is _____. I went to sleep last night at _____ P.M.
This morning I woke up at _____ A.M.

Today is _____. I went to sleep last night at _____ P.M.
This morning I woke up at _____ A.M.

Today is _____. I went to sleep last night at _____ P.M.
This morning I woke up at _____ A.M.

Today is _____. I went to sleep last night at _____ P.M.
This morning I woke up at _____ A.M.

The five physical activity codes (lying, sitting, standing, walking, and vigorous) have been calibrated using heart rate monitoring (Mckenzie, Sallis, & Nader, 1991) and validated using accelerometers (Scruggs et al., 2003). Walking and vigorous intervals were summed to indication MVPA. In addition, the number of individuals participating, defined by the number of individuals who were dressed out, in class are recorded. Each school observes activities during lessons on a selected number of randomly scheduled days.

SOFIT OBSERVER TRAINING, ASSESSMENT, AND RECALIBRATION

Five staff members are trained to conduct all observations. Training includes classroom lectures and discussion, videotaped assessment, and field practice. To become certified, the staff members must reach an interobserver agreement (IOA) criterion f = of 85% on all variables on precoded "gold-standard" videotaped lessons. The staff members are reassessed using this same criteria before each semester, and a review session is provided at the beginning of each semester to reduce interobserver drift and disagreement. This method of training was adopted from the M-SPAN study, a two-year middle-school physical education intervention (Mckenzie et al., 2004). M-SPAN performed a field-based interobserver reliability assessment of the SOFIT observation. The study used two observers, equipped with a y-adapter and two earphone jacks, who independently coded the same individual during the same lesson while being paced by a single tape recorder. The percent of IOA was calculated; overall IOAs were 83%, 95%, and 80% for individual activity, lesson content, and teacher behavior, respectively. The intraclass correlation for independent observers was 0.96 for MVPA minutes.

METABOLIC EQUIVALENT TO DETERMINE EXERCISE INTENSITY AND ENERGY EXPENDITURE

We can measure the intensity of exercise and the number of calories expended in physical activity by using the MET, which is a measure of energy expenditure equivalent to 1.2 kcal/kg/hour (Ainsworth et al., 2011; Ainsworth, Haskell, & Whitt, 2000).

Resting energy expenditure (REE) is considered 1 MET. Therefore, a 3-MET activity would require energy expenditure at a level equal to three times resting.

MVPA is any physical activity performed at an intensity level equal to or greater than 3 METS; roughly equivalent to brisk walking.

Vigorous physical activity (VPA) is any physical activity performed at an intensity level of 6 METS or greater, which is roughly equivalent to jogging.

One MET is equal to resting VO_2 (volume of oxygen used), which is approximately 3.5 mL (oxygen) per kilogram (body weight) per minute (American College of Sports Medicine [ACSM], 2010; Bar-Or & Rowland, 2004; Thompson et al., 2010).

$$\text{Resting } VO_2 \text{ (One MET)} = 3.5 \text{ mL} \times \text{kg} \times \text{minutes}$$

Thus, the energy cost of exercise can be described in multiples of resting VO_2 (i.e., METS), which simplifies the quantification of exercise energy requirement. For the purposes of obtaining a rough estimate of energy expenditure, however, we use the following formula to compute caloric expenditure during physical activity:

$$\text{Energy Expenditure (calories per minute)} = 0.0175 \text{ calories/kg/minute}$$
$$\times \text{MET} \times \text{body weight (kg)}$$

Example: The energy cost of cycling (less than 10 mph) is calculated to be 4 METS. The caloric expenditure for a 70-kg person cycling at this speed, for 1 hour, can be computed as follows:

$$\text{Energy Expenditure (calories per minute)} = 0.0175 \times 4 \text{ METS} \times 70 \text{ (kg)}$$
$$= 4.9 \text{ calories per minute}$$
$$= 4.9 \text{ calories per minute} \times 60 \text{ minutes}$$
$$= 294 \text{ calories expended}$$

PHYSICAL ACTIVITY SELF-REPORT QUESTIONNAIRES

There are several examples of physical activity rating self-report questionnaires, including the following: Godin Leisure-Time, Self-Administered Physical Activity Checklist (SAPAC), Physical Activity Questionnaire for Adolescents (PAQ-A), Youth Physical Activity Questionnaire (Y-PAQ), 3-Day Physical Activity Recall (3DPAR), and others (Corder et al., 2008).

The Godin–Shephard Leisure-Time Physical Activity Questionnaire (PAQ; Godin & Shephard, 1985) is a four-item self-reported recall of usual physical activities during a typical week. Individuals are asked to write how many times per week they engage in vigorous, moderate, and light intensity activity for 15 minutes or more. Examples of the types of activities are provided. A total score is derived by multiplying the frequency of each category by a standard MET (Vigorous × 9, Moderate × 5, and Light × 3). Individuals also are asked to report how many times they engage in activity long enough to make them sweat. Adequate reliability and validity have been reported (Sallis, 1993) with individuals as young as fourth graders.

Godin Leisure-Time Physical Activity Questionnaire

1. During a typical 7-day period (1 week), how many times on average do you do the following kinds of exercise for more than 15 minutes during your free time (write on each line the appropriate number):

Times per Week

a) STRENUOUS EXERCISE (HEART BEATS RAPIDLY)   _____

(e.g., running, jogging, hockey, football, soccer, squash, basketball, cross-country skiing, judo, roller skating, vigorous swimming, vigorous long-distance bicycling)

b) MODERATE EXERCISE (NOT EXHAUSTING)   _____

(e.g., fast walking, baseball, tennis, easy bicycling, volleyball, badminton, easy swimming, alpine skiing, popular and folk dancing)

c) MILD EXERCISE (MINIMAL EFFORT)   _____

(e.g., yoga, archery, fishing from river bank, bowling, horseshoes, golf, snowmobiling, easy walking)

2. During a typical 7-day period (1 week), in your leisure time, how often do you engage in any regular activity long enough to work up a sweat (heart beats rapidly)?

OFTEN	SOMETIMES	NEVER/RARELY
1. ☐	2. ☐	3. ☐

In this excerpt from the Godin Leisure-Time PAQ, the individual is asked to complete a self-explanatory, brief four-item query of usual leisure-time exercise habits.

CALCULATIONS

For the first question, weekly frequencies of strenuous, moderate, and light activities are multiplied by nine, five, and three, respectively. Total weekly leisure activity is calculated in arbitrary units by summing the products of the separate components, as shown in the following formula:

Weekly leisure activity score = (9 × Strenuous) + (5 × Moderate) + (3 × Light)

The second question is used to calculate the frequency of weekly leisure-time activities pursued "long enough to work up a sweat" (see questionnaire).

EXAMPLE

Strenuous = 3 times/week
Moderate = 6 times/week
Light = 14 times/week

Total leisure activity score = (9 × 3) + (5 × 6) + (3 × 14) = 27 + 30 + 42 = 99

SELF-REPORTED PHYSICAL ACTIVITY QUESTIONNAIRE

The self-reported PAQ determines total energy expenditure and the level of physical activity based on the MET method and the duration of different physical activities (Motl et al., 2004). The PAQ is administered to groups of students in a classroom setting. A trained staff member hands out the questionnaire to each student while students are seated at their desks in the classroom. He or she provides verbal instructions concerning the proper method with which to fill out the questionnaire. He or she will answer any questions asked by the students to increase the accuracy of the information contained in the form. Students are asked to raise their hand once they have completed the questionnaire. The staff member then will review the form with the student to ensure that all requested information has been inserted into the appropriate spaces on the form. The staff member will then collect the forms and transport them to the data center for analysis.

The 3DPAR is administered in a similar manner. An example of the questionnaire is below:

3-Day Physical Activity Recall: Sample Activity Time Sheet					
	Activity Number	Light	Moderate	Hard	Very Hard
7:00–7:30	Showering or bathing 22	X			
7:30–8:00	Getting ready 21	X			
8:00–8:30	Travel by walking 18		X		
8:30–9:00	Sitting in class 28	X			
9:00–9:30	Physical education class 26			X	

Source: Adapted from Motl et al., 2004.

SEDENTARY BEHAVIOR

Individuals should be asked to report the number of hours they spend in sedentary pursuits both before and after school (Eisenmann et al., 2011; Table 8.1). The sedentary activities assessed include television, video, computer, reading, homework, and telephone. The list of sedentary activities are taken from SAPAC (Sallis et al., 1995). Sedentary behavior from this measure is correlated with percent BMI in previous research (Crespo et al., 2001).

PHYSICAL ACTIVITY SOCIAL SUPPORT

The physical activity social support (PASS) scale (Edmundson, Parcel, Feldman, et al., 1996; Edmundson, Parcel, Perry, et al., 1996) is an 18-item measure that assesses perceived support for physical activity. Support from family, teachers, and friends is assessed in a yes–no format, and positive and negative social support subscales are derived.

INDIVIDUAL SELF-EFFICACY

The physical self-efficacy scale is used to measure an individual's like (or dislike) of physical activity and beliefs about his or her physical abilities, using seven items (i.e., "I am good at sports compared with my peers"). The items are rated on a five-point Likert scale, ranging from 1 = "I don't agree" to 5 = "I entirely agree." Acceptable results for reliability, validity, and norms have been reported (Losekam et al., 2010).

EXERCISE SELF-REGULATION QUESTIONNAIRE

The Exercise Self-Regulation Questionnaire (SRQ-E) assesses domain-specific individual differences in types of motivation or regulation (external, introjected, identified, and integrated). The SRQ-E is structured so that it asks one question and provides responses that represent the different forms of regulation. Individuals have to choose, for each one of the 16 items (four for each subscale), how they feel in a seven-point Likert scale, ranging from 1 (not at all true) to 7 (very true). Each scale is scored separately by averaging the responses to each of the subscale's items (range 4–28). Examples of items included in different regulations subscales, ordered from the least to the most fully internalized, are external regulation (e.g., "Because I feel like I have no choice about exercising; others make me do it"), introjected regulation (e.g., "Because I would feel bad about myself if I did not"), identified regulation (e.g., "Because it feels important to me personally to accomplish this goal"), and intrinsic regulation (e.g., "Because it is a challenge to accomplish my goal," or "Because it is fun") (Ryan & Connell, 1989).

FUNDAMENTAL MOVEMENT SKILL COMPETENCY

The Test of Gross Motor Development II (TGMD-2) is used to assess the individual's fundamental movement skill proficiency. The TGMD-2 is composed of six locomotor skills—run, gallop, hop, leap, horizontal jump, and slide—and six object-control skills—striking a stationary ball (strike), stationary basketball dribble (dribble), catch, stationary kick (kick), overhand throw (throw), and underhand roll (roll). These skills have been established as valid and reliable for individuals ages 3 to 20 years old (Ulrich, 2000). The test is administered following standardized procedures, instructions, and demonstrations in small groups (n ≤ 10) during baseline visit, follow-up visit, 6-month follow-up, and 1-year follow-up (Cliff et al., 2011).

DETAILED EXERCISE TESTING PROTOCOLS: MEASUREMENT OF FITNESS

Tailoring exercise recommendations to the individual needs of overweight children with comorbidities may require the administration of an exercise test to determine the aerobic fitness level (maximal oxygen uptake [peak VO_2]) of the obese child (Sothern, 2006). The maximal oxygen uptake (VO_2max) is an indicator of physical fitness level in both adult and youth populations (Astrand et al., 1986; Casaburi et al., 1989; McArdle & Magel, 1970; Mitchell & Blomqvist, 1971; Rowell, Taylor, & Wang, 1964). The maximal oxygen uptake indicates the functional capacity of the heart, lungs, and skeletal muscle and generally is assumed to be the single best indicator of physical fitness (Astrand et al., 1986). The VO_2max is determined by exercising a subject and determining O_2 intake and O_2 and CO_2 concentrations in expired air in a laboratory during a progressive exercise test using cycle ergometry or a treadmill (Ganley et al., 2011) All VO_2max tests should be supervised by trained and certified exercise physiologists and/or physicians. Cardiovascular responses to exercise stress can be evaluated by obtaining a value for (1) submaximal steady-state, or (2) peak or max exercise value (peak or max VO_2).

The criteria for achieving a peak VO_2 response in the pediatric population may not be similar to that of adults (Rowland et al., 1999). Obtaining a plateau in oxygen consumption in children often can be difficult. Several protocols, however, have been used and validated for pediatric exercise testing (Sothern, 2001; Sothern, Loftin, Blecker, et al., 1999, 2000). Unfortunately, limited guidance is available to assist health professionals in the selection of an appropriate exercise testing protocol for determining peak VO_2 in obese children and youth. Typically, exercise protocols at less strenuous treadmill speeds and inclines or cycle power outputs are utilized. In general, treadmill protocols yield higher values than cycle ergometry in normal weight youth. This is less clear in obese children especially under submaximal conditions.

One submaximal marker of aerobic fitness, ventilatory anaerobic threshold (VAT), may be particularly useful in assessing children with significant obesity, who may be less prone to provide an exhaustive effort during exercise testing (Rowland & Loftin, 2006). VAT is obtained during peak exercise testing by observing the point at which ventilation increases rapidly, indicating a shift from aerobic to anaerobic pathways. Once VAT is achieved, exhaustion soon follows. Thus, knowledge of VAT will provide an indication of exercise tolerance in obese youth. In fact, studies of VAT in obese children yield parallel findings to other more challenging indicators of aerobic fitness. Detailed instructions for administering exercise tests for obese children with varied levels of obesity and comorbid conditions follow. The results of these evaluations better inform the selection of appropriate physical activities for obese individuals.

CYCLE ERGOMETRY FITNESS TESTING

Cycle ergometry is shown to be suitable for obtaining VO_2max in children 11–14 years old (Loftin et al., 2004). Cycle ergometry is safer than other forms (i.e., treadmill) for testing obese patients and may be a more accurate means of assessing cardiovascular functional reserve in these subjects (Loftin et al., 2001). Participants using the cycle ergometer will experience increasing increments of resistance based on estimated maximum force output. The test will be terminated upon volitional exhaustion or if pedal rate drops 5 rpms below the protocol. The VO_2max will be accepted as the functional aerobic maximal capacity provided that appropriate criteria are met, including voluntary exhaustion, respiratory exchange ratio (RER) greater than 1.0, and maximum heart rate as specified by age (Rowland & Loftin, 2006). The heart rate will be monitored using a Polar Vantage XL heart rate monitor. Trained and certified exercise physiologists will supervise all VO_2max tests.

PHYSICAL WORK CAPACITY CYCLE TEST

The physical work capacity (PWC) protocol uses a 5-minute warm-up at 25 watts before maximal testing. The pedal rate should be held constant at 60 rpm throughout testing. The test should begin unloaded at 60 rpm for 2 minutes. After the 2 minutes, workload should increase by 29 watts (0.5 kg) every 2 minutes until 118 watts. From that point, power output should increase by 15 watts (0.25 kg) until volitional termination or a drop in pedal rate of 5 rpm.

LOFTIN–SOTHERN TEST

The Loftin–Sothern treadmill protocol is a modified Balke protocol, which includes a baseline standing measure and three submaximal, steady-state stages (Loftin et al., 2001, 2005; Sothern, 2001; Sothern, Loftin, Blecker, et al., 2000). The test was designed to observe baseline, submaximal, and maximal differences in specific metabolic and physiologic parameters between nonobese and obese children during weight-bearing exercise (walking). Subjects participate in a graded maximal exercise test using this protocol, which was adapted from Foster et al. (1995). All metabolic variables are determined by indirect calorimetry with a Sensormedics Measurement Cart No. 1 during submaximal and maximal exercise. Heart rate is determined by telemetry with a Polar Vantage Heart Rate Monitor, and blood pressure is calculated by indirect cuff sphygmomanometry during rest and exercise. Energy expenditure, VO_2, Ve, VCO_2, RER, and heart rate are determined during rest after a 4-hour period of fasting while standing unsupported. This is followed by three submaximal walking stages of 2.5 mph, 3.0 mph, and 3.5 mph, respectively. The subjects then walk at 3.5 mph with a 2% increase in grade every 2 minutes until maximal effort is achieved.

The VO_2max exercise testing as described is a relatively safe procedure if performed properly. Recent surveys of more than 2,000 clinical exercise testing laboratories with 600,000 tests performed show a death rate of approximately 0.5 per 10,000 exercise tests (ACSM, 2010). Major medical complications, such as myocardial infarction, ventricular fibrillation, dysrhythmias, asystole, or stroke, are most likely to occur in cardiac-diseased populations during diagnostic testing. Subjects will be screened medically for heart disease risk factors before testing.

A Sensormedics metabolic measurement cart model 2900C will be used to collect and assess ventilation (Ve), volume of oxygen (VO_2), oxygen uptake (VO_2 L/min and VO_2 mL/kg/min.), volume of carbon dioxide (VCO_2), RER, or respiratory quotient (RQ). Data will be collected every minute, and the oxygen and carbon dioxide analyzers will be calibrated with two different commercial gas mixtures (Tank 1: O_2 = 24%, CO_2 = 0%; Tank 2: O_2 = 16%, CO_2 = 4%) before and after testing. A summary of the protocol follows:

Pretest: Resting in a seated position for 30 minutes.
Fasting for 4 hours before the time of the test.
No vigorous activity for 48 hours before the test.

Baseline: Expired gases are collected with a metabolic measurement cart for 10 minutes while subject is standing, unsupported.

Submaximal: Expired gases are collected with a metabolic measurement cart during treadmill walking as follows:
2.5 mph for 5 minutes at 0% grade.
3.0 mph for 5 minutes at 0% grade.
3.5 mph for 5 minutes at 0% grade.

Maximal: Rate is 3.5 mph until test completion. Grade is increased 2% every 2 minutes until test completion.

Numerous other examples in studies recently were published using maximal exercise testing in children and adolescents. Potter et al. (2013) utilized cycle ergometry to obtain VO_2 peak in 11 overweight and 12 healthy weight children, approximately 11 years of age. After a 2-minute warm-up of unloaded pedaling, a power output of 30 W was initiated and then was increased by 12 Wmin_1 over a maximum duration of 15 minutes. The children performed the test until voluntary exhaustion. If a plateau in values was not reached, VO_2 peak was recorded as the highest 15-second moving average VO_2 during which at least two of the secondary criteria were met. In this case, the secondary criteria for the achievement of VO_2 peak were heart rate of B200 beats min_1 and a respiratory exchange ratio of X1.00. The children also demonstrated clear subjective symptoms of fatigue. Additional detailed protocols for assessing VO_2 peak or maximum in children and adolescents are found in several recent publications (Loftin et al., 2004, 2005, 2009; Loftin, Sothern, et al., 2007; Maffeis, 2008; Norman et al., 2005; Swain et al., 2010).

FIELD TESTING OF CARDIORESPIRATORY (AEROBIC) ENDURANCE

To estimate VO_2 peak or maximum in nonclinical settings, health care providers and educators may employ field testing to track the progress of their patients or students (Ganley et al., 2011). Acceptable methods for overweight and obese children include walking tests and the 20-minute shuttle run (California Department of Health, 2014). Detailed protocols are available in several publications (Beets & Pitetti, 2006; Coe et al., 2013; Joshi et al., 2012).

MUSCULAR STRENGTH AND ENDURANCE TESTING

Research over the years has sought to determine the role of maturation on the development of strength utilizing varied methods to control for differences in body size. The measurement of strength in developing youth, however, remains confounded by many factors (Croix, 2007). Accepted techniques to measure muscle forces include isometric or isokinetic dynamometers (Ganley et al., 2011). Isokinetic one-repetition maximum (1RM) tests are used in children and are shown to be safe in numerous studies. Caution should be executed, however, when administering this test especially in prepubertal children because these studies use carefully supervised protocols (Ganley et al., 2011). Detailed protocols for measuring muscular strength and endurance are available in numerous studies (Faigenbaum, Milliken, & Westcott, 2003; Shaibi et al., 2006) and in several fitness manuals (ACSM, 2010; Clark, Lucett, & Corn, 2008). An example of a protocol using an isokinetic dynamometer in children and adolescents follows:

EXAMPLE:

Subjects will be seated in a Cybex or Kin-Com isokinetic dynamometer and will perform the forward leg extension. The apparatus seat height will be adjusted to conform to the size of the subject. The subject will be strapped to the apparatus to prevent movement of adjacent body parts. Arms will move separately and measures will be recorded for three different exercise bouts. Likewise, legs will be assessed independently for three measures. The speed of movement will be set at low to moderate (60 degrees per second or 4–8 seconds per 180 degrees). Therefore, the tests described previously should provide a more accurate indication of change in muscular strength and endurance. Testing time should not exceed 45 minutes per subject. Possible side effects include delayed onset muscle soreness, which may occur 24–48 hours following testing. This condition is temporary and has not been shown to cause permanent damage to muscle fiber structure. The chance for injury during the movement with the weights will be minimized through the use of an individual spotter during testing. Additionally, the slow-to-moderate velocity for exercise movement will prevent the chance of musculoskeletal and, specifically, joint injuries.

MUSCULAR FLEXIBILITY TESTING

The measure of muscular flexibility is specific to the joint and usually is assessed using a goniometer or inclinometer (Ganley et al., 2011). Widespread application of this type of assessment is not practical, however. The sit-and-reach test is the most widely used field test of low-back and posterior-leg flexibility (Ganley et al., 2011). Although no general test exists as a measure of total body flexibility, the sit-and-reach test may be used to indirectly assess general flexibility as follows:

EXAMPLE:

The subject is instructed to remove his or her shoes and sit in front of a sit-and-reach box, which is 12 inches high and has a measured ruler atop it. The feet are placed flat against the front of the box with knees extended but not locked. The subject performs the test by reaching with both hands, one on top of the other and palms down, as far forward as possible making contact with the measuring scale. The test is performed three times with the highest score noted and recorded (Pollock, Wilmore, & Fox, 1984).

The Flex Test, which is detailed in Chapters 4 and 6 (Sothern, Gordon, & von Almen, 2006; Sothern, von Almen, & Schumacher, 2001), provides a useful assessment in overweight and obese children of muscular imbalances that may occur as a result of poor flexibility, such as the upper crossed syndrome (Janda, 1993).

MEASUREMENT OF RESTING METABOLISM: RESTING ENERGY EXPENDITURE AND RESPIRATORY QUOTIENT

The REE and the RQ (or fat oxidation) may be measured to determine resting metabolism. A reduced REE is a risk factor for weight gain. The RQ provides a measurement of fat oxidation, which is associated inversely with obesity. REE and RQ are measured under standardized conditions to observe both resting metabolism and fuel mix oxidation.

REE is determined by ventilated hood indirect calorimetry with the individual lying supine on a bed (Sothern, Loftin, et al., 2000). Individuals are instructed to fast for 12 hours and not to engage in vigorous physical activity for 24 hours before the test. Individuals are allowed to drink water before the test and rest in a recumbent position for 30 minutes before the start of each testing session. Parents accompany the children and a nonviolent cartoon video is shown to the children during the testing (Salbe et al., 1997). Metabolic measurements are taken continuously during the test. Expired gases are sampled and analyzed for O_2 and CO_2 concentrations using a Delatrac Metabolic Measurement Cart for a 20-minute period. REE then is calculated for each individual based on inspired and expired O_2 and CO_2 concentration (Fontainville, Dwyer, & Ravussin, 1992; Salbe et al., 1997). RQ is evaluated as an index of fat oxidation.

TANNER STAGING

Sexual maturity rating may be determined by a physician (trained in pediatric medicine) using methods from Falkner and Tanner (1979) in children and adolescents.

REFERENCES

Ainsworth, B. E., Haskell, W. L., Herrmann, S. D., Meckes, N., Bassett, D. R., Tudor-Locke, C., et al. (2011). 2011 compendium of physical activities. *Medicine and Science in Sports and Exercise*, 43(8), 1575–1581.

Ainsworth, B., Haskell, W., Whitt, M. (2000). Compendium of physical activities: an update of activity codes and MET intensities. *Medicine and Science in Sports and Exercise*, 32(9), S498–S516.

American College of Sports Medicine. (2010). *ACSM's Guidelines for Exercise Testing and Prescription* (8th ed.). Philadelphia, PA: Lippincott Williams & Wilkins.

Astrand, P. O., Hultman, E., Juhlin-Dannfelt, A., Reynolds, G. (1986). Disposal of lactate during and after strenuous exercise in humans. *Journal of Applied Physiology*, 61(1), 338–343.

Barlow, S. (2007). Expert Committee recommendations regarding the prevention, assessment and treatment of child and adolescent overweight and obesity: Summary report. *Pediatrics*, 120(Suppl 4), S164–S192.

Bar-Or, O., Rowland, T. (2004). *Pediatric Exercise Medicine: From Physiologic Principles to Health Care Application*. Champaign, IL: Human Kinetics.

Beets, M., Pitetti, K. (2006). Criterion-referenced reliability and equivalency between the pacer and 1-mile run/walk for high school students. *Journal of Physical Activity and Health*, 3(Suppl. 2), S21–S33.

Boye, K. R., Dimitriou, T., Manz, F., Schoenau, E., Neu, C., Wudy, S., Remer, T. (2002). Anthropometric assessment of muscularity during growth: Estimating fat-free mass with 2 skinfold-thickness measurements is superior to measuring mid-upper arm muscle area in healthy prepubertal children. *American Journal of Clinical Nutrition*, 76(3), 628–632.

Brambilla, P., Manzoni, P., Agostini, G., Beccaria, L., Ruotolo, G., Sironi, S., et al. (1999). Persisting obesity starting before puberty is associated with stable intraabdominal fat during adolescence. *International Journal of Obesity and Related Metabolic Disorders*, 23(3), 299–303.

Bray, G. A. (1987). Overweight is risking fate. Definition, classification, prevalence, and risks. *Annals of the New York Academy of Sciences*, 499, 14–28.

Bray, G. A., DeLany, J. P., Volaufova, J., Harsha, D. W., Champagne, C. (2002). Prediction of body fat in 12-y-old African American and white children: Evaluation of methods. *American Journal of Clinical Nutrition*, 76(5), 980–990.

California Department of Health. (2014). FitnessGram performance standards. Retrieved from http://www.cde.ca.gov/ta/tg/pf/documents/pft1314pfscharts.pdf.

Cameron, N., Griffiths, P. L., Wright, M. M., Blencowe, C., Davis, N. C., Pettifor, J. M., Norris, S. A. (2004). Regression equations to estimate percentage body fat in African prepubertal children aged 9 y. *American Journal of Clinical Nutrition*, 80(1), 70–75.

Casaburi, R., Spitzer, S., Haskell, R., Wasserman, K. (1989). Effect of altering heart rate on oxygen uptake at exercise onset. *Chest*, 95(1), 6–12.

Casanova Roman, M., Rodriguez Ruiz, I., Rico de Cos, S., Casanova Bellido, M. (2004). Body composition analysis using bioelectrical and anthropometric parameters. *Anales de Pediatria (Barcelona)*, 61(1), 23–31.

Catellier, D. J., Hannan, P. J., Murray, D. M., Addy, C. L., Conway, T. L., Yang, S., Rice, J. C. (2005). *Medicine and Science in Sports and Exercise*, 37(11 Suppl), S555–S562.

Centers for Disease Control and Prevention. (2010). Growth charts. http://www.cdc.gov/growthcharts.

Centers for Disease Control and Prevention. (2006). National Center for Health Statistics (NCHS). National Health and Nutrition Examination Survey Data (NHANES). Hyattsville, MD: U.S. Department of Health and Human Services.

Chumlea, C., Roche, R. (1979). Measurement descriptions and techniques. In T. Lohman, A. A. Roche, R. Martorell (Eds.), *Anthropometric Standardization Reference Manual*. Champaign, IL: Human Kinetics.

Clark, M., Lucett, S., Corn, R. (2008). *NASM Essentials of Personal Fitness Training* (3rd ed.). Baltimore, MD: Lippincott Williams & Wilkins.

Cliff, D. P., Okely, A. D., Morgan, P. J., Steele, J. R., Jones, R. A., Colyvas, K., Baur, L. A. (2011). Movement skills and physical activity in obese children: Randomized controlled trial. *Medicine and Science in Sports and Exercise*, 143(1), 90–100.

Coe, D., Peterson, T., Blair, C., Schutten, M., Peddie, H. (2013). Physical fitness, academic achievement, and socioeconomic status in school-aged youth. *Journal of School Health*, 83(7), 500–507.

Cook, S., Auinger, P., Huang, T. (2009). Growth curves for cardio-metabolic risk factors in children and adolescents. *Journal of Pediatrics*, 155(3), S6.e15–S6.e26.

Corder, K., Ekelund, U., Steele, R. M., Wareham, N. J., Brage, S. (2008). Assessment of physical activity in youth. *Journal of Applied Physiology*, 105(3), 977–987.

Corder, K., van Sluijs, E. M., Wright, A., Whincup, P., Wareham, N. J., Ekelund, U. (2009). Is it possible to assess free-living physical activity and energy expenditure in young people by self-report? *American Journal of Clinical Nutrition*, 89(3), 862–870.

Crespo, C. J., Smit, E., Troiano, R. P., Bartlett, S. J., Macera, C. A., Andersen, R. E. (2001). Television watching, energy intake, and obesity in US children: results from the third National Health and Nutrition Examination Survey, 1988–1994. *Archives of Pediatrics and Adolescent Medicine*, 155 (3), 360–365.

Croix, M. (2007). Advances in pediatric strength assessment: changing our perspective on strength development. *Journal of Sports Science and Medicine*, 6, 292–304.

Dowda, M., Pate, R. R., Sallis, J., Freedom, P. S. (1997). Accelerometer (CSA) count cut points for physical activity intensity ranges in youth 4 to 13. *Medicine and Science in Sports and Exercise*, 29(Suppl 5), S72.

Durnin, J., de Bruin, H., Feunekes, G. (1997). Skinfold thicknesses: Is there a need to be very precise in their location? *British Journal of Nutrition*, 77(1), 3–7.

Durnin, J. V., Womersley, J. (1974). Body fat assessed from total body density and its estimation from skinfold thickness: measurements on 481 men and women aged from 16 to 72 years. *British Journal of Nutrition*, 32(1), 77–97.

Edmundson, E., Parcel, G. S., Feldman, H. A., Elder, J., Perry, C. L., Johnson, C. C., Williston, B. J., Stone, E. J., Yang, M., Lytle, L., Webber, L. (1996). The effects of the Child and Adolescent Trial for Cardiovascular Health upon psychosocial determinants of diet and physical activity behavior. *Preventive Medicine*, 25(4), 442–454.

Edmundson, E., Parcel, G. S., Perry, C. L., Feldman, H. A., Smyth, M., Johnson, C. C., Layman, A., Bachman, K., Perkins, T., Smith, K., Stone, E. (1996). The effects of the child and adolescent trial for cardiovascular health intervention on psychosocial determinants of cardiovascular disease risk behavior among third-grade students. *American Journal of Health Promotion*, 10(3), 217–225.

Eisenkolbl, J., Kartasurya, M., Widhalm, K. (2001). Underestimation of percentage fat mass measured by bioelectrical impedance analysis compared to dual energy X-ray absorptiometry method in obese children. *European Journal of Clinical Nutrition*, 55(6), 423–429.

Eisenmann, J. C.; for the Subcommittee on Assessment in Pediatric Obesity Management Programs, National Association of Children's Hospital and Related Institutions (2011). Assessment of obese children and adolescents: A survey of pediatric obesity-management programs. *Pediatrics*, 129(Suppl 2), S51–S58.

Ellis, K. J., Shypailo, R. J., Pratt, J. A., Pond, W. G. (1994). Accuracy of dual-energy x-ray absorptiometry for body-composition measurements in children and adolescents. *American Journal of Clinical Nutrition*, 60 (5), 660–665.

Faigenbaum, A., Milliken, L., Westcott, W. (2003). Maximal strength testing in healthy children. *Journal of Strength and Conditioning Research*, 17(1), 162–166.

Falkner, F., Tanner, J. M. (1979). *Human Growth*. London: Bailliere Tindall.

Fernandez, J. R., Redden, D. T., Pietrobelli, A., Allison, D. B. (2004). Waist circumference in nationally representative samples of African-American, European-American, and Mexican-American children and adolescents. *Journal of Pediatrics*, 145(4), 439–444.

Fontainville, F. A., Dwyer, J., Ravussin, E. (1992). Resting metabolic rate and body composition in Pima Indian and Caucasian children. *International Journal of Obesity*, 16, 535–542.

Forbes, G. B. (1991). Exercise and body composition. *Journal of Applied Physiology*, 70(3), 994–997.

Friedl, K. E., DeLuca, J. P., Marchitelli, L. J., Vogel, J. A. (1992). Reliability of body-fat estimations from a four-compartment model by using density, body water, and bone mineral measurements. *American Journal of Clinical Nutrition*, 55 (4), 764–770.

Ganley, K., Paterno, M., Miles, C., Stout, J., Brawner, P., Girolami, G., Warran, M. (2011). Health-related fitness in children and adolescents. *Pediatric Physical Therapy*, 23(3), 208–220.

Godin, G., Shephard, R. J. (1985). Gender differences in perceived physical self-efficacy among older individuals. *Perceptual and Motor Skills*, 60(2), 599–602.

Goran, M. I., Driscoll, P., Johnson R., Nagy, T. R., Hunter, G. (1996). Cross-calibration of body-composition techniques against dual-energy X-ray absorptiometry in young children. *American Journal of Clinical Nutrition*, 63(3), 299–305.

Gordon S., Sothern, M. (2006). The role of the physician. In M. Sothern, S. Gordon, T. K. von Almen (Eds.), *Handbook of Pediatric Obesity: Clinical Management* (pp. 41–52). Boca Raton, FL: Taylor & Francis.

Gutin, B., Litaker, M., Islam, S., Manos, T., Smith, C., Treiber, F. (1996). Body-composition measurement in 9-11-y-old children by dual-energy X-ray absorptiometry, skinfold-thickness measurements, and bioimpedance analysis. *American Journal of Clinical Nutrition*, 63 (3), 287–292.

Hamill, P., Drizd, T., Johnson, T. (1979). Physical growth: National Center for Health Statistics percentiles. *American Journal of Clinical Nutrition*, 32, 607–629.

Jackson, A. S., Pollock, M. L. (1978). Generalized equations for predicting body density of men. *British Journal of Nutrition*, 40 (3), 497–504.

Jackson, A. S., Pollock, M. L., Graves, J. E., Mahar, M. T. (1988). Reliability and validity of bioelectrical impedance in determining body composition. *Journal of Applied Physiology*, 64(2), 529–534.

Janda, V. (1993). Muscle strength in relation to muscle length, pain and muscle imbalance. In K. Harms-Rindahl (Ed.), *Muscle Strength* (pp. 83–91). New York, NY: Churchill Livingstone.

Janz, K., Nielsen, D., Cassady, S., Cook, J., Wu, Y., Hansen, J. (1993). Cross-validation of the Alaughter skinfold equations for children and adolescents. *Medicine and Science in Sports and Exercise*, 25(9), 1070–1076.

Joshi, P., Bryan, C., Howat, H. (2012). Relationship of body mass index and fitness levels among schoolchildren. *Journal of Strength and Conditioning Research*, 26(4), 1006–1014.

Kowalski, K. C., Crocker, P. R. E., Kowalski, N. P. (1997). Convergent validity of the physical activity questionnaire for adolescents. *Pediatric Exercise Science*, 9, 342–352.

Krebs, N., Himes, J., Jacobson, D., Nicklas, T., Guilday, P., Styne, D. (2007). Assessment of child and adolescent overweight and obesity. *Pediatrics*, 120(Suppl 4), S193–S228.

Kwon, S., Janz, K., Burns, T., Levy, S. (2011). Association between light-intensity physical activity and adiposity in childhood. *Pediatric Exercise Science*, 23(2), 218–229.

Larson-Meyer, D. E., Newcomer, B. R., VanVrancken-Tompkins, C. L., Sothern, M. S. (2010). Feasibility of assessing muscle and liver lipid in prepubertal children. *Diabetes Technology and Therapeutics*, 12(3), 207–212.

Loftin, M., Heusel, L., Bonis, M., Sothern, M. (2005). Oxygen uptake kinetics and oxygen deficit in obese and normal weight adolescent females. *Journal of Sports Science and Medicine*, 4, 430–436.

Loftin, M. Nichols, J., Going, S., Sothern, M., Schmitz, K., Ring, K., Tuuri, G., Stevens, J. (2007). Comparison of the validity of anthropometric and bioelectric impedance equations to assess body composition in adolescent girls. *International Journal of Body Composition Research*, 5(1), 1–8.

Loftin, M., Sothern, M., Koss, C., Tuuri, G., VanVrancken, C., Kontos, A., Bonis, M. (2007). Energy expenditure and influence of physiologic factors during marathon running. *Journal of Strength and Conditioning Research*, 21(4), 1188–1191.

Loftin, M., Sothern, M., Trosclair, L., O'Hanlon, A., Miller, J., Udall, J. (2001). Scaling modes of VO_2 peak in obese and nonobese girls. *Obesity Research*, 9, 290–296.

Loftin, M., Sothern, M., Tuuri, G., Tompkins, C., Koss, C., Bonis, M. (2009). Gender comparison of physiologic and perceptual responses in recreational marathon runners. *International Journal of Sports Physiology and Performance*, 4, 307–316.

Loftin, M., Sothern, M., VanVrancken, C., Udall, J. (2003). Low heart rate peak in obese female youth. *Clinical Pediatrics*, 42(6), 505–510.

Loftin, M., Sothern, M., Warren, B., Udall, J. (2004). Comparison of VO_2 peak during treadmill and bicycle ergometry in severely overweight youth. *Journal of Sports Science and Medicine*, 3, 254–260.

Loftin, J., Strikmiller, P., Warren, B., Myers, L., Schroth, L., Pittman, P., Harsha, D., Sothern, M. (1998). Comparison and relationship of VO_2 peak and physical activity patterns in elementary and high school females. *Pediatric Exercise Science*, 10(2), 153–163.

Lohman, T. G. (1981). Skinfolds and body density and their relation to body fatness: A review. *Human Biology*, 53(2), 181–225.

Lohman, T., Roche, A. A., Martorell, R. (Eds.). (1988). *Anthropometric Standardization Reference Manual*. Champaign, IL: Human Kinetics.

Losekam, S., Goetzky, B., Kraeling, S., Rief, W., Hilbet, A. (2010). Physical activity in normal-weight and overweight youth: associations with weight teasing and self-efficacy. *Obesity Facts*, 3(4), 239–244.

Maffeis, C. (2008) Physical activity in the prevention and treatment of childhood obesity: Physio-pathologic evidence and promising experiences. *International Journal of Pediatric Obesity*, 3 (Suppl 2), 29–32.

Mazess, R. B., Barden, H. S., Bisek, J. P., Hanson, J. (1990). Dual-energy x-ray absorptiometry for total-body and regional bone-mineral and soft-tissue composition. *American Journal of Clinical Nutrition*, 51(6), 1106–1112.

McArdle, W. D., Magel, J. R. (1970). Physical work capacity and maximal oxygen uptake in treadmill and bicycle exercise. *Medicine and Science in Sports*, 2(3), 118–123.

McKenzie, T. L., Sallis, J. F., Nader, P. R. (1991). SOFIT: System for observing fitness instruction time. *Journal of Teaching in Physical Education*, 11, 195–205.

McKenzie, T. L., Sallis, J. F., Prochaska, J. J., Conway, T. L., Marshall, S. J., Rosengard, P. (2004). Evaluation of a two-year middle-school physical education intervention: M-SPAN. *Medicine and Science in Sports and Exercise*, 36(8), 1382–1388.

Mitchell, J. H., Blomqvist, G. (1971). Maximal oxygen uptake. *New England Journal of Medicine*, 284(18), 1018–1022.

Motl, R. W., Dishman, R. K., Dowda, M., Pate, R. R. (2004). Factorial validity and invariance of a self-report measure of physical activity among adolescent girls. *Research Quarterly for Exercise and Sport*, 75(3), 259–271.

Newton, R. L., Han, H., Sothern, M., Webber, L., Ryan, D. H., Williamson, D. A. (2011). Accelerometry measured ethnic differences in activity in rural adolescents. *Journal of Physical Activity and Health*, 8(2), 287–295.

Norman, A. C., Drinkard, B., McDuffie, J. R., Ghorbani, S., Yanoff, L. B., Yanovski, J. A. (2005). Influence of excess adiposity on exercise fitness and performance in overweight children and adolescents. *Pediatrics*, 115(6), e690–e696.

Parker, L., Reilly, J. J., Slater, C., Wells, J. C., Pitsiladis, Y. (2003). Validity of six field and laboratory methods for measurement of body composition in boys. *Obesity Research*, 11(7), 852–858.

Pollock, M. L., Wilmore, J. H., Fox, S. M. (1984). *Exercise in Health and Disease*. Philadelphia: W.B. Saunders.

Potter, C., Zakrzewski, J., Draper, S., Unnithan, V. (2013). The oxygen uptake kinetic response to moderate intensity exercise in overweight and non-overweight children. *International Journal of Obesity*, 37, 101–106.

Praphul, J., Bryan, C., Howat, H. (2012). Relationship of body mass index and fitness levels among schoolchildren. *Journal of Strength and Conditioning Research*, 26(4), 1006–1014.

Roche, A., Heymsfield, S. B., Lohman, T. G. (Eds.). (1996). *Human Body Composition*. Champaign, IL: Human Kinetics.

Rowell, L. B., Taylor, H. L., Wang, Y. (1964). Limitations to prediction of maximal oxygen intake. *Journal of Applied Physiology*, 19, 919–927.

Rowland, T., Kline, G., Goff, D., Martel, L., Ferrone, L. (1999). One-mile run performance and cardiovascular fitness in children. *Archives of Pediatrics and Adolescent Medicine*, 153(8), 845–849.

Rowland, T., Loftin, M. (2006). Exercise testing. In M. Sothern, S. Gordon, T. K. von Almen (Eds.), *Handbook of Pediatric Obesity: Clinical Management* (pp. 113–120). Boca Raton, FL: Taylor & Francis.

Ryan, R. M., Connell, J. P. (1989). Perceived locus of causality and internalization: examining reasons for acting in two domains. *Journal of Personality and Social Psychology*, 57(5), 749–761.

Salbe, A. D., Fontvieille, A. M., Harper, A. T., Ravussin, E. (1997). Low levels of physical activity in 5-year-old children. *Journal of Pediatrics*, 131(3), 423–429.

Sallis, J. F. (1993). Epidemiology of physical activity and fitness in children and adolescents. *Critical Reviews in Food Science and Nutrition*, 33 (4–5), 403–408.

Sallis, J. F., Berry, C. C., Broyles, S. L, McKenzie, T. L., Nader, P. R. (1995). Variability and tracking of physical activity over 2 yrs in young children. *Medicine and Science in Sports and Exercise*, 27(7), 1042–1049.

Scruggs, P. W., Beveridge, S. K., Eisenman, P. A., Watson, D. L., Schultz, B. B., Ransdell, L. B. (2003). Quantifying physical activity via pedometry in elementary physical education. *Medicine and Science in Sports and Exercise*, 35, 1065–1071.

Shaibi, G. Q., Cruz, M. L., Ball, G. D., Weigensberg, M. J., Salem, G. J., Crespo, N. C., Goran, M.I. (2006). Effects of resistance training on insulin sensitivity in overweight Latino adolescent males. *Medicine and Science in Sports and Exercise*, 38(7), 1208–1515.

Shypailo R., Butte, N., Ellis, K. (2008). DXA: Can it be used as a criterion reference for body fat measurements in children? *Obesity (Silver Spring, Md.)*, 16(2), 457–462.

Slaughter, M. H., Lohman, T. G., Boileau, R. A., Horswill, C. A., Stillman, R. J., Van Loan, M. D., Bemben, D. A. (1988). Skinfold equations for estimation of body fatness in children and youth. *Human Biology*, 60(5), 709–723.

Sloan, A. W. (1967). Estimation of body fat in young men. *Journal of Applied Physiology*, 23 (3), 311–315.

Sothern, M. (2001). Exercise as a modality in the treatment of childhood obesity. *Pediatric Clinics of North America*, 48(4), 995–1015.

Sothern, M. (2006). The business of pediatric weight management. In M. Sothern, S. Gordon, T. K. von Almen (Eds.), *Handbook of Pediatric Obesity: Clinical Management* (pp. 9–28). Boca Raton, FL: Taylor & Francis.

Sothern, M., Despeney, B., Brown, R., Suskind, R., Udall, J., Blecker, U. (2000). Lipid profiles of obese children and adolescents before and after significant weight loss: differences according to sex. *Southern Medical Journal*, 93, 278–282.

Sothern, M., Gordon, S., von Almen, T. K. (Eds.). (2006). *Handbook of Pediatric Obesity: Clinical Management*. Boca Raton, FL: Taylor & Francis.

Sothern, M., Loftin, M., Blecker, M., Suskind, R., Udall, J. (1999). Physiologic function and childhood obesity. *International Journal of Pediatrics*, 14(3), 1–5.

Sothern, M., Loftin, M., Blecker, U., Suskind, R., Udall, J. (2000). The impact of significant weight loss on maximal oxygen uptake in obese children and adolescents, *Journal of Investigative Medicine*, 48(6), 411–416.

Sothern, M., Loftin, M., Suskind, R., Udall, J. (1999). The impact of significant weight loss on resting energy expenditure in obese youth. *Journal of Investigative Medicine*, 47 (5), 222–226.

Sothern, M., von Almen, T. K., Schumacher, H. (2001). *Trim Kids: The Proven Plan That Has Helped Thousands of Children Achieve a Healthier Weight*. New York, NY: HarperCollins.

Steinberger, J., Jacobs, D., Raatz, S., Moran, A., Hong, C., Sinaiko, A. (2005). Comparison of body fatness measurements by BMI and skinfolds vs dual energy X-ray absorptiometry and their relation of cardiovascular risk factors in adolescents. *International Journal of Obesity (London)*, 29(11), 1346–1352.

Swain, K., Rosenkranz, S., Beckman, B., Harms, C. (2010). Expiratory flow limitation during exercise in prepubescent boys and girls: prevalence and implications. *Journal of Applied Physiology*, 108, 1267–1274.

Taylor, R., Williams, S., Grant, A., Ferguson, E., Taylor, B., Goulding, A. (2008). Waist circumference as a measure of trunk fat mass in children aged 3 to 5 years. *International Journal of Pediatric Obesity*, 3(4), 226–233.

Thompson, W., Bushman, B., Desch, J., Kravitz, L. (2010). *ACSM's Resources for the Personal Trainer* (3rd ed.). Philadelphia, PA: Lippincott Williams & Wilkins.

Treuth, M. S., Schmitz, K., Catallier, D. J., McMurray, D. M., Aleida, M. J., Going, S., Normna, J. E., Pate, R. (2004). Defining accelerometer thresholds for activity intensities in adolescent girls. *Medicine and Science in Sports and Exercise*, 36(7), 1259–1266.

Ulrich, D. A. (2000). *Test of Gross Motor Development II: Examiner's Manual*. Austin, TX: Pro-Ed.

von Almen, T. K., Sothern, M., Schumacher, H. (2006). Inter-disciplinary, interactive, group instruction. In M. Sothern, S. Gordon, T. K. von Almen (Eds.), *Handbook of Pediatric Obesity: Clinical Management*. Boca Raton, FL: Taylor & Francis.

Chapter 9

WHAT TO EXPECT

Regular physical activity is shown to lessen the burden of obesity-related comorbidities, including reductions in blood pressure, an increase in insulin sensitivity, and a decrease in hepatomegaly (Hassink et al., 2008; Martinez-Gomez et al., 2009; Shaibi et al., 2009; Sothern, 2004; Sothern et al., 1999a). Vigorous, intermittent physical activity is shown to reduce components of the metabolic syndrome in prepubertal children (Barbeau et al., 2007; Ben Ounis et al., 2010; Brambilla, Pozzobon, & Pietrobelli, 2011; Fedewa et al., 2013; Kahle et al., 1996; Nassis et al., 2005; Shaibi et al., 2006; Yu et al., 2005). Moreover, physical activity improves metabolic health in obese youth independent of adiposity change (Shaibi et al., 2009). Significant improvements in body composition are associated with exercise programs, including low- to moderate-intensity aerobic and high-repetition strength training (LeMura & Maziekas, 2002). Regular physical activity reduces depression and improves mental health (Pretty et al., 2005), and childhood obesity is associated with depression (Erickson et al., 2000). Developmentally appropriate physical activity improves motor performance (Ildiko et al., 2007) and cognition (Bergen, 2002) in youth, and regular aerobic exercise improves cognitive and function in overweight children (Davis et al., 2007; Davis et al., 2011). Regular participation in exercise reduces inflammatory cytokines (Radak, Chung, & Goto, 2008), and childhood obesity is associated with inflammation and asthma (Arshi et al., 2010; Goran & Sothern, 2005). Chronic exercise training increases skeletal muscle glycogen content and enhances fat oxidation, thus promoting fat as a fuel source over carbohydrates (Pedersen & Fischer, 2007; Tompkins et al., 2009). Furthermore, physical activity lifestyle changes positively alter satiety factors in youth (Balagopal et al., 2010). In contrast to these outcomes of regular physical activity, chronic sustained periods of muscular unloading (sitting, lying) reduce contractile stimulation and suppress muscle lipoprotein lipase activity, triglyceride and glucose uptake, and high-density lipoproteins production (Bey & Hamilton, 2003; Thomas et al., 2005).

METABOLIC HEALTH OUTCOMES AFTER PHYSICAL ACTIVITY AND EXERCISE TRAINING

The impact of physical activity on metabolic health depends on the type, intensity, and volume of activity pursued by the individual. It also depends on the genetic potential, gender and age, health, and current training status of the individual (Sothern, 2003, 2004; Sothern et al., 1999a). There is both an acute and chronic response of physical activity on metabolism. During an acute bout of exercise, metabolism is increased (1) during the actual physical activity, (2) immediately after the physical activity, (3) and for hours following physical activity (Hunter et al., 2006; Sothern, 2001; Wilmore & Costill, 1994). The prolonged impact of physical activity depends on the training status of the individual, the intensity of the exercise, and the duration of the exercise. Concerning the chronic response of physical activity, long-term exercise training is shown in numerous studies to (1) increase fat-free mass and reduce fat mass (Ballor & Keesey, 1991; Dao et al., 2004; Ildiko et al., 2007; Stiegler & Cunliffe, 2006; Yu et al., 2005) and visceral adipose tissue (Gutin et al., 2000), (2) improve oxidative capacity (Carter, Rennie, & Tarnopolsky, 2001), (3) increase resting metabolism (Haddock & Wilkin, 2006; Sothern et al., 1999b; Sothern, Loftin, Suskind, et al., 1999), (4) increase fat oxidation (Horowitz, 2001; Kanaley et al., 2001; Pedersen & Fischer, 2007; Talanian et al., 2007), (5) improve insulin sensitivity (Bell et al., 2007; Carrel et al., 2005; Fedewa et al., 2013; Nassis et al., 2005; Shaibi et al., 2006; Tompkins et al., 2009), and (6) control low-grade systemic inflammation (Stewart et al., 2007).

Key Points: Factors That Affect the Individual Response to Physical Activity

Genetic potential is complex and determined by many factors, such as the following:

- Mitochondria size and number
- Muscle fiber type

- Age and gender
- Health and medical history
- Current training status
  - Sedentary
  - Trained (specificity)

The genetic potential is complex and is determined by many factors. One of these factors, muscle fiber type, will determine each individual's response to varied exercise modalities (Sothern, 2001; Sothern, von Almen, & Schumacher, 2001). Muscle fibers within each body type generally are classified as slow twitch or fast twitch (Table 9.1). The percentage of each is determined genetically. Those with more slow-twitch muscles are better equipped to partake in moderate- to vigorous-intensity, long-duration exercises, such as basketball and soccer. Those with more fast-twitch muscles are well suited to high-intensity short-duration exercises, such as wrestling and power lifting. People with an equal number of both slow-twitch and fast-twitch fibers typically excel at middle-distance or moderate-intensity events, although they typically are competent in all types of sports or activities.

EXERCISE TRAINING AND FAT OXIDATION

The benefits of chronic exercise training to the ability of the body to use fat as a fuel (e.g., fat oxidation) are numerous. Endurance-trained muscle stores more glycogen and fat than untrained muscle (Byrne & Wilmore, 2001). In addition, as exercise training is continued, oxidative enzyme activity and free fatty acid levels increase (Hurley & Hagberg, 1998; Kelley et al., 1999). Over time, there is an increased use of fat as an energy source and a sparing of muscle and liver glycogen (Pedersen & Fischer, 2007; Talanian et al., 2007). Eventually, after 6–8 weeks of consistent exercise training, the lactate threshold increases, reflecting an improved ability to perform exercise aerobically at higher intensities (Tonkonogi et al., 2000). Once an individual reaches this status, fitness levels will be maintained as long as the training remains consistent.

Key Points: Reaching Genetic Potential

In formerly sedentary individuals, after consistent training, the following improvements in fitness may be expected:

Training Duration (weeks)	Percent Improvement in Fitness
6–12	~ 25%
12–24	~ 50%
24–36	~ 75%
36–52	~ 100%

After 1 year of consistent training, untrained individuals may reach their individual genetic potential.

Table 9.1   Classification of Muscle Fiber Types

Characteristic	Slow-twitch Type I	Fast-twitch (a) Type IIa	Fast-twitch (b) Type IIb
Aerobic capacity	High	Moderate	Low
Anaerobic capacity	Low	High	Highest
Oxidation	High	Moderate	Low
Glycolysis	Low	High	Highest
Force/size	Low	High	Highest
Fatigue time	Low	High	Highest

Source: From Sothern, M. S., *Pediatric Clinics of North America*, 48(4), 995–1015, 2001; Wilmore, J. H., Costill, D. L., *Physiology of Sport and Exercise*, Human Kinetics, Champaign, IL, 1994.

If training is discontinued, however, these improvements in metabolism, body composition, aerobic fitness, and muscular strength and endurance will begin to decline (Mujika & Padilla, 2000; Wilmore & Costill, 1994). Typically, strength gains will begin to deteriorate within a few days with approximately 3–4% reduction each day. To accompany this decline, the size and number of slow-twitch fibers, which are recruited for endurance-type activities, will be reduced as the muscles of the body atrophy. Fortunately, however, the ability of the muscles to perform endurance activities and the related oxidative enzyme activity does not begin to decline until 2 weeks after training ceases. This is closely followed by an increase in the respiratory quotient, indicating that the body is preferentially utilizing carbohydrates over fat fuel stores, an indication that fat oxidation is lower. After 4 weeks of detraining, muscle glycogen stored in the muscles with be reduced by approximately 40% (Wilmore & Costill, 1994).

Key Points: Move It or Lose It

- The effect of chronic exercise is reversed if training ceases:
  - Protein synthesis ↓ within 6 hours
  - Strength ↓ 3–4% per day.
  - Area and percentage of slow twitch fibers ↓ as muscles atrophy
  - Muscle endurance performance and oxidative enzyme activity ↓ after 2 weeks.
  - Respiratory quotient (RQ) ↑
  - Muscle glycogen ↓ 40% after 4 weeks

Sources: Adapted from Mujika & Padilla, 2000; Wilmore & Costill, 1994.

COGNITIVE, EMOTIONAL, AND PHYSICAL HEALTH OUTCOMES OF REGULAR PHYSICAL ACTIVITY

Physical fitness in youth is associated with better cognitive functioning and improved academic performance (Castelli et al., 2007; Davis et al., 2007, 2011; Grissom, 2005; London & Castrechini, 2011). In younger children, unstructured playtime promotes increased cognitive abilities (Bergen, 2002). And, during active play, which is typically vigorous, intermittent physical activity is shown to reduce components of the metabolic syndrome in prepubertal children (Barbeau et al., 2007; Kahle et al., 1996; Nassis et al., 2005; Yu et al., 2005). There are numerous positive physical and emotional outcomes to engaging in physical activity outdoors (Kuo & Taylor, 2004; Pretty et al., 2005; Taylor & Kuo, 2009). Time outdoors is associated with greater physical activity and lower overweight prevalence in 10- to 12-year-old girls and boys (Cleland et al., 2008). In addition, children who play outdoors less than 30 minutes per day or watch more than 2.5 hours per day of television are more likely to have vitamin D insufficiency (Absoud et al., 2011; Ganji et al., 2011; Ly et al., 2011). Vitamin D levels are shown to be insufficient in 35% of children 4–18 years of age. Vitamin D is associated with childhood obesity, insulin resistance, high cholesterol, and high blood pressure. Thus, one additional positive outcome to participation in outdoor play is the positive impact on vitamin D insufficiency.

Key Points: Benefits of Outdoor Play in Nature

There are many additional benefits of engaging in outdoor play in nature:

- Promotes creativity and imagination while building dexterity and physical strength
- Encourages healthy brain development
- Improves self-advocacy skills
- Improves social skills: working in groups, sharing, negotiating, resolving conflicts
- Improves symptoms of attention deficit–hyperactivity disorder
- Improves well-being and problem solving

Sources: Adapted from Brender, Burke, & Glass, 2005; Ginsburg et al., 2007; Kuo & Taylor, 2004; Taylor & Kuo, 2009.

Imaginative play is shown to improve social cognition, increase inventiveness, enhance language development, encourage the use of symbols, improve comprehension skills, and provide opportunities for children to imitate and interpret adult behavior (Bergen, 2002; Guddemi & Eriksen, 1992; Perry, 2003; Singer & Singer, 2000). Furthermore, recent research also indicates that sedentary school time is associated with increased symptoms of attention deficit–hyperactivity disorder (ADHD) (Tsujii et al., 2007), and before school physical activity is shown to reduce ADHD symptoms and improve cognitive, motor, social, and behavioral functioning in kindergarten through third-grade students with ADHD (Smith et al., 2011). Thus, after increasing daily developmentally appropriate physical activity, children will experience numerous positive outcomes relating to improved academic school performance, social functioning, and self-advocacy, in addition to cardiopulmonary and metabolic health improvements.

BIOCHEMICAL, ANTHROPOMETRIC, BEHAVIORAL, AND FITNESS OUTCOMES RELATED TO PHYSICAL ACTIVITY

In overweight and obese children when physical activity is combined with diet and behavioral counseling, the following short-term outcomes are observed:

- Reduced percent fat
- Maintenance of resting energy expenditure
- Improved relative fitness
- Reduced total cholesterol and LDL
- Maintained growth velocity
- Decreased insulin resistance
- Decreased leptin
- Decreased estradiol

(Brown et al., 2000; Dao et al., 2004; Eisenmann et al., 2011; Escobar et al., 1999; Savoye et al., 2007; Sothern, Gordon, & von Almen, 2006; Sothern, Despeney, Brown, et al., 2000; Sothern & Gordon, 2005; Sothern, Loftin, Suskind, et al., 1999; Sothern, Udall, Suskind, et al., 2000; U.S. Preventive Services Task Force, 2010).

There are few long-term weight loss trials in overweight and obese children. Of these, data demonstrate maintenance of weight loss 5 and 10 years later (Position of the American Dietetic Association, 2006).

Research examining the independent contribution of aerobic or resistance exercise to improved weight status and metabolic health in numerous studies demonstrates improved health outcomes (VanVrancken-Tompkins, Sothern, & Bar-Or, 2006; Tables 9.2 and 9.3).

In particular, frequent vigorous exercise periods are shown to be associated with decreased abdominal fat in youth (Barbeau et al., 2007). In children with diabetes, physical activity may

Table 9.2 Results of Long-Term Childhood Obesity Studies

Authors	Age (years)	Intervention	Outcome
Epstein et al., 1990	6–12	Parent–child	−19.7% @ 10 years
Braet, Van Winckel, & Van Leeuwen, 1997	9–12	Behavioral vs. advice	−17.3% @ 4.5 years
Nuutinen & Knip, 1992	6–15	Group vs. individual	−11.7% @ 5 years
Epstein et al., 1990	6–12	Parental obesity	NS @ 10 years
Epstein, 1993	6–12	Exercise + diet	NS @ 10 years
Epstein et al., 1994	6–12	Lifestyle exercise	−15.3% @ 10 years

Note: NS = nonsignificant change.

Table 9.3 Effects of Strength and Aerobic Training in Short-Term Studies on Health Outcomes

• Percent fat	↓	
• Bone mineral density	↑	
• Visceral adipose tissue	↓	
• Oxygen uptake (VO$_2$): relative/kg		↑
• Total cholesterol and LDL		↓
• Insulin sensitivity		↑
• Insulin resistance		↓
• Strength (1RM)	↑	
• Cardiovascular fitness		↑
• Fat oxidation and HDL		↑

Sources: Adapted from Barbeau, P., et al., *Obesity (Silver Spring, Md.)*, 15(8), 2077–2085, 2007; Ben Ounis et al., *Acta Paediatrica*, 99(11), 1679–1685, 2010; Dao, H. H., et al., *International Journal of Obesity and Related Metabolic Disorders*, 28(2), 290–299, 2004; Shaibi, G. Q., et al., *Medicine and Science in Sports and Exercise*, 38(7), 1208–1215, 2006; Sothern, M. S., Gordon, S. T., von Almen, T. K., *Handbook of Pediatric Obesity: Clinical Management*, Taylor & Francis, Boca Raton, FL, 2006; Yu, C. C., et al., *Journal of Strength and Conditioning Research*, 19(3), 667–672, 2005.
Note: 1RM = one-repetition maximum; HDL = high-density lipoprotein; LDL = low-density lipoprotein

improve insulin sensitivity and glucose uptake in skeletal muscle (Fedewa et al., 2013; Tompkins et al., 2009). Aerobic-based physical activity lasting 40–60 minutes daily for a minimum of 4 months is shown to enhance insulin sensitivity, and this may reduce the risk for type 2 diabetes (Fedewa et al., 2013; Tompkins et al., 2009). Resistance training may increase skeletal muscle mass, therefore increasing whole-body glucose disposal capacity. A 16-week resistance-training program significantly increased insulin sensitivity in overweight Latino adolescent males at risk for type 2 diabetes. Overweight Latino adolescent males (N = 22) were randomly assigned to 2-week resistance training (RT = 11) or a nonexercising control (C = 11) for 16 weeks. Strength was assessed by one-repetition maximum (1RM), lean and fat mass by dual-energy x-ray absorptiometry (DEXA), and insulin sensitivity by the frequently sampled intravenous glucose tolerance test with minimal modeling. Significant increases were found in strength (p < .05) and insulin sensitivity in the RT compared with the C group (45.1±7.3% in the RT group vs. −0.9±12.9% in controls [p < .01]). Results remained significant after adjusting for fat and lean mass (p < .05) (Shaibi et al., 2006). In another study, strength training was shown to improve lean muscle and bone mineral content. Obese, prepubertal children around 10 years old were randomized to (1) diet alone (n = 41; the control group) or (2) diet plus strength training (n = 41; the training group). The training group participated in 75-minute strength exercises three times each week. After 6 weeks, the children in the training group showed significantly larger increases in (1) lean body mass (+0.8 kg [2.4%] vs. +0.3 kg [1.0%], p < .05) than the control group, and (2) total bone mineral content (+46.9 g [3.9%] vs. +33.6 g [2.9%], p < .05) than the control group (Yu et al., 2005).

CURRENT U.S. EVIDENCE-BASED RECOMMENDATIONS FOR PHYSICAL ACTIVITY

EVIDENCE-BASED RECOMMENDATIONS FOR PHYSICAL ACTIVITY IN SCHOOL-AGE YOUTH

A panel of experts convened under a contract with the Divisions of Nutrition and Physical Activity and Adolescent and School Health of the Centers for Disease Control and

Prevention to review and evaluate existing evidence on the influence of physical activity on several health and behavior outcomes in youth. They concluded that data were strong for beneficial effects of physical activity on musculoskeletal health, several components of cardiovascular health, adiposity in overweight youth, and blood pressure (Strong et al., 2005). The U.S. Department of Health and Human Services (U.S. DHHS, 2008) identified physical activity as a means to reduce anxiety and depression as well as promote positive mental health, improve concentration, memory, and classroom behavior. The U.S. DHHS recommends that children and adolescents should do 60 minutes or more of physical activity daily. The majority of the 60 minutes or more should be either moderate- or vigorous-intensity aerobic physical activity and should include vigorous activity at least 3 days a week. Furthermore, muscle strengthening and bone strengthening should be included in the 60 minutes or more at least 3 days a week. It also recognized that it is important to encourage young people to participate in physical activities that are age appropriate, enjoyable, and offer variety (U.S. DHHS, 2008).

Key Points: U.S. Recommendations for Physical Activity in Youth

School-age youth should participate daily in 60 minutes or more of moderate- to vigorous-intensity physical activity that is developmentally appropriate, is enjoyable, and involves a variety of activities.

Sources: Adapted from Strong et al., 2005; U.S. DHHS, 2008.

During the preschool years, general movement activities, such as jumping, throwing, running, climbing, are recommended. Before entering puberty (6–9 years), children should engage in more specialized and complex movements and anaerobic activities, such as tag, games, and recreational sports. Once the child enters puberty (10–14 years), he or she may participate in organized sports and other activities that provide skill development. Adolescents (15–18 years) are able to participate in more structured health and fitness activities, which will promote the refinement of skills (Strong et al., 2005; U.S. DHHS, 2008). Following are the minimum recommendations for intensity, duration, and frequency for school-age youth:

Key Points: Evidence-Based Recommendations for Physical Activity in School-Age Youth

Intensity: 5–8 metabolic equivalents (moderate to vigorous) are needed to derive the most health benefits, such as active outdoor play, brisk walking, or cycling

Duration: 60 minutes per day; cumulative, not necessarily sustained

Frequency: daily

Sources: Adapted from Strong et al., 2005; U.S. DHHS, 2008.

RECOMMENDATIONS FOR OUTDOOR PLAY
The American Academy of Pediatrics recommends more outdoor play to achieve the following:

- Promote healthy emotional and physical development
- Increase vitamin D levels
- Replace screen time indoors
- Increase overall physical activity
- Reduce the risk of attention problems

(Christakis et al., 2004; Ginsburg, American Academy of Pediatrics Committee on Communications, & American Academy of Pediatrics Committee on Psychosocial Aspects of Child and Family Health, 2007).

The most successful outdoor play experiences involve the child's free choice, which is self-motivated, enjoyable, and process oriented. Natural experiences, such as collecting leaves, throwing stones in a pond, jumping over small brush or logs, and building sandcastles, challenge the child's imagination and reasoning abilities (Clements, 2004; Sothern et al., 2001, 2006).

EVIDENCE-BASED RECOMMENDATIONS FOR PHYSICAL ACTIVITY: PHYSICALLY INACTIVE SCHOOL-AGE YOUTH

Strong et al. (2005) and the U.S. DHHS (2008) have recommended that physically inactive children and adolescents take an incremental approach to reach the 60 minutes per day recommendation, increasing overall physical activity by 10% each week. Progressing too quickly may be counterproductive and could lead to injury. The American Heart Association (Daniels et al., , 2009) has recommended that overweight children be given realistic, easily obtainable physical activity goals and should not be compared with normal weight peers. In addition, exercise prescriptions for obese children should involve family support as well as activities that are doable, are fun, and develop participatory skills (Hassink et al., 2008).

SUMMARY OF EVIDENCE-BASED STUDIES INCLUDING EXERCISE IN OVERWEIGHT CHILDREN

On the basis of the summary of evidence, following are recommendations for future research:

- Sufficient research is needed to routinely recommend exercise in combination with diet and behavioral counseling.
- More research is needed to support recommending exercise alone.
- More research is needed to support reducing sedentary behaviors as opposed to increasing physical activity.

(American Dietetic Association, 2006; Eisenmann, 2011; Kitzmann et al., 2010).

According to the U.S. Preventive Services Task Force (2010), there is adequate evidence for multicomponent, moderate- to high-intensity behavioral interventions for obese children ages 6 years and older. Multicomponent interventions include dietary, physical activity, and behavioral counseling. Research confirms that there is adequate evidence that potential harms resulting from these mulitcomponent behavioral interventions are small. Furthermore, the American Heart Association (2009) has suggested that the complex and multiple factors causing pediatric obesity warrant a multidisciplinary, collaborative approach, which will engage professionals across multiple disciplines. Furthermore, the association has proposed that a national effort is warranted, including research, health, advocacy, education, media, and consumer advertising.

LIFESTYLE RECOMMENDATIONS BY WEIGHT CLASSIFICATION

The following lifestyle recommendations for the management of obesity are classified by weight in youth ages 7–18 years (Tables 9.4–9.7).

Table 9.4 Recommendations for Healthy Weight Youth

Weight classification	Healthy weight (5th–84th percentile BMI)
Level of behavioral treatment	Receive support in maintaining or establishing healthy lifestyle (prevention) behaviors
Dietary counseling	Family nutrition education and parent training emphasizing appropriate food portions, reduced sugar and saturated fat, increased fruits and vegetables, and recommended dairy and fiber intake
Physical activity	Limit screen time; recommended physical activity requirements: 60 minutes of daily moderate to vigorous physical activity (3 days per week of vigorous activity) and bone- and muscle-strengthening activities

Sources: Adapted from Barlow, *Pediatrics*, 120(Suppl 4), S164–S192, 2007; Sothern, Gordon, & von Almen, *Handbook of Pediatric Obesity*, Taylor & Francis, Boca Raton, FL, 2006.
Note: Guidelines should be readjusted every 10–15 weeks based on evaluation results.

Table 9.5   Recommendations for Overweight Youth

Weight classification	Overweight (85th–94th percentile BMI)
Level of behavioral treatment	Some children should receive prevention counseling (if no evidence of health risk), whereas others (evidence of health risk) should receive more-active interventions
Dietary counseling	Family nutrition education and parent training in combination with portion control methods or balanced calorie meal plans emphasizing appropriate food portions, reduced sugar and saturated fat, increased fruits and vegetables, and recommended dairy and fiber intake
Physical activity	Limit screen time; incremental approach to increase physical activity volume; weight-bearing aerobic activities (e.g., field sports, tennis, jump rope); pacing skills; parent training; fitness education

Sources: Adapted from Barlow, *Pediatrics*, 120(Suppl 4), S164–S192, 2007; Sothern, Gordon, & von Almen, *Handbook of Pediatric Obesity*, Taylor & Francis, Boca Raton, FL, 2006.
Note: Guidelines should be readjusted every 10–15 weeks based on evaluation results.

Table 9.6   Recommendations for Obese Youth

Weight classification	Obese (≥95th percentile BMI)
Level of behavioral treatment	Most children considered obese should be advised to focus on weight control practices
Dietary counseling	Family nutrition education and parent training in combination with balanced hypocaloric diets emphasizing appropriate food portions, reduced sugar and saturated fat, increased fruits and vegetables, recommended dairy and fiber intake, and low–glycemic index diet
Physical activity	Limit screen time; incremental approach to increase physical activity volume; alternate between weight-bearing and non-weight-bearing activities (e.g., swimming, cycling, seated or lying circuit training); parent training; fitness education

Sources: Adapted from Barlow, *Pediatrics*, 120(Suppl 4), S164–S192, 2007; Sothern, Gordon, & von Almen, *Handbook of Pediatric Obesity*, Taylor & Francis, Boca Raton, FL, 2006.
Note: Guidelines should be readjusted every 10–15 weeks based on evaluation results.

Table 9.7   Recommendations for Severely Obese Youth

Weight classification	Severely obese (>120% of 95th BMI or absolute BMI >35 kg/m²)
Level of behavioral treatment	Other emotional and dietary concerns must be addressed
Dietary counseling	Family nutrition education and parent training in combination with altered macronutrient dietary approaches as follows: low–glycemic index diet, Atkins diet, protein modified fast diet followed by balanced hypocaloric diet
Physical activity	Limit screen time; incremental approach to increase physical activity volume; non-weight-bearing activities (e.g., swimming, cycling, seated or lying circuit training); parent training; fitness education

Sources: Adapted from Barlow, *Pediatrics*, 120(Suppl 4), S164–S192, 2007; Kelly et al., *Circulation*, 128(15), 1689–1712; Sothern, Gordon, & von Almen, *Handbook of Pediatric Obesity*, Taylor & Francis, Boca Raton, FL, 2006.
Note: Guidelines should be readjusted every 10–15 weeks based on evaluation results.

Absoud, M., Cummins, C., Lim, M. J., Wassmer, E., Shaw, N. (2011). Prevalence and predictors of vitamin D insufficiency in children: A Great Britain population based study. *PloS One*, 6(7), e22179.

American Dietetic Association. (2006). Position of the American Dietetic Association: Individual-, family-, school-, and community-based interventions for pediatric overweight. *Journal of the American Dietetic Association*, 106(6), 925–945.

Arshi, M., Cardinal, J., Hill, R. J., Davies, P. S., Wainwright, C. (2010). Asthma and insulin resistance in children. *Respirology*, 15(5), 779–784.

Balagopal, P. B., Gidding, S. S., Buckloh, L. M., Yarandi, H. N., Sylvester, J. E., George, D. E., et al. (2010). Changes in circulating satiety hormones in obese children: A randomized controlled physical activity-based intervention study. *Obesity*, 18(9), 1747–1753.

Ballor, D. L., Keesey, R. E. (1991). A meta-analysis of the factors affecting exercise-induced changes in body mass, fat mass and fat-free mass in males and females. *International Journal of Obesity*, 15(11), 717–726.

Barbeau, P., Johnson, M. H., Howe, C. A., Allison, J., Davis, C. L., Gutin, B., et al. (2007). Ten months of exercise improves general and visceral adiposity, bone, and fitness in black girls. *Obesity (Silver Spring, Md.)*, 15(8), 2077–2085.

Barlow, S. (2007). Expert Committee recommendations regarding the prevention, assessment and treatment of child and adolescent overweight and obesity: Summary report. *Pediatrics*, 120(Suppl 4), S164–S192.

Bell, L. M., Watts, K., Siafarikas, A., Thompson, A., Ratnam, N., Bulsara, M., et al. (2007). Exercise alone reduces insulin resistance in obese children independently of changes in body composition. *Journal of Clinical Endocrinology and Metabolism*, 92(11), 4230–4235.

Ben Ounis, O., Elloumi, M., Makni, E., Zouhal, H., Amri, M., Tabka, Z., et al. (2010). Exercise improves the ApoB/ApoA-I ratio, a marker of the metabolic syndrome in obese children. *Acta Paediatrica*, 99(11), 1679–1685.

Bergen, D. (2002). The role of pretend play in children's cognitive development. *Early Childhood Research and Practice*, 4(1), 13.

Bey, L., Hamilton, M. T. (2003). Suppression of skeletal muscle lipoprotein lipase activity during physical inactivity: A molecular reason to maintain daily low-intensity activity. *Journal of Physiology*, 551(Pt 2), 673–682.

Brambilla, P., Pozzobon, G., Pietrobelli, A. (2011). Physical activity as the main therapeutic tool for metabolic syndrome in childhood. *International Journal of Obesity* (2005), 35(1), 16–28.

Brender, E., Burke, A., Glass, R. M. (2005). JAMA patient page: Vitamin D. *JAMA*, 294(18), 2386.

Brown, R., Sothern, M., Suskind, R., Udall, J., Blecker U. (2000). Racial differences in the lipid profiles of obese children and adolescents before and after significant weight loss. *Clinical Pediatrics*, 39, 427–431.

Byrne, H. K., Wilmore, J. H. (2001). The relationship of mode and intensity of training on resting metabolic rate in women. *International Journal of Sport Nutrition and Exercise Metabolism*, 11(1), 1–14.

Carrel, A. L., Clark, R. R., Peterson, S. E., Nemeth, B. A., Sullivan, J., Allen, D. B. (2005). Improvement of fitness, body composition, and insulin sensitivity in overweight children in a school-based exercise program: A randomized, controlled study. *Archives of Pediatrics and Adolescent Medicine*, 159(10), 963–968.

Carter, S. L., Rennie, C., Tarnopolsky, M. A. (2001). Substrate utilization during endurance exercise in men and women after endurance training. *American Journal of Physiology, Endocrinology, and Metabolism*, 280(6), E898–E907.

Castelli, D. M., Hillman, C. H., Buck, S. M., Erwin, H. E. (2007). Physical fitness and academic achievement in third- and fifth-grade students. *Journal of Sport and Exercise Psychology*, 29(2), 239–252.

Christakis, D. A., Ebel, B. E., Rivara, F. P., Zimmerman, F. J. (2004). Television, video, and computer game usage in children under 11 years of age. *Journal of Pediatrics*, 145(5), 652–656.

Cleland, V., Crawford, D., Baur, L. A., Hume, C., Timperio, A., Salmon, J. (2008). A prospective examination of children's time spent outdoors, objectively measured physical activity and overweight. *International Journal of Obesity*, 32(11), 1685–1693.

Clements, R. (2004). An investigation of the status of outdoor play. *Contemporary Issues in Early Childhood*, 5(1), 68–80.

Daniels, S. R., Jacobson, M. S., McCrindle, B. W., Eckel, R. H., Sanner, B. M. (2009). American Heart Association childhood obesity research summit: Executive summary. *Circulation*, 119(15), 2114–2123.

Dao, H. H., Frelut, M. L., Oberlin, F., Peres, G., Bourgeois, P., Navarro, J. (2004). Effects of a multidisciplinary weight loss intervention on body composition in obese adolescents. *International Journal of Obesity and Related Metabolic Disorders*, 28(2), 290–299.

Davis, C. L., Tomporowski, P. D., Boyle, C. A., Waller, J. L., Miller, P. H., Naglieri, J. A., et al. (2007). Effects of aerobic exercise on overweight children's cognitive functioning: A randomized controlled trial. *Research Quarterly for Exercise and Sport*, 78(5), 510–519.

Davis, C. L., Tomporowski, P. D., McDowell, J. E., Austin, B. P., Miller, P. H., Yanasak, N. E., et al. (2011). Exercise improves executive function and achievement and alters brain activation in overweight children: A randomized, controlled trial. *Health Psychology*, 30(1), 91–98.

Donnelly, J. E., Lambourne, K. (2011). Classroom-based physical activity, cognition, and academic achievement. *Preventive Medicine*, 52(Suppl 1), S36–S42.

Eisenmann, J. C.; for the Subcommittee on Assessment in Pediatric Obesity Management Programs, National Association of Children's Hospital and Related Institutions (2011). Assessment of obese children and adolescents: A survey of pediatric obesity-management programs. *Pediatrics*, 129(Suppl 2), S51–S58.

Epstein, L. H. (1993). Methodological issues and ten-year outcomes for obese children. *Annals of the New York Academy of Science*, 13, 237–249.

Epstein, L. H., Valoski, A., Wing, R. R., McCurley, J. (1990). Ten-year follow-up of behavioral, family-based treatment for obese children. *JAMA*, 264(19), 2519–2523.

Epstein, L. H., Valoski, A., Wing, R. R., McCurley, J. (1994). Ten-year outcomes of behavioral family-based treatment for childhood obesity. *Health Psychology*, 13(5), 373–383.

Erickson, S. J., Robinson, T. N., Haydel, K. F., Killen, J. D. (2000). Are overweight children unhappy? Body mass index, depressive symptoms, and overweight concerns in elementary school children. *Archives of Pediatrics and Adolescent Medicine*, 154(9), 931–935.

Escobar, O., Mizuma, H., Sothern, M., Blecker, U., Udall, J., Suskind R., Hilton, C., Vargas, A. (1999). Hepatic insulin clearance increases after natural weight loss in obese children and adolescents. *American Journal of the Medical Sciences*, 317(5), 282–286.

Fedewa, M., Gist, N., Evans, E., Dishman, R. (2013). Exercise and insulin resistance in youth: A meta-analysis. *Pediatrics*, 133(1), 1–12.

Ganji, V., Zhang, X., Shaikh, N., Tangpricha, V. (2011). Serum 25-hydroxyvitamin D concentrations are associated with prevalence of metabolic syndrome and various cardiometabolic risk factors in U.S. children and adolescents based on assay-adjusted serum 25-hydroxyvitamin D data from NHANES 2001-2006. *American Journal of Clinical Nutrition*, 94(1), 225–233.

Ginsburg, K. R., American Academy of Pediatrics Committee on Communications, American Academy of Pediatrics Committee on Psychosocial Aspects of Child and Family Health. (2007). The importance of play in promoting healthy child development and maintaining strong parent-child bonds. *Pediatrics*, 119(1), 182–191.

Goran, M., Sothern, M. (Eds.). (2005). *Handbook of Pediatric Obesity: Etiology, Pathophysiology, and Prevention*. Boca Raton, FL: Taylor & Francis.

Grissom, J. (2005). Physical fitness and academic achievement. *Journal of Exercise Physiology*, 8, 11–25.

Guddemi, M., Eriksen, A. (1992). Designing outdoor learning environments for and with children. *Dimensions of Early Childhood*, 20(4), 15–24.

Gutin, B., Barbeau, P., Litaker, M. S., Ferguson, M., Owens, S. (2000). Heart rate variability in obese children: Relations to total body and visceral adiposity, and changes with physical training and detraining. *Obesity Research*, 8(1), 12–19.

Haddock, B. L., Wilkin, L. D. (2006). Resistance training volume and post exercise energy expenditure. *International Journal of Sports Medicine*, 27(2), 143–148.

Hassink, S. G., Zapalla, F., Falini, L., Datto, G. (2008). Exercise and the obese child. *Progress in Pediatric Cardiology*, 25(2), 153–157.

Horowitz, J. F. (2001). Regulation of lipid mobilization and oxidation during exercise in obesity. *Exercise and Sport Sciences Reviews*, 29(1), 42–46.

Hunter, G. R., Byrne, N. M., Gower, B. A., Sirikul, B., Hills, A. P. (2006). Increased resting energy expenditure after 40 minutes of aerobic but not resistance exercise. *Obesity (Silver Spring, Md.)*, 14(11), 2018–2025.

Ildiko, V., Zsofia, M., Janos, M., Andreas, P., Dora, N. E., Andras, P., et al. (2007). Activity-related changes of body fat and motor performance in obese seven-year-old boys. *Journal of Physiological Anthropology*, 26(3), 333–337.

Kahle, E. B., Zipf, W. B., Lamb, D. R., Horswill, C. A., Ward, K. M. (1996). Association between mild, routine exercise and improved insulin dynamics and glucose control in obese adolescents. *International Journal of Sports Medicine*, 17(1), 1–6.

Kanaley, J. A., Weatherup-Dentes, M. M., Alvarado, C. R., Whitehead, G. (2001). Substrate oxidation during acute exercise and with exercise training in lean and obese women. *European Journal of Applied Physiology*, 85(1-2), 68–73.

Kelley, D. E., Goodpaster, B., Wing, R. R., Simoneau, J. A. (1999). Skeletal muscle fatty acid metabolism in association with insulin resistance, obesity, and weight loss. *American Journal of Physiology*, 277(6 Pt 1), E1130–E1141.

Kelly, A. S., Barlow, S. E., Rao, G., Inge, T. H., Hayman, L. L., Steinberger, J., et al. (2013). Severe obesity in children and adolescents: Identification, associated health risks, and treatment approaches—A scientific statement from the American Heart Association. *Circulation*, 128(15), 1689–1712.

Kitzmann, K. M., Dalton, W. T., III, Stanley, C. M., Beech, B. M., Reeves, T. P., Buscemi, J., et al. (2010). Lifestyle interventions for youth who are overweight: A meta-analytic review. *Health Psychology*, 29(1), 91–101.

Kuo, F. E., Taylor, A. F. (2004). A potential natural treatment for attention-deficit/hyperactivity disorder: Evidence from a national study. *American Journal of Public Health*, 94(9), 1580–1586.

LeMura, L. M., Maziekas, M. T. (2002). Factors that alter body fat, body mass, and fat-free mass in pediatric obesity. *Medicine and Science in Sports and Exercise*, 34(3), 487–496.

London, R. A., Castrechini, S. (2011). A longitudinal examination of the link between youth physical fitness and academic achievement. *Journal of School Health*, 81(7), 400–408.

Ly, N. P., Litonjua, A., Gold, D. R., Celedon, J. C. (2011). Gut microbiota, probiotics, and vitamin D: Interrelated exposures influencing allergy, asthma, and obesity? *Journal of Allergy and Clinical Immunology*, 127(5), 1087–1096.

Martinez-Gomez, D., Tucker, J., Heelan, K. A., Welk, G. J., Eisenmann, J. C. (2009). Associations between sedentary behavior and blood pressure in young children. *Archives of Pediatrics and Adolescent Medicine*, 163(8), 724–730.

Mujika, I., Padilla, S. (2000). Detraining: Loss of training-induced physiological and performance adaptations. Part I: Short term insufficient training stimulus. *Sports Medicine*, 30(2), 79–87.

Nassis, G. P., Papantakou, K., Skenderi, K., Triandafillopoulou, M., Kavouras, S. A., Yannakoulia, M., et al. (2005). Aerobic exercise training improves insulin sensitivity without changes in body weight, body fat, adiponectin, and inflammatory markers in overweight and obese girls. *Metabolism*, 54(11), 1472–1479.

Nuutinen, O., Knip, M. (1992). Weight loss, body composition and risk factors for cardiovascular disease in obese children: Long-term effects of two treatment strategies. *Journal of the American College of Nutrition*, 11(6), 707–714.

Pedersen, B., Fischer, C. (2007). Physiological roles of muscle-derived interleukin-6 in response to exercise. *Current Opinion in Clinical Nutrition and Metabolic Care*, 10, 256–271.

Perry, J. (2003). Making sense of outdoor pretend play. *Young Children*, 58(3), 26–30.

Pretty, J., Peacock, J., Sellens, M., Griffin, M. (2005). The mental and physical health outcomes of green exercise. *International Journal of Environmental Health Research*, 15(5), 319–337.

Radak, Z., Chung, H. Y., Goto, S. (2008). Systemic adaptation to oxidative challenge induced by regular exercise. *Free Radical Biology and Medicine*, 44(2), 153–159.

Savoye, M., Shaw, M., Dziura, J., Tamborlane, W. V., Rose, P., Guandalini, C., et al. (2007). Effects of a weight management program on body composition and metabolic parameters in overweight children: A randomized controlled trial. *JAMA*, 297(24), 2697–2704.

Shaibi, G. Q., Cruz, M. L., Ball, G. D., Weigensberg, M. J., Salem, G. J., Crespo, N. C., et al. (2006). Effects of resistance training on insulin sensitivity in overweight Latino adolescent males. *Medicine and Science in Sports and Exercise*, 38(7), 1208–1215.

Shaibi, G. Q., Michaliszyn, S. B., Fritschi, C., Quinn, L., Faulkner, M. S. (2009). Type 2 diabetes in youth: A phenotype of poor cardiorespiratory fitness and low physical activity. *International Journal of Pediatric Obesity*, 4(4), 332–337.

Singer, D., Singer, J. (2000). *Make-Believe Games and Activities for Imaginative Play*. Washington, DC: Magination Press.

Smith, A. L., Hoza, B., Linnea, K., McQuade, J. D., Tomb, M., Vaughn, A. J., et al. (2011). Pilot physical activity intervention reduces severity of ADHD symptoms in young children. *Journal of Attention Disorders*, 17(1), 70–82.

Sothern, M. (2001). Exercise as a modality in the treatment of childhood obesity. *Pediatric Clinics of North America*, 48(4), 995–1015.

Sothern, M. (2004). Obesity prevention in children: Physical activity and nutrition. *Nutrition*, 20 (7-8), 704–708.

Sothern, M., Despeney, B., Brown, R., Suskind, R., Udall, J., Blecker, U. (2000). Lipid profiles of obese children and adolescents before and after significant weight loss: differences according to sex. *Southern Medical Journal*, 93, 278–282.

Sothern, M., Gordon, S. (2003). Prevention of obesity in young children: A critical challenge for the medical professional. *Clinical Pediatrics*, 42(2), 101–111.

Sothern, M., Gordon, S. (2005). Family-based weight management in the pediatric health care setting. *Obesity Management*, 1(5), 197–202.

Sothern, M., Gordon, S., von Almen, K. (2006). *Handbook of Pediatric Obesity: Clinical Management.* Boca Raton, FL: Taylor & Francis.

Sothern, M., Loftin, M., Blecker, M., Suskind R., Udall, J. (1999a). Health benefits of physical activity in children and adolescents: Implications for chronic disease prevention. *European Journal of Pediatrics*, 158, 271–274.

Sothern, M., Loftin, M., Blecker, M., Suskind R., Udall, J. (1999b). Physiologic function and childhood obesity. *International Journal of Pediatrics*, 14(3), 1–5.

Sothern, M., Loftin, M., Suskind, R., Udall, J. (1999). The impact of significant weight loss on resting energy expenditure in obese youth. *Journal of Investigative Medicine*, 47(5), 222–226.

Sothern, M., Udall, J. Suskind, R., Vargas, A., Blecker, U. (2000). Weight loss and growth velocity in obese children after very low calorie diet, exercise and behavior modification. *Acta Paediatrica*, 89(9), 1036–1043.

Sothern, M., von Almen, T. K., Schumacher, H. (2001). *Trim Kids: The Proven Plan That Has Helped Thousands of Children Achieve a Healthier Weight.* New York, NY: HarperCollins.

Sothern, M., von Almen, K., Schumacher, R. D., Suskind, R., Blecker, U. A. (1999). Multidisciplinary approach to the treatment of childhood obesity. *Delaware Medical Journal*, 71(6), 255–261.

Stewart, L. K., Flynn, M. G., Campbell, W. W., Craig, B. A., Robinson, J. P., Timmerman, K. L., et al. (2007). The influence of exercise training on inflammatory cytokines and C-reactive protein. *Medicine and Science in Sports and Exercise*, 39(10), 1714–1719.

Stiegler, P., Cunliffe, A. (2006). The role of diet and exercise for the maintenance of fat-free mass and resting metabolic rate during weight loss. *Sports Medicine (Auckland, N.Z.)*, 36(3), 239–262.

Strong, W. B., Malina, R. M., Blimkie, C. J., Daniels, S. R., Dishman, R. K., Gutin, B., et al. (2005). Evidence based physical activity for school-age youth. *Journal of Pediatrics*, 146(6), 732–737.

Talanian, J. L., Galloway, S. D., Heigenhauser, G. J., Bonen, A., Spriet, L. L. (2007). Two weeks of high-intensity aerobic interval training increases the capacity for fat oxidation during exercise in women. *Journal of Applied Physiology*, 102(4), 1439–1447.

Taylor, A. F., Kuo, F. E. (2009). Children with attention deficits concentrate better after walk in the park. *Journal of Attention Disorders*, 12(5), 402–409.

Tsujii, N., Okada, A., Kaku, R., Kuriki, N., Hanada, K., Matsuo, J., et al. (2007). Association between activity level and situational factors in children with attention deficit/hyperactivity disorder in elementary school. *Psychiatry and Clinical Neurosciences*, 61(2), 181–185.

Tompkins, C., Soros, A., Sothern, M., Vargas, A. (2009). Effects of physical activity on diabetes management and lowering risk for type 2 diabetes. *American Journal of Health Education*, 40(5), 286–290.

U.S. Department of Health and Human Services. (2008). Physical activity guidelines for Americans. Retrieved June 25, 2009, from http://www.health.gov/paguidelines.

U.S. Preventive Services Task Force. (2010). Screening for obesity in children and adolescents: US preventive services task force recommendation statement. *Pediatrics*, 125(2), 361–367.

VanVrancken-Tompkins, C., Sothern, M., Bar-Or, O. (2006). Strengths and weaknesses in the response of the obese child to exercise. In M. Sothern, S. Gordon, T. K. von Almen (Eds.), *Handbook of Pediatric Obesity: Clinical Management.* Boca Raton, FL: Taylor & Francis.

Wilmore, J. H., Costill, D. L. (1994). *Physiology of Sport and Exercise.* Champaign, IL: Human Kinetics.

Yu, C. C., Sung, R. Y., So, R. C., Lui, K. C., Lau, W., Lam, P. K., et al. (2005). Effects of strength training on body composition and bone mineral content in children who are obese. *Journal of Strength and Conditioning Research,* 19(3), 667–672.

Chapter 10

FUTURE TRENDS IN EXERCISE RESEARCH IN OVERWEIGHT AND OBESE YOUTH

Healthy People 2020 identifies a need to decrease the proportion of children considered obese from 10.7% in 2002–2008 to 9.6% by 2020 (U.S. Centers for Disease Control and Prevention [CDC], 2012; U.S. Department of Health and Human Services, 2008). Childhood obesity health effects include, but are not limited to, type 2 diabetes, coronary artery disease, asthma, and mental health conditions (Rahman, Cushing, & Jackson, 2011; Strong et al., 2005). Not only are these children affected concurrently, obese children are more likely to be obese adults and consequently may suffer an even greater number and severity of health conditions (Guo & Chumlea, 1999; Nader et al., 2006; Whitaker et al., 1997). The aggressiveness of the childhood obesity epidemic is undeniable. Overall, obesity has the potential to decrease the life expectancy by 2–5 years by mid-century if efforts to slow the epidemic are not successful (Olshansky, Passaro, & Hershow, 2005). Furthermore, a report by the American Public Health Association determined that the national health cost associated with overweight and obesity is approximately $142 billion. This estimation includes health care costs, lost wages due to illness and disability, and future earnings lost by premature death (Rahman et al., 2011). Costs are projected to reach between $860 and $956 billion by the year 2030, accounting for 15.8–17.6% of total health care spending (Wang et al., 2008).

Sedentary behaviors are shown to promote obesity in children and adolescents, but the majority of youth in the United States do not participate in the recommended amount of moderate to vigorous physical activity (MVPA) (Hills, King, & Armstrong, 2007; Tomporowski, Lambourne, & Okumura, 2011). Data from recent studies on children's exercise report that approximately 40% of school-age boys and 60% of school-age girls have been performing the recommended 60 minutes of moderate intensity physical activity daily (Field, 2011). Physical activity is an undisputed need in human life. Researchers agree that humans have an evolutionary derived and genetically primed need for regular physical activity to maintain a healthy lifestyle and prevent chronic disease and even death (Hills et al., 2007). Physical activity has an effect on many components of the human body, including the development of tissues, fat, skeletal muscle, and bone, which are all imperative to the growth and maturation of a child (Hills et al., 2007). Evidence reveals that appropriate levels of physical activity among children and youth, including sufficient time in MVPA, are related positively to increased on-task classroom behavior, cognitive development, and academic performance (Siedentop, 2009).

PRIMARY TARGETS FOR EXERCISE RESEARCH IN OVERWEIGHT AND OBESE CHILDREN

Although there has been much progress in the field of exercise and childhood obesity, there are still many inconsistencies. More adequately powered, high-quality research is needed to determine the long-term effects of exercise in children who are overweight or obese and, therefore, at risk for becoming overweight adults with related comorbidities (Epstein & Wrotniak, 2010). Thus far, obesity prevention interventions in children are potentially effective and, where examined, have not caused adverse outcomes or increased health inequalities (Waters et al., 2011). A recent Cochrane review of interventions to prevent childhood obesity concluded that more translational research is needed. Moreover, inconsistencies need to be eliminated and interventions should be evaluated for sustainability. Furthermore, studies should be examined carefully to ensure equitable outcomes (Waters et al., 2011). As such, interventions, which can be incorporated easily into ongoing medical practice and existing operating systems, should be examined for feasibility and sustainability (Waters et al., 2011). Currently, the range of feasible and effective interventions for use in reducing the risk of childhood obesity is exhaustive. It remains unclear, however, which specific intervention components are most effective in promoting a healthy weight while also being cost-effective (Waters et al., 2011). The majority of interventions fail to report the costs of the intervention. Potential cost effectiveness is an important aspect to consider when health practitioners determine the best use of the available resources in a community or school setting (Leung et al., 2012). Furthermore, level of exposure to the intervention, adherences, study design, and subsequent reporting may limit the effectiveness of interventions (van Sluijs, McMinn, & Griffin, 2007). Another challenge to assessing the impact, particularly when considering translation into practice, is the limited measures of long-term sustainability of the intervention's impact (Leung et al., 2012). A systematic review by Leung et al. (2012) found that only 5 out of 12 studies incorporated postintervention follow-up measures, which reported no more than 12 months' follow-up.

Despite well-established efficacy, few childhood obesity programs including exercise are available to the public. The majority of programs are limited to tertiary care centers, are available only to research participants, or have costs or limited accessibility, which prohibit their use for the general population. There remains a critical need for accessible treatments of childhood obesity, which are shown to be effective. Health care professionals recognize that community interventions may dilute the treatment effects seen in specialized clinics, but the reality remains that community-based intervention greatly enhances the scalability of treatment (Foster et al., 2012).

SCHOOL ENVIRONMENT
HEALTH AND PHYSICAL EDUCATION IN ELEMENTARY AND SECONDARY SCHOOLS

Schools may be an effective venue for intervention to improve physical inactivity in overweight and obese children and adolescents, especially disadvantaged children. School-based interventions alone will not be sufficient to solve the problem, yet it is unlikely that the current trends in childhood overweight and obesity can be reversed without the inclusion of more effective school-based programming (Leatherdale, 2010). Children spend approximately 6 hours a day at school, and resources—such as physical education programs—are already in place (Budd & Volpe, 2006). Physical education may be the only setting in which some children, particularly those from poor families, can get vigorous physical activity and learn important generalizable movement skills (Mckenzie, 2007). Given that the Institute of Medicine recommends that children expend approximately 50% of daily energy at school, school-based physical activity provides an important opportunity to not only provide physical activity but also to shape an individual's physical activity habits. The provision of quality daily physical education to all students has long been promoted by physical education professionals (i.e., the National Association for Sport and Physical Education), but more recently, external agencies and organizations, such as the American Academy of Pediatrics, American Heart Association, American College of Sports Medicine, CDC, and the U.S. DHHS, have recognized the importance of physical education (Mckenzie et al., 2004). In 2004, the World Health Organization recognized school-based intervention as the most cost-effective investment a state or nation can make to simultaneously improve both education and health (McKenzie, 2007). And, this can occur without compromising academic performance, as there is no evidence that time spent in physical education or physical activity has a negative influence on student achievement; research indicates that it is the contrary. Evidence reveals that appropriate levels of physical activity among children and youth, including sufficient time in MVPA, are positively related to increased on-task classroom behavior, cognitive development, and academic performance (Siedentop, 2009).

School-based interventions aimed to increase physical activity and reduce sedentary behavior have the ability to help children maintain a healthy weight, but results remain inconsistent (Brown & Summerbell, 2008). Presently, there is insufficient evidence for the benefits of school-based physical activity programs on childhood overweight and obesity because of methodological concerns that limit the validity of and comparability between programs (Kropski, Keckley, & Jensen, 2008). Future studies should incorporate sound study designs with adequate power, evaluation protocols that assess short- and long-term weight outcomes, valid analyses of physical activity outcomes, and discussion of process outcomes and cost-effectiveness analysis.

To effectively promote physical activity on school campuses and to encourage it in communities beyond the school day requires an understanding of the modifiable school- and student-level factors associated with overweight and obesity. This knowledge is critical for informing future programs and policies. A review by van Stralen and colleagues (2011) consistently found self-efficacy and intention as mediators of intervention effects on physical activity in school-age children. To optimally inform future interventions, research should examine whether interventions strategies are specific to the targeted mediator of behavior change. The authors suggested that the use of taxonomies to examine intervention strategy effectiveness with regard to specific mediators will provide relevant information for future interventions. Research also should evaluate and intervene on external factors within the school environment that may affect the student. Leatherdale (2010) found that school-level differences, including the physical environment, instruction and programs, supportive social environment and community partnerships, accounted for 5.4% of the variability in the odds of a student being overweight.

Intervening within existing physical education programs may be a cost-effective and beneficial strategy for increasing physical activity in a large number of children and adolescents (O'Malley et al., 2009). Based on estimates, expanding existing physical education instruction time nationwide to a level at which every child in kindergarten gets at least 5 hours of physical education per week could decrease the prevalence of overweight among girls by 4.2 percentage points (43%) and the prevalence of children who are at risk for overweight by 9.2 percentage points (Datar & Sturm, 2004). Few relationships, however, have been found between physical education interventions and body mass index (BMI), specifically. This may be due to students altering their behaviors outside of school or simply that, although physical education interventions raise energy expenditure, it is not enough to affect weight (O'Malley et al., 2009). Mckenzie (2007) suggested that physical educators will need to develop skills that are not typically taught in undergraduate physical education teacher education (PETE) programs. Furthermore, to prepare physical educators for expanded public health roles, PETE programs should include more content that specifically focuses on children's behavioral and psychological responses to exercise and physical activity, including correlates of childhood physical activity, ecological models, and environmental engineering. It is further suggested that PETE programs increase the diversity of field experiences and develop promotion, advocacy, and politicking skills in the physical educators (Mckenzie, 2007).

Once feasible and effective obesity interventions are identified, widespread diffusion should become a priority. Owen et al. (2006) identified that the lack of dissemination and diffusion of evaluation research and policy advocacy is one of the factors limiting the impact of evidence-based physical activity interventions on public health. For example, although several effective physical education programs, such as SPARK (Sports Play, and Active Recreation for Kids) and CATCH (Coordinated Approach to Child Health) are available, few systematic efforts have documented the extent of their dissemination and diffusion into physical education practice (Owen et al., 2006). Before pursuing strategies further, it is necessary to identify and learn from the existing strategies and limitations already present in the scientific literature.

BEFORE-, DURING-, AND AFTER-SCHOOL OPPORTUNITIES
Research confirms that interschool programs provide important opportunities for youth to be active, particularly for children who lack the time, skills, or confidence to play in other organized sporting activities. Children living in rural or lower socioeconomic status areas where access to community recreational facilities may be limited also benefit (Leatherdale, 2010). In addition, after-school time often is referred to as the "critical hours" because it is a time when young people engage in a substantial proportion of their leisure time activity

and is predictive of overall physical activity patterns (Atkin et al., 2011). To date, however, findings indicate that interventions to promote physical activity delivered in after-school settings have been ineffective. Potential moderators of intervention effectiveness include sample characteristics, study quality, or theoretical framework employed (Atkin et al., 2011). Furthermore, even studies with positive effects on physical activity failed to report long-term follow-up; thus, it is not possible to determine whether changes were maintained beyond the intervention time frame. A systematic review of interventions to promote physical activity in school-age children located in after-school settings reported inconsistent findings, primarily because of weaknesses in methodology or implementation (Atkin et al., 2011). Further research is needed to determine effective intervention strategies to promote physical activity in school settings outside of mandated class-time. To effectively use these "critical hours," interventions should target physical activity alone rather than targeting weight gain prevention or diet and activity together (Atkin et al., 2011).

Free, unstructured playtime also contributes to the amount of physical activity children engage in each day. According to the American Academy of Pediatrics (Milteer et al., 2012), free play allows children to use their creativity and imagination while building dexterity and physical strength. In addition, free play contributes to healthy brain development by providing opportunities for children to learn to work in groups, share, negotiate, resolve conflicts, and learn self-advocacy skills. Unfortunately, research suggests that both parents and children do not relate playful activities to physical activity, and they perceive them as different constructs. Play is considered fun and physical activity as organized activity, which requires time, transportation, and other barriers (Curtis, Hinckson, & Water, 2012). Since the 1970s, children have lost approximately 12 hours a week of free time, including a 25% decrease in play and a 50% decrease in outdoor play time (McCurdy et al., 2010).

Recently, the American Academy of Pediatrics (Murray, Ramstetter, & Council on School Health Executive Committee, 2013) published a position statement in support of recess. The report emphasized that recess has cognitive, emotional, physical, and social benefits for children, yet schools are reducing recess to accommodate additional time for academic subjects. Ironically, minimizing or eliminating recess may be counterproductive for academic improvement. Recess is shown to have the following benefits:

- Cognitive/Academic Benefits
  - Develops constructs and cognitive understanding through interaction
  - Improves attention and productivity in the classroom
- Social and Emotional Benefits
  - Provides social and emotional peer interaction that develops communication and coping skills
- Physical Benefits
  - Provides time to practice movement and motor skills
  - Gives children joy
  - Helps children get the recommended 60 minutes of MVPA

It is further recommended that recess occur at regular intervals and provide sufficient time for children to regain their focus before further instruction. Structuring recess will sacrifice many social and emotional benefits and the time for children to make personal choices. Thus, it is also recommended that schools adhere to the following:

- Provide appealing equipment that will promote free play.
- Avoid using structured recess as a substitute for physical education.

Research indicates that boys are more physically active during recess than girls (Ridgers et al., 2012). There is a need to determine why adolescent boys, in particular, are more active than girls during recess, as this will inform intervention strategies targeting this setting. Furthermore, research is needed to determine whether specific types of equipment, such as the overall availability of unfixed equipment during recess, are associated with higher levels of physical activity. Ridgers and colleagues (2012) found that providing access to different facilities during recess or lunchtime at school may benefit physical activity. In addition, schools should be encouraged to have a written programming policy that includes recess to promote more consistent scheduling to increase daily physical activity levels for children and adolescents. On the basis of scientific research, withholding recess for punitive or academic reasons would be counterproductive to the intended outcomes and may have unintended consequences in regards to children's acquisition of important life skills (Murray et al., 2013).

COMMUNITY AND RECREATIONAL SETTINGS: THE BUILT ENVIRONMENT

Research is needed to move beyond behavioral approaches targeting individual children to developing exercise interventions that focus on the environment, policy, and community aspects (Nixon et al., 2012). To date, few interventions have focused on changing the physical environment that shapes children's health behavior and development. Primarily, research needs to first increase the evidence base that informs policy makers about the benefits of changing the built environment to promote physical activity in youth. Examining the effects of the neighborhood environment is the first step. The neighborhood represents the broader social and community context that influences individual behavior, such as physical activity and sedentary behavior. Neighborhood conditions are modifiable through social policies (Singh et al., 2008). Numerous studies have examined the role of neighborhood characteristics in explaining variations in physical activity and obesity levels in adults, yet similar studies are far more limited in children (Singh, Siahpush, & Kogan, 2010). Certain factors in the built environment encourage active travel and outdoor play, such as connected streets, sidewalks, and access to recreational facilities (McCurdy et al., 2010). Conversely, the absence of playgrounds, green space, and sidewalks discourages play. In a recent investigation, it was shown that children who lived within a kilometer of a park that contained playground equipment were almost five times more likely to be of a healthier weight than children without access to playgrounds (McCurdy et al., 2010). Additionally, studies performed in children have found a significant relationship among crime rates, decreased outdoor activity and obesity (Molnar et al., 2004; Singh et al., 2008, 2010). Therefore, it is plausible to suggest that neighborhood crime events, especially violent crime, are significant environmental barriers to outdoor physical activity and affect neighborhood safety perceptions. Furthermore, children living in a favorable social environment have greater overall physical activity, more days of vigorous exercise and physical education in school, and more free time movement activities (Franzini et al., 2009).

There is a movement toward a comprehensive overall strategy for increasing physical activity and combating obesity, including both public and private efforts and a mixture of top-down and bottom-up approaches (Huang, Grimm, & Hammond, 2011). The majority of interventions to date have been designed to influence individual knowledge, skills, attitudes, beliefs, and behaviors. The top-down approach, however, influences policies, encourages environmental change, or helps change social norms that facilitate individual behavior change. Top-down approaches primarily are driven by the government and primary sector, whereas bottom-up approaches are defined as being driven by academia, community-based organizations, grassroots organizations, or private organizations (Huang et al., 2011). Huang et al. (2011) emphasized the top-down approach as a vision of a more comprehensive approach to obesity prevention. In addition to policy change, the top-down approach can provide support for bottom-up or individual-based interventions to increase their scalability and provide a wider reach in a population. Ultimately, the sustainability, scalability, and reach of interventions are key considerations for future childhood obesity interventions (Huang et al., 2011).

FAMILY AND HOME ENVIRONMENT

Family-based behavioral interventions are effective approaches for treating childhood obesity, especially pediatric obesity (Holm et al., 2012). Parents and family play an integral role in shaping a developing child's physical activity behaviors. It is especially important to target families with young children, as the social influence of a family over health behaviors wanes as children reach adolescence and become increasingly exposed to messages from peers and the media

(Knowlden & Sharma, 2012). Despite this, only two randomized controlled trials targeting pediatric obesity in the context of the family and home environment were performed in the United States from 2001 to 2011 and only nine interventions were performed worldwide (Knowlden & Sharma, 2012). Many studies determined that targeting parents alone was more effective than targeting both parents and children. Furthermore, only three of these interventions relied on behavioral and social theory to drive behavior change even though theory-based interventions offer many advantages over atheoretical interventions (Knowlden & Sharma, 2012).

Parents and family participation is integral to clinic-based childhood obesity treatment, especially when considering the benefits of role-modeling positive behaviors (Leung et al., 2012). Studies examining childhood obesity prevention interventions identify a supportive family environment as an effective method to promote positive behaviors targeted through intervention (Leung et al., 2012). Target populations, intervention strategies, and evaluations, however, have not remained consistent in this area of research (van Sluijs, Kriemler, & McMinn, 2011). Earlier reviews demonstrate that family-based interventions may be more effective in a home setting. Interventions typically include self-monitoring and goal-setting techniques for specific lifestyle changes. These strategies, however, have not been further validated in recent research (van Sluijs et al., 2011). These and other previously identified strategies, including the use of pedometers, graded tasks, and providing performance feedback, should be further explored and tested, using high-quality research methods with longer follow-up (Sluijs et al., 2011). Furthermore, additional research is needed to examine the extent to which parental change in physical activity affects child behaviors. Moreover, research should examine whether this relationship is due to parents and children engaging in activities together or due to other factors. Studies should identify other influential factors, such as parents working with their children to set goals for family physical activity (Holm et al., 2012). Additional factors, such as socioeconomic status, parent employment status, and family structure also may moderate the influence of parents on their child's change in physical activity (Holm et al., 2012).

Sung-Chan et al. (2012) reviewed the 35-year evolution of family-based childhood obesity interventions and identified four major types: (1) behavioral approach, (2) behavioral approach plus parent education, (3) family therapy, and (4) family therapy plus family-based psychoeducation. The behavioral approach consistently achieved greater outcomes than the other three types. The authors concluded that more family-based interventions should consider the use of the behavioral approach to family-based lifestyle interventions with parent education on parenting style (Sung-Chan et al., 2012). A systematic review performed by Nixon et al. (2012) found that obesity prevention interventions were more successful with high parental involvement and the following behavior change strategies: (1) developing skills and behavioral capability, (2) developing self-efficacy, (3) educating parents and children about the benefits of a healthy lifestyle, and (4) modeling. Furthermore, the authors suggested the use of effective behavior change strategies, rather than the use of specific behavioral models. Sung-Chan and colleagues (2012) concluded that studies also need to further identify the family components that potentially mediate treatment effects, such as family dynamics, family functioning, competence, resilience, and worldview (Sung-Chang et al., 2012). Perhaps even more important is the finding that none of the 15 randomized controlled trials considered gender and culture, two factors that may moderate the effect of family-based behavioral interventions on physical activity among children (Sung-Chan et al., 2012).

FACTORS THAT INHIBIT EXERCISE IN OVERWEIGHT AND OBESE YOUTH

Future research should account for the physiologic and psychological challenges overweight and obese children face to maintain regular physical activity as compared with their normal weight counterparts (Sothern, 2001, 2004; Sothern et al., 2006; VanVrancken-Tompkins, Sothern, & Bar-Or, 2006). Overall, an overweight or obese child has different physical fitness, defined as an attribute that includes fitness components, such as cardiorespiratory endurance, muscle strength and endurance, flexibility, and body composition (Bovet, Auguste, & Burdette, 2007; Brambilla, Pozzobon, & Pietrobelli, 2011; Joshi et al., 2012; Maffeis et al., 1993; Nemet et al., 2003; Pascal, Auguste, & Burdette, 2007; Salvadori et al., 1999). In a study aimed to establish whether inactivity is the cause of fatness or whether the opposite is the case, Metcalf and colleagues (2011) determined that percent body fat (BF%) was predictive of changes in physical activity over 3 years, but physical activity levels were not predictive of subsequent changes in BF% during the same period. In addition, Pascal et al. (2007) examined whether physical fitness was different in children in the lowest and the highest weight categories as compared with children with normal weight and found a strong inverse relationship between excess body fat and physical fitness. The association was particularly present for physical fitness tests involving agility and movability as compared with assessments relying more on strength (Pascal et al., 2007). A review by Schultz, Anner, and Hills (2009) identified several physiological differences that may cause heavier children to be more physically inactive. The authors suggested that exercise can cause musculoskeletal pain in overweight children and that the extra energy costs of moving a greater body mass results in breathlessness and fatigue during exercise sooner than their normal weight counterparts.

In addition, studies have shown that normal weight children have a greater level of gross motor coordination over time than their obese or overweight counterparts (Cliff, Okely, & Morgan, 2012; D'Hondt et al., 2012). Adequate levels of motor competence and functional motor skills are essential to a child's development but, more important, are the foundation for an active lifestyle (D'Hondt et al., 2012). Exercise interventions should include strategies to improve motor skills to eliminate the increasingly widening gap in performance between overweight and obese children and their normal weight counterparts. Enhanced motor skill coordination likely will promote regular participation in physical activity among overweight and obese children (Cliff et al., 2012; D'Hondt et al., 2012).

In addition to physiological differences, children who suffer from overweight or obesity face greater psychological challenges when engaging in physical activity. Regardless of their physical ability, overweight and obese children face social stressors, such as weight teasing and decreased self-efficacy, which result in greater levels of physical inactivity. Studies consistently demonstrate that overweight and obese youth are less physically active, perceive physical activity more negatively, and find sedentary activity more reinforcing than physical activities when compared with normal weight youth (Salvy et al., 2012). Overweight and obese youth often are teased by their peers because of their physical appearances. Moreover, they routinely are subjected to peer rejection, ostracism, and physical and verbal victimization, and these actions result in decreased physical activity in overweight, obese, and normal weight youth (Losekam et al., 2010; Salvy et al., 2012). Research indicates that weight criticism during physical activity and other verbal, physical, and relational manifestations of victimization are shown to be predictive of increased depressive symptoms, time spent alone, and feelings of loneliness. When criticized during physical activity, children experience a reduction in sports enjoyment and perceive their ability relative to their peers more negatively; this results in less overall physical activity (Salvy et al., 2012). Thus, the actual experience of engaging in physical activity, if not carefully structured and monitored, may promote negative outcomes. It may be that overweight and obese children should first obtain the skills necessary to successfully participate in individual goal-based sports. Then, after time, they can be mainstreamed gradually into team-based activities with healthy weight youth (Sothern, 2004; Sothern et al., 2006). Additional research is needed to determine the most optimal setting to promote positive experiences while engaging in physical activity in overweight and especially significantly obese children and adolescents (Salvy et al., 2012).

EVALUATING EXERCISE OUTCOMES: WEIGHT BIAS AND DEVELOPMENTAL ISSUES

The effects of adiposity need to be considered when interpreting physiologic and metabolic findings during exercise testing of overweight and obese children and adolescents (Rowland &

Loftin, 2006). During tests to determine performance in distance exercise events, especially in those utilizing weight-bearing activities (walking, jogging, running), the resulting time will be modified by body fat content (Bovet et al., 2007; Loftin et al., 2001). Excess fat also negatively affects endurance performance during exercise testing (Rowland & Loftin, 2006). This observation is particularly present for physical fitness tests involving agility and ambulation in contrast to those requiring muscular strength and endurance (Bovet et al., 2007). Allometric scaling of VO_2 peak reduces the bias associated with excess fat during exercise testing in overweight and obese youth. Loftin and colleagues (2001) examined obese versus nonobese youth and reported that adjusting VO_2 peak for stature and mass reduced the difference of 50% found in the ratio method to 10% (allometric method). More recently, an equivocal finding was observed when determining the relationship between VO_2max and insulin resistance in children (Ahn, McMurray, & Harrell, 2013). In this instance, the authors recommended that aerobic fitness be expressed in units per kilogram of fat-free mass to eliminate the confounding effect of fat mass when examining associations between VO_2max and insulin resistance.

In summary, research indicates that there is a significant weight bias associated with the reduced endurance performance and lower VO_2max per kilogram observed in overweight and obese children (Loftin et al., 2001, 2003, 2004, 2005; Maffeis, 2008; Sothern, 2001; Sothern et al., 1999, 2006; VanVrancken et al., 2006). These deficiencies likely are not the result of a depressed cardiac functional reserve (Bar-Or & Rowland, 2004; Daniels et al., 2009; Drinkard et al., 2007; Goran et al., 2000; Norman et al., 2005; Sothern, 2001; VanVrancken-Tompkins et al., 2006). Thus, at the beginning of an exercise program, specific recommendations for frequency, intensity, and duration do not necessarily need to focus on the improvement of cardiovascular fitness. Rather, lower intensity exercise, which may be more comfortable for obese children, can provide opportunities for increasing caloric expenditure and improving body composition (Brambilla et al., 2011; Rowland & Loftin, 2006). This observation recently was supported in a review by Brambilla and colleagues (2011), which examined physical activity as a therapeutic tool for obesity-related metabolic syndrome. On the basis of decades of research, the authors concluded that exercise prescriptions in overweight and obese youth should consider a multistep strategy. In this case, sedentary activities initially are replaced with light-intensity activities that are enjoyable and unstructured, and then intensity gradually increases over time in such a way that goals to include 60 minutes of MVPA eventually are met (U.S. DHHS, 2008; Strong et al., 2005; Sothern, 2001, 2004;

Table 10.1   Physical Activity for Metabolic Syndrome: Label for Use in Childhood

Label	Information/Details
Description of the drug	Any body movement produced by skeletal muscles that results in energy expenditure
Clinical pharmacology	Effect on insulin sensitivity and substrate disposal; regular use induces changes in enzyme function and mitochondrial activity
Indications	Metabolic health maintenance and treatment, any condition requiring an increase of energy expenditure, improvement of vascular function
Contraindications	None
Warnings	Modulate according to gender and age categories, endurance training is not recommended in young children, suggested use in small groups
Precautions	Hypoglycemia in diabetes mellitus type 1, risk for water and salt losses in particular climate conditions
Adverse effects	Musculoskeletal disorders, hypertension (limited to activities with high workload)

Source: Adapted from Brambilla, P., Pozzobon, G., & Pietrobelli, A., *International Journal of Obesity*, 35(1), 16–28, 2011. With permission.

Sothern, von Almen, & Schumacher, 2001; Sothern et al., 2006). One of the more provocative recommendations of the article was the proposal to consider physical activity as a therapeutic agent for the prevention and management of obesity-related metabolic syndrome, a precursor to type 2 diabetes. As such, Table 10.1 summarizes the authors' recommendations for physical activity and its "label for use in childhood" for metabolic syndrome in clinical settings. In further support of this recommendation, results from a recent meta-analysis by Fedewa and colleagues (2014) concluded that exercise training in youth should be included in efforts to prevent and treat type 2 diabetes.

SUMMARY

It is clear from the available scientific evidence that increased physical activity and prescribed structured exercise are necessary for the primary, secondary, and tertiary prevention of obesity in youth. Interventions should target parents, include the involvement of family members, and be delivered in community, school, and family home environments. In younger children, large amounts of intermittent MVPA that simulates "free play" are needed to prevent the onset of obesity. In older children, numerous opportunities for MVPA are needed to reach a minimum goal of 60 minutes per day. This minimal goal, however, is likely not adequate to reverse obesity in older children. Moreover, opportunities to participate in free play and structured exercise remain limited despite an emphasis from the medical community at large to provide safe and accessible environments to encourage such opportunities. Although many questions concerning the mechanistic role of exercise to the amelioration of obesity remain unanswered, solution-based research, which considers social, environmental, and behavioral factors, is the next logical step to promoting physical activity and reducing obesity in youth.

REFERENCES

Ahn, B., McMurray, R., Harrell, J. (2013) Scaling of VO$_2$max and its relationship with insulin resistance in children. *Pediatric Exercise Science,* 25(1), 43–51.

Atkin, A., Gorely, T., Biddle, S., Cavill, N., Foster, C. (2011). Interventions to promote physical activity in young people conducted in the hours immediately after school: A systematic review. *International Journal of Behavioral Medicine,* 18, 176–187.

Bar-Or, O., Rowland, T. W. (2004). *Pediatric Exercise Medicine: From Physiologic Principles to Health Care Application.* Champaign, IL: Human Kinetics.

Bovet, P., Auguste, R., Burdette, H. (2007). Strong inverse association between physical fitness and overweight in adolescents: a large school-based survey. *International Journal of Behavioral Nutrition and Physical Activity,* 4, 24.

Brambilla, P., Pozzobon, G., Pietrobelli, A. (2011). Physical activity as the main therapeutic tool for metabolic syndrome in childhood. *Journal of Obesity,* 35(1), 16–28.

Brown, T., Summerbell, C. (2008). Systematic review of school-based interventions that focus on changing dietary intake and physical activity levels to prevent childhood obesity: an update to the obesity guidance produced by the national institute for health and clinical experience. *Obesity Reviews,* 10, 110–141.

Budd, G., Volpe, S. (2006). School-based obesity prevention: Research, challenges, and recommendations. *Journal of School Health,* 76(10), 485–495.

Cliff, D. P., Okely, A. D., Morgan, P. J. (2011). Movement skills and physical activity in obese children: Randomized controlled trial. *Medicine and Science in Sports and Exercise,* 43(1), 90–100.

Curtis, A. D., Hinckson, E. A., Water, T. C. (2012). Physical activity is not play: Perceptions of children and parents from deprived areas. *New Zealand Medical Journal,* 125(1365), 38–47.

Daniels, S. R., Jacobson, M. S., McCrindle, B. W., Eckel, R. H., Sanner, B. M. (2009). American Heart Association childhood obesity research summit: Executive summary. *Circulation,* 119(15), 2114–2123.

Datar, A., Sturm, R. (2004). Physical education in elementary school and body mass index: Evidence from the early childhood longitudinal study. *American Journal of Public Health,* 94(9), 1501–1506.

D'Hondt, E., Deforche, B., Gentier, I., De Bourdeaudhuij, I., Vaeyens, R., Philippaerts, R., Lenoir, M. (2012). A longitudinal analysis of gross motor coordination in overweight and obese children versus normal-weight peers. *International Journal of Obesity,* 1–7. Doi: 10.1038/ijo.2012.55 [Epub ahead of print]

Drinkard, B., Roberts, M. D., Ranzenhofer, L. M., Han, J. C., Yanoff, L. B., Merke, D. P., et al. (2007). Oxygen-uptake efficiency slope as a determinant of fitness in overweight adolescents. *Medicine and Science in Sports and Exercise,* 39(10), 1811–1816.

Epstein, L., Wrotniak, B. (2010). Future directions for pediatric obesity treatment. *Obesity,* 18(Suppl 1), S8–S12.

Fedewa, M., Gist, N., Evans, E., Dishman, R. (2014). Exercise and insulin resistance in youth: A meta-analysis. *Pediatrics,* 133(1), 1–12.

Foster, G., Sundal, D., McDermott, C., Jelalian, E., Lent, M., Vojta, D. (2012). Feasibility and preliminary outcomes of a scalable, community-based treatment of childhood obesity. *Pediatrics,* 130(4), 652–659.

Franzini L, Elliott, M., Cuccaro, P., Schuster, M., Gilliland, J., Grunbaum, J., Franklin, F., Tortolero, S. (2009). Influences of physical and social neighborhood environments on children's physical activity and obesity. *American Journal of Public Health,* 2009; 99(2), 271–278.

Goran, M., Fields, D. A., Hunter, G. R., Herd, S. L., Weinsier, R. L. (2000). Total body fat does not influence maximal aerobic capacity. *International Journal of Obesity and Related Metabolic Disorders,* 24(7), 841–848.

Guo, S. S., Chumela, W. (1999). Tracking of body mass index in children in relation to overweight in adulthood. *American Journal of Clinical Nutrition* 70, 145–148.

Hills, A., King, N., Armstrong, T. (2007). The contribution of physical activity and sedentary behaviors to the growth and development of children and adolescents. *Sports Medicine,* 37(6), 533–545.

Holm, K., Wyatt, H., Murphy, J., Hill, J., Odgen, L. (2012). Parental influence on child change in physical activity during a family-based intervention for child weight gain prevention. *Journal of Physical Activity and Health,* 9, 661–669.

Huang, T., Grimm, B., Hammond, R. (2011). A systems-based typological framework for understanding the sustainability, scalability and reach of childhood obesity interventions. *Children's Health Care,* 40(3), 253–266.

Joshi, P., Bryan, C., Howat, H. (2012). Relationship of body mass index and fitness levels among schoolchildren. *Journal of Strength and Conditioning Research,* 26(4), 1006–1014.

Knowlden, A., Sharma, M. (2012). Systematic review of family and home-based interventions targeting paediatric overweight and obesity. *International Association for the Study of Obesity,* 13, 499–508.

Kropski, J., Keckley, P., Jensen, G. (2008). School-based obesity prevention programs: An evidence-based review. *Obesity*, 16(5), 1009–1018.

Leatherdale, S. (2010). The association between overweight and school policies on physical activity: A multilevel analysis among elementary school youth in the play-on study. *Health Education Research*, 25(6), 1061–1073.

Leung, M. M., Agaronov, A., Grytsenko, K., Yeh, M. C. (2012). Intervening to reduce sedentary behaviors and childhood obesity among school-age youth: A systematic review of randomized trials. *Journal of Obesity*, 685430.

Loftin, M., Heusel, L., Bonis, M., Sothern, M. (2005). Oxygen uptake kinetics and oxygen deficit in obese and normal weight adolescent females. *Journal of Sports Science and Medicine*, 4, 430–436.

Loftin, M., Sothern, M., VanVrancken, C., Udall, J. (2003). Low heart rate peak in obese female youth. *Clinical Pediatrics*, 42(6), 505–510.

Loftin, M., Sothern, M., Warren, B., Udall, J. (2004). Comparison of VO_2 peak during treadmill and bicycle ergometry in severely overweight youth. *Journal of Sports Science and Medicine*, 3, 254–260.

Loftin, M., Sothern, M., Trosclair, L., O'Hanlon, A., Miller, J., Udall, J. (2001). Scaling VO(2) peak in obese and non-obese girls. *Obesity Research*, 9(5), 290–296.

Losekam, S., Goetzky, B., Kraeling, S., Rief, W., Hilbert, A. (2010). Physical activity in normal-weight and overweight youth: Associations with weight teasing and self-efficacy. *Obesity Facts*, 3, 239–244.

Maffeis, C. (2008) Physical activity in the prevention and treatment of childhood obesity: Physio-pathologic evidence and promising experiences. *International Journal of Pediatric Obesity*, 3(Suppl 2), 29–32.

Maffeis, C., Schutz, Y., Schena, F., Zaffanello, M., Pinelli, L. (1993). Energy expenditure during walking and running in obese and nonobese prepubertal children. *Pediatrics*, 123(2), 193–199.

McCurdy, L., Winterbottom, K., Mehta, S., Roberts, J. (2010). Using nature and outdoor activity to improve children's health. *Current Problems in Pediatric and Adolescent Health Care*, 40(6), 1102–1117.

Mckenzie, T. (2007). The preparation of physical educators: A public health persepctive. *Quest*, 59(4), 345–357. Retrieved from http://www.tandfonline.com/doi/pdf/10.1080/0033629 7.2007.10483557.

Mckenzie, T., Sallis, J., Prochaska, J., Conway, T., Marshall, S., Rosengard, P. (2004). Evaluation of a two-year middle-school physical education intervention: M-span. *Medicine and Science in Sports and Exercise*, 4, 1382–1388.

Milteer, R. M., Ginsburg, K. R., Council on Communications and Media, Committee on Psychosocial Aspects of Child and Family Health. (2012). The importance of play in promoting healthy child development and maintaining strong parent-child bond: Focus on children in poverty. *Pediatrics*, 129(1), e204–e213.

Metcalf, B., Hosking, J., Jeffrey, A., Voss, L., Henley, W., Wilkin, T. (2011). Fatness leads to inactivity, but inactivity does not lead to fatness: a longitudinal study in children (earlybird 45). *Archives of Disease in Childhood*, 96, 942–947.

Molnar, B. E., Gortmaker, S. L., Bull, F. C., Buka, S. L. (2004). Unsafe to play? Neighborhood disorder and lack of safety predict reduced physical activity among urban children and adolescents. *American Journal of Health Promotion*, 18(5), 378–386.

Murray, R., Ramstetter, C., Council on School Health Executive Committee. (2013). The crucial role of recess in school. *American Academy of Pediatrics*, 131(1), 183–188.

Nader, P. R., O'Brien, M., Houts, R., Bradley, R., Belsky, J., Crosnoe, R., et al. (2006). Identifying risk for obesity in early childhood. *Pediatrics*, 118(3), e594–e601.

Nemet, D., Wang, P., Funahashi, T., Matsuzawa, Y., Tanaka, S., Engelman, L., Cooper, D. M. (2003). Adipocytokines, body composition, and fitness in children. *Pediatric Research*, 53(1), 148–152.

Nixon, C., Moore, H., Douthwaite, W., Gibson, E., Vogele, C., Kreichauf, S., Wildgruber, A., Manios, Y. (2012). Identifying effective behavioral models and behavior change strategies underpinning preschool- and school-based obesity prevention interventions aimed at 4-6 year-olds: a systematic review. *Obesity Reviews*, 13(Suppl 1), 106–117.

Norman, A., Drinkard, B., McDuffie, J., Ghorbani, S., Yanoff, L., Yanovski, J. (2005). Influence of excess adiposity on exercise fitness and performance in overweight children and adolescents. *Pediatrics*, 115(6), 690–696.

Olshansky, S., Passaro, D., Hershow, R., Layden, J., Carnes, B., Brody, J., et al. (2005). A potential decline in life expectancy in the United States in the 21st century. *New England Journal of Medicine*, 352, 1138–1145.

O'Malley, P., Johnston, L., Delva, J., Terry-McElrath, Y. (2009). School physical activity environment related to student obesity and activity: a national study of schools and students. *Journal of Adolescent Health*, 45, 71–81.

Owen, N., Glanz, K., Sallis, J., Kelder, S. (2006). Evidence-based approaches to dissemination and diffusion of physical activity interventions. *American Journal of Preventive Medicine*, 31(4S), 35–44.

Pascal, B., Auguste, R., Burdette, H. (2007). Strong inverse association between physical fitness and overweight in adolescents: A large school-based survey. *International Journal of Behavioral Nutrition and Physical Activity*, 4(24), 1479–1488.

Rahman, T., Cushing, R. A., Jackson, R. J. (2011). Contributions of built environment to childhood obesity. *Mount Sinai Journal of Medicine*, 78, 49–57.

Ridgers, N., Salmon, J., Parrish, A., Stanley, R., Okely, A. (2012). Physical activity during school recess: A systematic review. *American Journal of Preventive Medicine*, 43(2), 320–328.

Salvadori, A., Fanari, P., Fontana, M., Buotempi, L., Saezza, A., Baudo, S., Miserocchi, G., Longhini, E. (1999). Oxygen uptake and cardiac performance in obese and normal subjects during exercise. *Respiration*, 66, 25–33.

Salvy, S., Bowker, J., Germeroth, L., Barkley, J. (2012). Influence of peers and friends on overweight/obese youths' physical activity. *American College of Sports Medicine*, 40(3), 127–132.

Schultz, S., Anner, J., Hills, A. (2009). Paediatric obesity, physical activity and the musculoskeletal system. *Obesity Reviews*, 10(5), 576–582.

Siedentop, D. (2009). National plan for physical activity: Education sector. *Journal of Physical Activity and Health*, 6(Suppl 2), S168–S180.

Singh, G. K., Kogan, M. D., Siahpush, M., van Dyck, P. C. (2008). Independent and joint effects of socioeconomic, behavioral, and neighborhood characteristics on physical inactivity and activity levels among U.S. children and adolescents. *Journal of Community Health*, 33, 206–216.

Singh, G. K., Siahpush, M., Kogan, M. D. (2010). Neighborhood socioeconomic conditions, built environments, and childhood obesity. *Health Affairs*, 29(3), 503–512.

Sothern, M. (2001). Exercise as a modality in the treatment of childhood obesity. *Pediatric Clinics of North America*, 48(4), 995–1015.

Sothern, M. (2004). Obesity prevention in children: Physical activity and nutrition. *Nutrition*, 20(7–8), 704–708.

Sothern, M., Loftin, M., Blecker, M., Suskind R., Udall, J. (1999). Physiologic function and childhood obesity. *International Journal of Pediatrics*, 14(3), 1–5.

Sothern, M., VanVrancken-Tompkins, C., Brooks, C., Thélin, C. (2006). Increasing physical activity in overweight youth in clinical settings. In M. Sothern, S. Gordon, T. K. von Almen (Eds.), *Handbook of Pediatric Obesity: Clinical Management* (pp. 173–188). Boca Raton, FL: Taylor & Francis.

Sothern, M., von Almen, T. K., Schumacher, H. (2001). *Trim Kids: The Proven Plan That Has Helped Thousands of Children Achieve a Healthier Weight.* New York, NY: HarperCollins.

Sung-Chan, P., Sung, Y., Zhao, X., Brownson, R. (2012). Family-based models for childhood-obesity intervention: a systematic review of randomized controlled trials. *Obesity Reviews,* 1–13.

Tomporowski, P., Lambourne, K., Okumura, M. (2011). Physical activity interventions and children's mental function: An introduction and overview. *Preventive Medicine,* 52, 1–15.

U.S. Centers for Disease Control and Prevention. (2012). Overweight and obesity: Consequences. Retrieved June 9, 2012, from http://www.cdc.gov/obesity/childhood/basics.html.

U.S. Department of Health and Human Services. (2008). Physical activity guidelines for Americans. Retrieved June 25, 2009, from http://www.health.gov/paguidelines.

van Sluijs, E., Kriemler, S., McMinn, A. (2011). The effect of community and family interventions on young people's physical activity levels: a review of reviews and updated systematic review. *British Journal of Sports Medicine,* 45, 914–922.

van Sluijs, E. M., McMinn, A. M., Griffin, S. J. (2007) Effectiveness of interventions to promote physical activity in children and adolescents: Systematic review of controlled trials. *British Medical Journal,* 335(7622), 703.

van Stralen, M., Yildirim, M., Velde, S., Brug, J., van Mechelen, W., Chinapaw, M. (2011). What works in school-based energy balance behaviour interventions and what does not? A systematic review of mediating mechanisms. *International Journal of Obesity,* 35, 1251–1265.

VanVrancken-Tompkins, C., Sothern, M., Bar-Or, O. (2006). Strengths and weaknesses in the response of the obese child to exercise. In M. Sothern, S. Gordon, T. K. von Almen (Eds.), *Handbook of Pediatric Obesity: Clinical Management.* Boca Raton, FL: Taylor & Francis.

Wang, Y., Beydoun, M., Liang, L., Caballero, B., Kumanyika, S. (2008). Will all Americans become overweight or obese? Estimating the progression and cost of the US obesity epidemic. *Obesity,* 16(10), 2323–2330.

Waters, E., de Silva-Sanigorski, A., Hall, B. J., Brown, T., Campbell, K. J., Gao, Y., Armstrong, R., Prosser, L., Summerbell, C. D. (2011). Interventions for preventing obesity in children. *Cochrane Database System Review,* 12, CD001871.

Whitaker, R. C., Wright, J. A., Pepe, M. S., Seidel, K. D., Dietz, W. H. (1997). Predicting obesity in young adulthood from childhood and parental obesity. *New England Journal of Medicine,* 337(13), 869–873.

INDEX

Page numbers followed by a "t" or "f" indicate that the entry is included in a table or figure